PLANS OF CARE FOR
SPECIALTY PRACTICE

Noncardiac Critical Care Nursing

PLANS OF CARE FOR
SPECIALTY PRACTICE

Noncardiac Critical Care Nursing

LINDA G. WAITE, RN, MN, CCRN
JOANNE M. KRUMBERGER, RN, MSN, CCRN

KATHY V. GETTRUST, RN, BSN ~ *Series Editor*
Case Manager
Midwest Medical Home Care
Milwaukee, Wisconsin

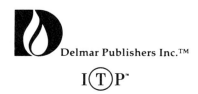
Delmar Publishers Inc.™
I(T)P™

NOTICE TO THE READER

Publisher does not warrant or guarantee any of the products described herein or perform any independent analysis in connection with any of the product information contained herein. Publisher does not assume, and expressly disclaims, any obligation to obtain and include information other than that provided to it by the manufacturer.

The reader is expressly warned to consider and adopt all safety precautions that might be indicated by the activities described herein and to avoid all potential hazards. By following the instructions contained herein, the reader willingly assumes all risks in connection with such instructions.

The publisher makes no representations or warranties of any kind, including but not limited to, the warranties of fitness for particular purpose or merchantability, nor are any such representations implied with respect to the material set forth herein, and the publisher takes no responsibility with respect to such material. The publisher shall not be liable for any special, consequential or exemplary damages resulting, in whole or in part, from the readers' use of, or reliance upon, this material.

Delmar publishing team:
Publisher: David C. Gordon
Administrative Editor: Patricia Casey
Associate Editor: Elisabeth F. Williams
Project Editor: Danya M. Plotsky
Production Coordinator: Mary Ellen Black
Art and Design Coordinator: Megan K. DeSantis
                            Timothy J. Conners

For information, address

Delmar Publishers Inc.
3 Columbia Circle, Box 15015
Albany, NY 12212-5015

COPYRIGHT © 1994 BY DELMAR PUBLISHERS INC.

The trademark ITP is used under license.

All rights reserved. No part of this work covered by the copyright hereon may be reproduced or used in any form, or by any means—graphic, electronic, or mechanical including photocopying, recording, taping, or information storage and retrieval systems—without written permission of the publisher.

Printed in the United States of America
Published simultaneously in Canada
by Nelson Canada,
a division of The Thomson Corporation

1 2 3 4 5 6 7 8 9 10 XXX 00 99 98 97 96 95 94

Library of Congress Cataloging-in-Publication Data

Waite, Linda G.
  Noncardiovascular critical care nursing / Linda G. Waite, Joanne M. Krumberger.
    p. cm.—(Plans of care for specialty practice)
  Includes index.
  ISBN 0-8273-5985-3
  1. Intensive care nursing. 2. Nursing care plans.
I. Krumberger, Joanne M. II. Title. III. Series.
  [DNLM: 1. Critical Care—nurses' instruction. 2. Patient Care
Planning—nurses' instruction. WY 154 W145n 1994]
  RT120.I5W35 1994
  610.73'61—dc20
  DNLM/DLC
  for Library of Congress   93-23541
                                                                         CIP

TABLE OF CONTENTS

PREFACE xi
SERIES INTRODUCTION xiii
LIST OF TABLES xix

ENDOCRINE CARE

1. Acute Adrenal Crisis — 3
   Fluid volume deficit, Altered tissue perfusion—cardiovascular and peripheral, Altered thought processes, Activity intolerance
2. Diabetic Ketoacidosis — 13
   Fluid volume deficit, Electrolyte imbalance, Ineffective breathing pattern, Altered thought processes
3. Disturbances of Antidiuretic Hormone (ADH) — 22
   Fluid volume deficit, Fluid volume excess
4. Hyperglycemic Hyperosmotic Nonketotic Coma — 30
   Fluid volume deficit, Electrolyte imbalance, Altered thought processes
5. Hypoglycemic Crisis — 35
   Altered nutrition—less than body requirements, Altered thought processes
6. Myxedema Coma — 41
   Fluid volume excess, Decreased cardiac output, Hypothermia, Altered thought processes, Ineffective breathing pattern, Activity intolerance
7. Thyroid Storm — 51
   Decreased cardiac output, Hyperthermia, Ineffective breathing pattern, Activity intolerance, Altered thought processes

GASTROINTESTINAL CARE

8. Abdominal Aortic Aneurysm — 63
   Altered tissue perfusion—central and peripheral, High risk for injury—aneurysmal rupture, High risk for injury—embolic, Acute pain, Knowledge deficit
9. Abdominal Surgery — 70
   Acute pain, High risk for fluid volume deficit, Impaired gas exchange, High risk for infection, Altered nutrition—Less than body requirements
10. Peritonitis — 78
    Acute pain, Fluid volume deficit, High risk for infection, Ineffective breathing pattern/impaired gas exchange

11   Acute Gastrointestinal Bleed   86
Fluid volume deficit, High risk for impaired gas exchange, Altered tissue perfusion—central and peripheral, Knowledge deficit

12   Acute Pancreatitis   96
Fluid volume deficit, Acute pain, Altered nutrition—less than body requirements, Electrolyte imbalance, Impaired gas exchange

13   Fulminant Hepatic Failure   104
Fluid volume deficit, Altered nutrition—less than body requirements, Altered thought processes, Ineffective breathing pattern, High risk for impaired skin integrity

HEMATOLOGICAL CARE

14   Anaphylaxis   119
Ineffective breathing pattern, Decreased cardiac output

15   Disseminated intravascular coagulation   125
Altered tissue perfusion—central and peripheral, High risk for injury, High risk for impaired tissue integrity, High risk for decreased cardiac output, High risk for impaired gas exchange

16   Human Immunodeficiency Virus   134
Impaired gas exchange, Decreased cardiac output, High risk for infection, Altered sensory perception, Impaired skin integrity, Altered nutrition—less than body requirements, Diarrhea, Activity intolerance, Ineffective individual coping

NEUROLOGICAL CARE

17   Acute Spinal Cord Injury   151
Decreased cardiac output, Ineffective breathing pattern, Impaired physical mobility, Altered sensory perception—tactile, Ineffective thermoregulation, Bowel incontinence, Urinary retention, Ineffective individual coping

18   Cerebral Aneurysm   165
Altered tissue perfusion—cerebral, High risk for fluid volume excess, Impaired physical mobility

19   Guillain-Barré Syndrome   174
Ineffective breathing pattern, Impaired physical mobility, Decreased cardiac output, Altered sensory perception, Altered bowel/urinary elimination, High risk for impaired skin integrity

20   Head Trauma   186
Altered tissue perfusion—cerebral, Impaired physical mobility, High risk for injury

21   Increased Intracranial Pressure   191
Altered tissue perfusion—cerebral, Impaired gas exchange, Ineffective airway clearance, Impaired physical mobility, Altered sensory perception, High risk for injury

22   Intracranial Infections   209
Altered thought processes, Altered tissue perfusion—cerebral, Impaired physical mobility, High risk for injury

23 Myasthenia Crisis — 218
Ineffective breathing pattern, Ineffective airway clearance, Impaired physical mobility, Altered cardiac output

24 Status Epilepticus — 226
Altered tissue perfusion—cerebral and cardiopulmonary, Impaired gas exchange, Altered tissue perfusion—renal, High risk for injury

PULMONARY CARE

25 Acute Respiratory Distress Syndrome — 237
Impaired gas exchange, Ineffective breathing pattern, Impaired airway clearance, Decreased cardiac output

26 Acute Respiratory Failure — 246
Ineffective breathing pattern, Impaired gas exchange, Ineffective airway clearance, Anxiety, Altered nutrition—less than body requirements

27 Chest Trauma — 258
Impaired gas exchange, Ineffective breathing pattern, Ineffective airway clearance, Acute pain, High risk for fluid volume deficit, High risk for decreased cardiac output

28 Mechanical Ventilation — 269
Ineffective breathing pattern, Impaired gas exchange, Ineffective airway clearance, Dysfunctional ventilatory weaning response, Fluid volume excess, Decreased cardiac output, High risk for infection, Anxiety, Altered nutrition—less than body requirements

29 Pulmonary Embolism — 287
Impaired gas exchange, Altered tissue perfusion—pulmonary, Acute pain, High risk for decreased cardiac output

30 Respiratory Acidosis — 297
Ineffective breathing pattern, Decreased cardiac output

31 Respiratory Alkalosis — 303
Acid-base imbalance, Ineffective breathing pattern

32 Status Asthmaticus — 308
Ineffective breathing pattern, Impaired gas exchange, Anxiety

33 Thoracic Surgery — 316
Ineffective breathing pattern, Impaired gas exchange, Ineffective airway clearance, Acute pain, High risk for injury—hemorrhage, Altered nutrition—less than body requirements

RENAL CARE

34 Acute Renal Dialysis — 329
Fluid volume deficit, High risk for injury (peritoneal dialysis), High risk for injury (hemodialysis/continuous renal replacement therapy)

35 Acute Renal Failure — 338
Altered urinary elimination, Fluid volume excess, Fluid volume deficit, High risk for infection, Activity intolerance, Impaired skin integrity

36	Disturbances of Calcium	350
	Hypercalcemia	
	Electrolyte imbalance—hypercalcemia, Altered urinary elimination	
	Hypocalcemia	
	Electrolyte imbalance—hypocalcemia, Decreased cardiac output, High risk for impaired gas exchange	
37	Disturbances of Magnesium	363
	Hypermagnesemia	
	Decreased cardiac output, Ineffective breathing pattern, Activity intolerance	
	Hypomagnesemia	
	Decreased cardiac output, Activity intolerance	
38	Disturbances of Phosphate	374
	Hyperphosphatemia	
	Decreased cardiac output, Activity intolerance	
	Hypophosphatemia	
	Decreased cardiac output, Ineffective breathing pattern, Activity intolerance	
39	Disturbances of Potassium	385
	Hyperkalemia	
	Decreased cardiac ouput, Activity intolerance	
	Hypokalemia	
	Decreased cardiac output, Activity intolerance, High risk for ineffective breathing pattern	
40	Disturbances of Sodium	397
	Hypernatremia	
	Fluid volume deficit, Altered thought processes	
	Hyponatremia	
	Fluid volume excess, Altered thought processes	
41	Disturbances of Water Balance	406
	Primary Water Excess	
	Fluid volume excess, Impaired gas exchange	
	Primary Water Deficit	
	Fluid volume deficit	
42	Metabolic Acidosis	413
	Decreased cardiac output, Altered thought processes	
43	Metabolic Alkalosis	418
	Acid-base imbalance, Ineffective breathing pattern	

MISCELLANEOUS

44	Drug Intoxication	425
	Ineffective breathing pattern, Altered thought processes, Decreased cardiac output, Ineffective individual coping, High risk for injury, High risk for self-directed violence	
45	Hypovolemic Shock	438
	Fluid volume deficit, Impaired gas exchange, Decreased cardiac output, Altered tissue perfusion	

46	Psychosocial Care	447
	Anxiety, Sleep pattern disturbance, Ineffective individual coping, Hopelessness, Powerlessness, Altered sensory perception (overload), *Altered sensory perception* (deprivation), *Altered thought processes, Altered family processes, Spiritual*	
47	Septic Shock	465
	Altered tissue perfusion, Impaired gas exchange, Altered cardiac output	

APPENDICES: COMMON NURSING DIAGNOSES

A:	Altered Nutrition—Less Than Body Requirements	475
B:	Knowledge Deficit	483
C:	High Risk for Injury	487
D:	Normal Laboratory Values	491
	Normal Hemodynamic Values	493
	Normal Arterial Blood Gas (ABG) Values	493

INDEX 495

PREFACE

The purpose of this book is to provide experienced, practicing critical care nurses with an easy-to-use resource to facilitate the planning of care for noncardiac critically ill patients. Comprehensive, state-of-the-art data for the most commonly seen disorders are presented, providing a framework for nurses to plan individualized patient care. Elements of the text that facilitate ease of use include (1) organization of content by systems (2) separation of widely applicable diagnoses into appendices, (3) inclusion of the physiological cause for specific clinical manifestations, (4) integration of collaborative and independent interventions, and (5) provision of scientific rationale for the more complex interventions. Nurses who are just entering critical care practice and/or nursing students with clinical experiences in critical care may also find this book useful.

For the most part, frequency of interventions are omitted from the text. Most critical care units establish standards that dictate the minimum frequency of certain assessments and/or interventions, that is, vital signs and assessments every two hours; cardiac output every four hours. The patient's condition and/or the implementation of specific interventions dictates whether these frequencies need to be modified. An unstable patient on vasoactive drips may require vital signs every fifteen minutes. A patient with decreasing mental status may require neurological checks every hour. A patient just given a diuretic will need urine output measured every hour to assess the adequacy of the response. Because the patient's condition can change so rapidly, setting specific time lines would be misleading. The experienced critical care nurse adjusts the frequency of assessments and interventions based on standards, patient condition, and the need to assess response to prescribed therapies.

Four nursing diagnoses have been dealt with separately in the Appendices: Altered Nutrition–Less Than Body Requirements; Knowledge Deficit; High Risk for Injury and Laboratory, Hemodynamic and Arterial Blood Gas Values. These diagnoses are applicable to all critically ill patients. Nutrition, an area often neglected, is a high priority in critically ill patients who are stressed and require all the healing powers they possess. Research has shown that adequate nutrition and survival rates are linked. Critical care nurses teach their patients constantly: about the critical care environment, about the current plan of care, about the long-term implications of their illness. Risk for injury in the critical care environment is a constant concern due to the use of multiple invasive and noninvasive monitoring devices and the frequency of altered mental status in patients.

Psychosocial diagnoses have been dealt with in a separate chapter and not within each disorder to avoid repetition and because of their importance and wide range of applicability. This allows experienced critical care nurses to select and apply psychosocial diagnoses as appropriate for their patient(s).

For the most part, patients are not discharged home from a critical care unit but, rather, are transferred to a less acute area prior to discharge. It may be difficult prior to transfer to predict the extent of patient disability and/or discharge destination. Although teaching regarding the patient's diagnosis, it's implications, and patient progress are ongoing elements of nursing care, research has also found that very little teaching done during the intensive phase of critical illness is retained by patients. For this reason the primary focus for "discharge planning" by the critical care nurse becomes continuity of care, that is, communicating appropriate data to the nursing unit to which the patient is transferred after the critical phase of illness/injury is past. Each patient is different and responds differently to critical illness and/or injury, both physically and psychologically. Thus, this section of each chapter remains consistent throughout the book, emphasizing important areas to be dealt with and communicated to transfer units. Where appropriate, more detailed discharge needs, specific for a particular disorder, may be found under appropriate diagnoses and/or rationales within each chapter. This again allows the critical care nurse to individualize data collected related to continuity of care.

In today's cost conscious critical care environment, an up-to-date and ready reference to assist in the development of appropriate, individualized plans of care for specific disorders is invaluable. This book provides such a resource.

SERIES INTRODUCTION

Scientific and technological developments over the past several decades have revolutionized health care and care of the sick. These rapid and extensive advancements of knowledge have occurred in all fields, necessitating an ever-increasing specialization of practice. For nurses to be effective and meet the challenge in today's specialty settings, the body of clinical knowledge and skill needs to continually expand. *Plans of Care for Specialty Practice* has been written to aid the practicing nurse in meeting this challenge. The purpose of this series is to provide comprehensive, state-of-the-art plans of care and associated resource information for patient situations most commonly seen within a specialty that will serve as a standard from which care can be individualized. These plans of care are based on the profession's scientific approach to problem solving—the nursing process. Though the books are primarily written as a guide for frontline staff nurses and clinical nurse specialists practicing in specialty settings, they have application for student nurses as well.

DOCUMENTATION OF CARE

The Joint Commission on Accreditation of Healthcare Organizations (JCAHO) assumes authority for evaluating the quality and effectiveness of the practice of nursing. In 1991, the JCAHO developed its first new nursing care standards in more than a decade. One of the changes brought about by these new standards was the elimination of need for every patient to have a handwritten or computer-generated care plan in his or her chart detailing all or most of the care to be provided. The Joint Commission's standard that describes the documentation requirements stipulates that nursing assessments, identification of nursing diagnoses and/or patient care needs, interventions, outcomes of care, and discharge planning be permanently integrated into the clinical record. In other words, the nursing process needs to be documented. A separate care plan is no longer needed; however, planning and implementing care must continue as always, but using whatever form of documentation that has been approved by an institution. *Plans of Care for Specialty Practice* can be easily used with a wide variety of approaches to documentation of care.

ELEMENTS OF THE PLANS OF CARE

The chapter title is the presenting situation, which represents the most commonly seen conditions/disorders treated within the specialty setting. It may be a medical diagnosis (e.g., diabetes mellitus), a syndrome (e.g., acquired immunodeficiency syndrome), a surgical procedure (e.g., mastectomy), or a diagnostic/therapeutic procedure (e.g., thrombolytic therapy).

An opening paragraph provides a definition or concise overview of the presenting situation. It describes the condition and may contain pertinent physiological/psychological bases for the disorder. It is brief and not intended to replace further investigation for comprehensive understanding of the condition.

Etiologies

A listing of causative factors responsible for or contributing to the presenting situation is provided. This may include predisposing diseases, injuries or trauma, surgeries, microorganisms, genetic factors, environmental hazards, drugs, or psychosocial disorders. In presenting situations where no clear causal relationship can be established, current theories regarding the etiology may be included.

Clinical Manifestations

Objective and subjective signs and symptoms which describe the particular presenting situation are included. This information is revealed as a result of a health history and physical assessment and becomes part of the data base.

Clinical/Diagnostic Findings

This component contains possible diagnostic tests and procedures which might be done to determine abnormalities associated with a particular presenting situation. The name of the diagnostic procedure and the usual abnormal findings are listed.

Nursing Diagnosis

The nursing management of the health problem commences with the planning care phase of the nursing process. This includes obtaining a comprehensive history and physical assessment, identification of the nursing diagnoses, expected outcomes, interventions, and discharge planning needs.

Diagnostic labels identified by NANDA through the Tenth National Conference in April 1992 are being used throughout this series. (Based on North American Nursing Diagnosis Association, 1992. *NANDA Nursing Diagnoses: Definitions and Classification 1992.*) We have also identified new diagnoses not yet on the official NANDA list. We endorse NANDA's recommendation for nurses to develop new nursing diagnoses as the need arises and we encourage nurses using this series to do the same.

"Related to" Statements

Related to statements suggest a link or connection to the nursing diagnosis and provide direction for identifying appropriate nursing interventions. They are termed contributing factors, causes, or etiologies. There is frequently more than one related to statement for a given diagnosis. For example, change in job, marital difficulties, and impending surgery may all be "related to" the patient's nursing diagnosis of anxiety.

There is disagreement at present regarding inclusion of pathophysiological/medical diagnoses in the list of related to statements. Frequently, a medical diagnosis does not provide adequate direction for nursing care. For example, the nursing diagnosis of chronic pain related to rheumatoid arthritis does not readily suggest specific nursing interventions. It is more useful for the nurse to identify specific causes of the chronic pain such as inflammation, swelling, and fatigue; these in turn suggest more specific interventions. In cases where the medical diagnosis provides the best available information, as occurs with the more medically oriented diagnoses such as decreased cardiac output or impaired gas exchange, the medical terminology is included.

Defining Characteristics
Data collection is frequently the source for identifying defining characteristics, sometimes called signs and symptoms or patient behaviors. These data, both subjective and objective, are organized into meaningful patterns and used to verify the nursing diagnosis. The most commonly seen defining characteristics for a given diagnosis are included and should not be viewed as an all-inclusive listing.

Risk Factors
Nursing diagnoses designated as high risk are supported by risk factors that direct nursing actions to reduce or prevent the problem from developing. Since these nursing diagnoses have not yet occurred, risk factors replace the listing of actual defining characteristics and related to statements.

Patient Outcomes
Patient outcomes, sometimes termed patient goals, are observable behaviors or data which measure changes in the condition of the patient after nursing treatment. They are objective indicators of progress toward prevention of the development of high-risk nursing diagnoses or resolution/modification of actual diagnoses. Like other elements of the plan of care, patient outcome statements are dynamic and must be reviewed and modified periodically as the patient progresses. Assigning realistic "target or evaluation dates" for evaluation of progress toward outcome achievement is crucial. Since there are so many considerations involved in when the outcome could be achieved (e.g., varying lengths of stay, individual patient condition), these plans of care do not include evaluation dates; the date needs to be individualized and assigned using the professional judgment and discretion of the nurse caring for the patient.

Nursing Interventions
Nursing interventions are the treatment options/actions the nurse employs to prevent, modify, or resolve the nursing diagnosis. They are driven by the related to statements and risk factors and are selected based on the outcomes to be achieved. Treatment options should be chosen only if they apply realistically to a specific patient condition. The nurse also needs to determine frequencies for each intervention based on professional judgment and individual patient need.

We have included independent, interdependent, and dependent nursing interventions as they reflect current practice. We have not made a distinction between these kinds of interventions because of institutional differences and increasing independence in nursing practice. The interventions that are interdependent or dependent will require collaboration with other professionals. The nurse will need to determine when this is necessary and take appropriate action. The interventions include assessment, therapeutic, and teaching actions.

Rationales

The rationales provide scientific explanation or theoretical bases for the interventions; interventions can then be selected more intelligently and actions can be tailored to each individual's needs.

The rationales provided may be used as a quick reference for the nurse unfamiliar with the reason for a given intervention and as a tool for patient education. These rationales may include principles, theory, and/or research findings from current literature. The rationales are intended as reference information and, as such, should not be transcribed into the permanent patient record. A rationale is not provided when the intervention is self-explanatory.

Discharge Planning/Continuity of Care

Because stays in acute care hospitals are becoming shorter due to cost containment efforts, patients are frequently discharged still needing care; discharge planning is the process of anticipating and planning for needs after discharge. Effective discharge planning begins with admission and continues with ongoing assessment of the patient and family needs. Included in the discharge planning/continuity of care section are suggestions for follow-up measures, such as skilled nursing care; physical, occupational, speech, or psychiatric therapy; spiritual counseling, social service assistence; follow-up appointments, and equipment/supplies.

References

A listing of references appears at the conclusion of each plan of care or related group of plans. The purpose of the references is to cite specific work used and to specify background information or suggestions for further reading. Citings provided represent the most current nursing theory and/or research bases for inclusion in the plans of care.

Clinical Clips

Interspersed throughout the books are brief pieces of information related to the particular specialty. The intent is to blend some concept or theory tidbits with the practical nature of the books. This information not only may enrich the nurse's knowledge base but also may be used in the dissemination of patient education information.

A Word About Family

The authors and editors of this series recognize the vital role that family and/or other significant people play in the recovery of a patient. Isolation from the family unit during hospitalization may disrupt self-concept and feelings of security. Family members, or persons involved in the patient's care, must be included in the teaching to ensure that it is appropriate and will be followed. In an effort to constrain the books' size, the patient outcome, nursing intervention, and discharge planning sections usually do not include reference to the family or other significant people; however, the reader can assume that they are to be included along with the patient whenever appropriate.

Any undertaking of the magnitude of this series becomes the concern of many people. I specifically thank all of the very capable nursing specialists who authored or edited the individual books. Their attention to providing state-of-the-art information in a quick, usable form will provide the reader with current reference information for providing excellent patient care.

The editorial staff, particularly Patricia E. Casey and Elisabeth F. Williams, and production people at Delmar Publishers have been outstanding. Their frank criticism, comments, and encouragement have improved the quality of the series.

Finally, but most importantly, I thank my husband, John, and children, Katrina and Allison, for their sacrifices and patience during yet another publishing project.

Kathy V. Gettrust
Series Editor

LIST OF TABLES

17.1	Levels and Consequent Results of Spinal Injury
17.2	Types of Incomplete Cord Transection
21.1	Pathologic Reflexes
21.2	Respiratory Patterns Related to Brain Pathology
21.3	Glasgow Coma Scale
21.4	Intracranial Pressure Monitoring Devices
21.5	Intracranial Pressure Waveforms

Endocrine Care

▼

ACUTE ADRENAL CRISIS

The adrenal cortex is responsible for the secretion of glucocorticoids (primarily cortisol) and mineralcorticoids (primarily aldosterone). Cortisol release is regulated by adrenocorticotropic hormone (ACTH) from the anterior pituitary gland, which in turn is controlled by corticotropin releasing factor from the hypothalamus. Cortisol influences glucose, protein and fat metabolism; has anti-inflammatory actions and psychic effects; and plays a major role in regulating the stress response. Aldosterone is regulated by the renin-angiotensin system and its major role is in regulating potassium and sodium levels and water balance. Disease of the adrenal gland may be due to either destruction of the adrenal gland itself (primary disease) or a disorder of the hypothalamic-pituitary-adrenal system (secondary disease).

Acute adrenal crisis is a life-threatening state of acute suppression or absolute lack of secretion of cortisol and/or aldosterone. Deficiency of glucocorticoids is particularly serious because cortisol's role in the body's defense mechanisms and response to stress is essential for life.

ETIOLOGIES

- Primary mechanisms (Addison's disease): destruction of the adrenal gland secondary to
  - –autoimmune disorders
  - –granulomatous infiltrations
  - –adrenal hemorrhage
  - –irradiation
  - –infarction
  - –metastasis
  - –infections: tuberculosis, fungal disease, cytomegalovirus (AIDS)
  - –bilateral adrenalectomy

These disorders result in a deficit of both glucocorticoids (cortisol) and mineralcorticoids (aldosterone).

- Secondary mechanisms: suppression of adrenocorticotropic hormone (ACTH) and/or corticosteroid secretion secondary to
  - –long-term steroid use
  - –pituitary and hypothalamic disorders

These disorders result in a deficit of glucocorticoids (cortisol).

- Acute crisis
  - most commonly occurs in patients currently on or recently withdrawn from corticosteroid therapy who are stressed in some way
  - can also occur in any patient with chronic adrenal insufficiency who does not receive adequate hormone replacement during stress

CLINICAL MANIFESTATIONS

- Cardiovascular: Hypovolemia, decreased vascular tone, and hyperkalemia produce
  - dysrhythmias
  - CO < 4 L/min
  - CVP < 2 mmHg
  - hypotension
  - weak rapid pulse
  - possible hemodynamic collapse and shock
  - cold, pale skin
  - CI < 2.5 L/min/m^2
  - PCWP < 8 mmHg
  - tachycardia
- Electrical: Hyperkalemia produces
  - prolonged QT interval
  - long PR interval
  - widened QRS
  - first-degree heart block
  - decreased P amplitude
  - peaked T waves
  - ventricular dysrhythmias
- Gastrointestinal: Decreased digestive enzymes, intestinal motility, and digestion produce
  - abdominal pain
  - nausea and vomiting
  - diarrhea
  - anorexia
  - weight loss
- Renal: Decreased circulating volume and hypotension produce decreased urine output.
- Skin: Increased ACTH and melanotic stimulating hormone (primary disease only) produce hyperpigmentation, especially in the creases of the hands and on the soles of the feet.
- Neurological: Hypoglycemia, decreased protein metabolism, hyponatremia, and hypovolemia produce
  - emotional lability
  - headaches
  - mental confusion
  - apathy
  - fatigue and weakness
  - lethargy
  - depression

  NOTE: Look for patients at risk, with predisposing factors or physical findings associated with chronic adrenal insufficiency.

CLINICAL/DIAGNOSTIC FINDINGS

- Decreased glucocorticoids produce
  - decreased plasma cortisol (normal values vary)
  - hypoglycemia (<60 mg/dL)
  - increased ACTH (primary)

- −decreased ACTH (secondary)
- −BUN > 20 mg/dL
- −anemia (Hgb < 13 g/dL)
- −eosinophilia (>350/mm³)
- −lymphocytosis (>4000/mm³)

NOTE: Plasma cortisol values normally fluctuate during a 24-hr period and increase with stress. If the value is *normal* in a stressed individual, it is considered inappropriately low.

- Decreased aldosterone produces
  - −hyperkalemia (>5.0 mEq/L)
  - −hyponatremia (<135 mEq/L)
  - −metabolic acidosis (pH < 7.35)
- Decreased volume produces
  - −hypercalcemia (>10.5 mg/dL)
  - −hyperuricemia (>6 mg/dL for women; >7 mg/dL for men)

NOTE: Because of the life-threatening nature of this condition, the patient is initially treated based on clinical manifestations, that is, before lab results can confirm the diagnosis. Dexamethasone (Decadron) is given in the interim since it will not interfere with serum cortisol levels.

NURSING DIAGNOSIS: FLUID VOLUME DEFICIT

Related To aldosterone deficiency producing loss of sodium and water

Defining Characteristics
CO < 4 L/min
CVP < 2 mmHg
Dry mucous membranes
Hyponatremia (<135 mEq/L)
Skin cool, pale, and dry
Urine output < 30 mL/hr

CI < 2.5 L/min/m²
PCWP < 8 mmHg
Hyperkalemia (>5 mEq/L)
Hypotension
Tachycardia

Patient Outcomes
Adequate fluid balance is maintained/restored, as evidenced by:
- blood pressure within 10 mmHg of patient baseline
- CO 4–8 L/min; CI 2.5–4 L/min/m²
- CVP 2–10 mmHg; PCWP 8–12 mmHg
- heart rate 60–100 bpm
- pink, moist mucous membranes
- serum sodium 135–145 mEq/L
- serum potassium 3.5–5.0 mEq/L
- warm, pink skin
- urine output > 30 mL/hr

Nursing Interventions	Rationales
Assess for peripheral indicators of fluid balance: mucous membranes, skin turgor, and thirst	Dry mucous membranes, poor skin turgor, and increased thirst are indicators of fluid volume deficit.
Monitor/document cardiovascular status: vital signs with orthostatic changes, hemodynamics, and peripheral pulses.	Increased respiratory rate, increased heart rate, decreased blood pressure, and/or orthostatic changes; low CVP, PCWP, CO/CI, and MAP and weak peripheral pulses indicate persistent hypovolemia.
Monitor and record fluid balance: daily weight and intake and output.	
Monitor heart rhythm (EKG) continuously and document any changes.	Decreased aldosterone can produce hyperkalemia and decreased volume can produce hypercalcemia either of which may cause dysrhythmias.
Monitor potassium and sodium.	Aldosterone deficiency can produce hyperkalemia and hyponatremia. Return of these values to normal reflects adequate hormone and fluid replacement. Correction will minimize cardiac dysrhythmias (hyperkalemia), altered mental status (hyponatremia), and water loss.
Monitor renal function: BUN, creatinine, hourly urine output, specific gravity, urine sodium, and potassium.	These measures indicate the adequacy of hormone and fluid volume replacement. Blood urea nitrogen and creatinine reflect renal function and their increase forewarns of prolonged decreased renal perfusion from hypovolemia. A low urine output and high specific gravity show decreased renal perfusion and inadequate fluid replacement.

Nursing Interventions	Rationales
Administer intravenous fluids and electrolytes as prescribed until signs and symptoms of hypovolemia stabilize. Monitor for signs of fluid overload: increased CVP, increased PCWP, adventitious lung sounds, jugular venous distention, and signs of respiratory distress.	Initially 5% dextrose in normal saline is given rapidly to reverse hypoglycemia and dehydration. The patient must be monitored closely to prevent fluid overload, particularly if there is underlying cardiac disease.
Avoid abrupt changes in position (to upright) until fluid balance is restored.	During hypovolemia, orthostatic changes can produce dizziness and syncope.
Prevent adrenal crisis by ensuring patients at risk receive exogenous cortisol in stress states.	Patients with chronic adrenal insufficiency should be instructed to double their dose of steroids with minor stress or contact their physician with severe stress.

NURSING DIAGNOSIS: ALTERED TISSUE PERFUSION—CARDIOVASCULAR AND PERIPHERAL

Related To
- Decreased effectiveness of catecholamines
- Decreased vascular tone
- Hypovolemia

Defining Characteristics
Confusion
CO < 4 L/min
CVP < 2 mmHg
Hypotension
SvO_2 < 70%
Weak, thready peripheral pulses

Cool, clammy skin
CI < 2.5 L/min/m^2
PCWP < 8 mmHg
Urine output < 30 mL/hr
SVR < 800 dyn/s/cm^{-5}

Patient Outcomes
Central and peripheral perfusion and hemodynamics are stable, as evidenced by
- blood pressure within 10 mmHg of patient baseline
- MAP > 60 mmHg
- CO 4–8 L/min; CI 2.5–4.0 L/min/m^2
- CVP 2–10 mmHg; PCWP 8–12 mmHg
- SVR 800–1200 dyn/s/cm^{-5}
- peripheral pulses that are palpable to patient baseline

- sensorium that returns to patient baseline
- warm, dry skin
- urine output > 30 mL/hr
- SvO_2 70–90%

Nursing Interventions	Rationales
Monitor/record changes in mental status, that is, anxiety, confusion, lethargy, coma, and personality changes.	Cortisol deficiency and hyponatremia can produce changes in mental status. Hypovolemia may also produce changes in mental status due to decreased cerebral perfusion. A worsening of mental status may indicate inadequate hormone and/or volume replacement.
Monitor/record heart rate, respiratory rate, and blood pressure.	Heart rate and respiratory rate will be elevated as long as tissue perfusion is low. Blood pressure will be low until vasodilatation and low volume are corrected by administration of intravenous hormone and fluids.
Monitor/record CVP, PCWP, and SvO_2 if available.	A low CVP and PCWP will indicate the patient is still hypovolemic. A low SvO_2 indicates inadequate tissue perfusion and oxygen transport.
Monitor/record cardiac output (CO)/cardiac index (CI) and systemic vascular resistance (SVR).	Cardiac output is a major determinant of tissue perfusion. A low CO/CI indicates volume and hormone replacement is not yet adequate. A low SVR indicates continued decreased vascular tone (vasodilatation) and hypoperfusion.
Monitor peripheral circulation status and record: Inspect skin, noting color and temperature; check quality of peripheral pulses and capillary refill time (CRT).	Cool, clammy, pale skin, weak peripheral pulses, or increased CRT indicate decreased circulating volume and peripheral perfusion.

Nursing Interventions	Rationales
Note hourly changes in urine output. Record specific gravity.	Urine output reflects kidney perfusion. A low urine output and high specific gravity indicate inadequate volume and hormone replacement.
Administer scheduled doses of intravenous glucocorticoids (hydrocortisone, 100–300 mg IV immediately and an additional 100 mg in IV solution every 6–8 hr until stable), assess patient response, and assess for side effects.	Since low cortisol levels are responsible for the acute signs and symptoms, they should disappear with administration of hydrocortisone. Possible side effects from glucocorticoid administration include hyperglycemia, fluid and electrolyte imbalances, congestive heart failure, hypertension, and nausea and vomiting.

NURSING DIAGNOSIS: ALTERED THOUGHT PROCESSES

Related To
- Decreased glucose levels
- Decreased perfusion
- Decreased protein metabolism
- Decreased sodium

Defining Characteristics
Confusion
Emotional lability
Hypoglycemia (<60 mg/dL)
Hyponatremia (<135 mEq/L)
Lethargy

Patient Outcomes
- Sensorium returns to patient baseline.
- Serum glucose and sodium levels are within normal range.

Nursing Interventions	Rationales
Assess level of consciousness, ability to speak, and response to stimuli and/or commands.	The hypoglycemia, decreased perfusion, and hyponatremia resulting from adrenal crisis can produce changes in level of consciousness and neurological response.

Nursing Interventions	Rationales
Observe for behavioral responses, orientation, confusion, and irritability.	Same as for the first intervention above.
Monitor serum glucose and sodium levels.	Glucose is the primary energy source for the brain; thus hypoglycemia can produce altered mental status. Hyponatremia produces an extracellular hypoosmolar state causing water to move into brain cells, which can produce cerebral edema and altered mental status.
Minimize effects of environment on mental status: 1. Provide for consistent caregivers when possible. 2. Encourage family/significant other to stay with patient. 3. Minimize stressful situations. 4. Promote sleep and rest. 5. Reorient as needed. 6. Explain all procedures and cares. 7. Orient to immediate environment and equipment.	The stresses of the critical care environment (sensory overload, sensory deprivation, and sleep deprivation) can aggravate mental status changes produced physiologically. Taking preventive measures may minimize the environmental effects.
Administer and assess effects of prescribed drugs.	As corticosteroids are replaced, mental status should clear.

NURSING DIAGNOSIS: ACTIVITY INTOLERANCE

Related To
- Use of endogenous protein for energy needs
- Loss of skeletal muscle mass

Defining Characteristics
Early fatigue
Exertional dyspnea
Weakness

Patient Outcomes
The patient will demonstrate increased tolerance to physical activity, as evidenced by

- the return of blood pressure, heart rate, and respiratory rate to baseline within 4 min of activity.
- the patient verbalizing decreased fatigue.

Nursing Interventions	Rationales
Assess muscle strength and need for assistance.	
Assess for causes of fatigue, that is, treatments, medications, inadequate nutrition, and inadequate sleep.	
Monitor patient response to activity: blood pressure, respiratory rate, heart rate, and heart rhythm before, during, and after activity. Note tachycardia, dysrhythmias, dyspnea, pallor, diaphoresis, dizziness, or fatigue.	Heart rate, blood pressure, and respiratory rate should return to baseline within 4 min after activity.
Provide passive/active range-of-motion exercises to patient if bedridden	Range-of-motion exercises maintain blood flow, muscle tone, and flexibility.
Increase activity gradually. Terminate if there are signs or symptoms of intolerance.	
Schedule activities to decrease energy expenditure. Space with rest periods.	
Provide supplemental oxygen during activity.	Oxygen administration can increase exercise tolerance.

DISCHARGE PLANNING/CONTINUITY OF CARE

- Assess need for/type of long-term care and follow-up.
- If the discharge destination is home, assess existing supports and the need for assistance.
- Determine coping deficits/support needs and institute assistance measures.
- Determine knowledge deficits/teaching needs; document and institute a teaching plan.
- Refer patient to social services as appropriate.

- Communicate coping deficits/support needs and knowledge deficits/teaching needs to the unit accepting the patient on transfer.

REFERENCES

Chin, R. & Zekan, J. M. (1990). Adrenal insufficiency. *Problems in Critical Care, 4*(3), 312–324.

Epstein, C. D. (1992). Adrenocortical insufficiency in the critically ill patient. *AACN Clinical Issues in Critical Care Nursing, 3*(3), 705–713.

Knowlton, A. I. (1989). Adrenal insufficiency in the intensive care setting. *Journal of Intensive Care Medicine, 4*(1), 35–45.

Lee, L. M. & Gumowski, J. (1992). Adrenocortical insufficiency: A medical emergency. *AACN Clinical Issues in Critical Care Nursing, 3*(2), 319–330.

Longcope, C. (1991). Hypoadrenal crisis. In J. M. Rippe, R. S. Irwin, J. S. Alpert, & M. P. Fink (Eds.), *Intensive Care Medicine* (2nd ed., pp. 983–987). Boston, MA: Little, Brown.

Reasner, C. A. (1990). Adrenal disorders. *Critical Care Nursing Quarterly, 13*(3), 67–73.

▼

DIABETIC KETOACIDOSIS

Diabetic ketoacidosis (DKA), a common complication of insulin-dependent diabetes mellitus (IDDM), results from sustained relative or absolute insulin deficiency. In DKA, uptake of glucose by muscle cells is decreased, production of glucose by the liver is increased, and the metabolism of free fatty acids into ketone bodies within the liver is increased. The physiological result is a disorder manifested by hyperglycemia, uncontrolled lipolysis (decomposition of fat), ketogenesis (production of ketone bodies), ketonemia, negative nitrogen balance, fluid loss, electrolyte imbalance, and acid-base imbalance. Developing over several hours or days, fluid loss and ketoacidosis may be severe enough to produce shock and coma. The mortality rate for this disorder ranges from 2 to 18%.

ETIOLOGIES

- Most common:
  - initial presentation of previously undiagnosed patient with diabetes mellitus
  - Type I insulin-dependent diabetic who omits insulin dose or decreases dose, does not adhere to diabetic diet, has uncontrolled diabetes with inadequate insulin coverage, and experiences severe stress without adequate adjustment of insulin
  - Type II NIDDM with coexistent severe medical problems or stress
- Stressors
  - infections: pneumonia, sepsis, urinary tract, upper respiratory, meningitis, pancreatitis, cholecystitis
  - severe stress: infection, trauma, surgery, acute illness, pregnancy
- Less common
  - drugs that impair glucose metabolism: thiazide diuretics, phenytoin, steroids, epinephrine, psychotropics, analgesics, beta blockers
  - endocrine disorders: hyperthyroidism, Cushing's disease, pheochromocytoma
  - Alcohol intoxication, salicylate intoxication

CLINICAL MANIFESTATIONS

- Presentation: polyuria, polydipsia, weakness, abdominal pain, nausea, vomiting
- Cardiovascular: Hypovolemia from hyperglycemic osmotic diuresis produces
  - –tachycardia
  - –CVP < 2 mmHg
  - –hypothermia
  - –weak peripheral pulses
  - –CO < 4 L/min
  - –hypotension
  - –PCWP < 8 mmHg
  - –pale, moist, cool skin
  - –CI < 2.5 L/min/m^2
- Pulmonary: Metabolic acidosis and increased ketones can produce
  - –Kussmaul respirations
  - –acetone breath
- Neurological: Hypovolemia and acidosis can produce
  - –confusion
  - –lethargy
  - –headache
  - –decreased tendon reflexes
  - –delirium
  - –visual disturbances
  - –coma
- Gastrointestinal: Acidosis and dehydration produce
  - –nausea and vomiting
  - –polydipsia
  - –abdominal pain
  - –anorexia
  - –weight loss
- Renal: Hyperglycemia produces polyuria.

CLINICAL/DIAGNOSTIC FINDINGS

- Uncontrolled glucose produces
  - hyperglycemia (350–750 mg/dL)
  - hyperosmolality (>295 mOsm/L)
  - increased urine glucose
- Ketoacidosis produces
  - arterial pH < 7.35 (commonly <7.1)
  - serum bicarbonate < 15 mmol/L
  - anion gap > 20 mmol/L
  - serum and urine ketones
- Osmotic diuresis produces
  - hemoconcentration: increased hematocrit, BUN, leukocytosis
  - normal, elevated, or decreased potassium but body stores that are depleted regardless of level
  - normal or elevated sodium depending on hydration
  - initial hypermagnesemia, then hypomagnesemia (total body stores depleted)
  - hypophosphatemia (phosphate < 2.5 mg/dL)

Diabetic Ketoacidosis 15

NURSING DIAGNOSIS: FLUID VOLUME DEFICIT

Related To
- Osmotic diuresis
- Vomiting
- Total body water loss

Defining Characteristics

Hypotension	Tachycardia
CVP < 2 mmHg	PCWP < 8 mmHg
CO < 4 L/min	CI < 2.5 L/min/m^2
Dry mucous membranes	Poor skin turgor
Weak peripheral pulses	Weight loss

Patient Outcomes

Adequate fluid balance is maintained/restored, as evidenced by
- blood pressure within 10 mmHg patient baseline
- heart rate 60–100 bpm
- CVP 2–10 mmHg; PCWP 8–12 mmHg
- CO 4–8 L/min; CI 2.5–4 L/min/m^2
- normal skin turgor
- moist mucous membranes
- weight return to patient baseline

Nursing Interventions	Rationales
Monitor vital signs for hypotension, tachycardia, and increased respiratory rate.	Fluid deficit produces hypotension, tachycardia, and increased respiratory rate. Hypotension, if prolonged, can produce other complications such as acute renal failure and must be corrected rapidly.
Monitor hemodynamic measurements for low CVP/PCWP and low CO/CI.	Fluid volume deficit produces low CVP, PCWP, CO and CI. Low CO/CI, if prolonged, can produce other complications such as acute renal failure.
Monitor peripheral indicators of fluid deficits: peripheral pulses, skin turgor, and mucous membranes.	Weak, thready pulses, poor skin turgor, and dry mucous membranes indicate fluid volume deficit.

16 Endocrine Care

Nursing Interventions	Rationales
Monitor/document fluid balance: intake and output, hourly urine output, and daily weight.	Decreased urine output (<30mL/hr) reflects decreased renal perfusion due to inadequate volume replacement. If decreased renal perfusion is prolonged, acute renal failure may develop. Hourly monitoring is required to evaluate the adequacy of fluid replacement.
Monitor neurological status closely during fluid administration	Hypovolemia severe enough to produce hypotension, hypernatremia, and low cardiac output can result in neurological signs such as confusion, lethargy, delirium, and drowsiness. These signs should resolve with treatment of DKA. If these signs become worse during treatment, it may indicate fluid overload and cerebral edema.
Initiate intravenous fluid administration as prescribed, monitoring for signs and symptoms of fluid overload: increased heart rate, increased blood pressure, jugular venous distention, fine crackles, c/o SOB, increased CVP/PCWP, and increased weight over baseline.	Initially, isotonic saline is administered rapidly (1–2 L in the first few hours) to correct the fluid volume deficit. Close monitoring of vital signs and hemodynamics must occur to prevent fluid overload.

NURSING DIAGNOSIS: ELECTROLYTE IMBALANCE
Related To
- Lack of insulin
- Acid-base imbalance
- Fluid shifts
- Vomiting

Defining Characteristics

Hyperglycemia (>350 mg/dL)
Potassium < 3.5 mEq/L
Magnesium < 1.5 mg/dL
Serum bicarbonate < 21 mEq/L
Sodium < 135 mEq/L
Phosphate < 2.5 mg/dL
pH < 7.35

Patient Outcomes

Serum glucose and electrolyte values will return to normal range.

Nursing Interventions	Rationales
Evaluate the patient for a precipitating cause.	The precipitating cause of DKA (underlying illness, improper insulin administration, drugs, etc.) must be identified and treated to prevent ongoing and future problems with serum glucose control.
Monitor blood glucose every hour via a glucose meter.	While receiving insulin, glucose can drop rapidly and dextrose should be added to intravenous fluids when the blood sugar reaches 250–300 mg/dL (see the last intervention in this part).
Monitor serum electrolytes every 2 hr until stable, especially potassium, magnesium, and phosphorus.	The serum potassium level may initially be high, but body stores of potassium are depleted due to movement of potassium out of the cells and diuresis. Magnesium and phosphorus are also lost in the osmotic diuresis.
Monitor for signs and symptoms of hypokalemia: flat/inverted T waves, depressed ST segment, confusion, fatigue, irritability, and paresthesias.	Potassium plays a major role in maintaining neuromuscular and cardiac function. Hypokalemia can produce life-threatening dysrhythmias.
Monitor for signs and symptoms of hypomagnesemia: tremors, muscle cramps, dysrhythmias, confusion, paresthesias, and EKG changes.	Magnesium is important for neuromuscular transmission, muscle contraction, and myocardial function. Deficits can produce cardiac and neuromuscular compromise.

Nursing Interventions	Rationales
Monitor for signs and symptoms of hypophosphatemia: tremors, paresthesias, weakness, mental status changes, GI symptoms, and decreased myocardial and respiratory function.	Phosphorus is essential for muscle contraction and nerve transmission. Severe hypophosphatemia (<1.0 mg/100 mL) can produce severe myocardial depression and respiratory failure.
Monitor arterial pH and administer sodium bicarbonate if pH < 7.10.	Sodium bicarbonate should be administered with restraint since the pH will correct itself as insulin is given and the blood sugar returns to normal, halting the production of ketoacids. Though its administration remains controversial, administration should be considered if the patient demonstrates neurological or cardiovascular complications. Monitor the pH closely for the development of metabolic alkalosis.
Titrate insulin therapy according to glucose level, monitoring the patient for signs and symptoms of hypoglycemia.	
Replace electrolytes as needed per protocols according to serum measurements.	Critical care units frequently have protocols for administration of electrolytes such as potassium and magnesium based on serum values. Specific cautions for administration are described under the specific electrolyte disorder in Section 6.
Add glucose to maintenance IVs once blood sugar is 250–300 mg/dL.	Dropping glucose levels too rapidly can cause fluid shifts between the brain and serum due to differences in osmolality resulting in cerebral edema.

NURSING DIAGNOSIS: INEFFECTIVE BREATHING PATTERN

Related To
- Metabolic acidosis
- Decreased level of consciousness

Defining Characteristics

Kussmaul respirations (increased rate and depth)
Decreased $PaCO_2$ (<35 torr)
Altered mental status

Patient Outcomes

An effective breathing pattern will be maintained/restored, as evidenced by:

- normal respiratory rate and pattern
- $PaCO_2$ 35–45 torr
- return of patient's normal mentation

Nursing Interventions	Rationales
Assess respiratory status every 2 hr: airway and breathing effort and use of accessory muscles; rate and depth of respiration; breath sounds; and ABGs as ordered and prn and correlate results with clinical exam.	The metabolic acidosis in DKA produces increased rate and depth of respirations as a method of compensation. Respirations should normalize as arterial pH normalizes. However, rapid administration of fluid, especially in patients with compromised cardiac function, can produce fluid collection in the lungs and worsen breathing patterns.
Support airway as appropriate: airway, supplementary oxygen, suctioning, or endotracheal intubation.	
Position patient for ease of respiratory effort, that is, head of bed elevated.	
Minimize activity to decrease oxygen need.	
Prevent aspiration in patients with impaired level of consciousness: head of bed elevated and nasogastric decompression.	Patients with DKA may experience nausea and vomiting. If they also have an impaired level of consciousness, they may be unable to adequately protect their airway from aspiration. The risk should be evaluated and preventive measures taken.

NURSING DIAGNOSIS: ALTERED THOUGHT PROCESSES

Related To
- Hyperglycemia
- Electrolyte imbalance
- Acidosis

Defining Characteristics
Confusion
Drowsiness
Lethargy
Coma

Patient Outcomes
The patient will return to baseline mentation.

Nursing Interventions	Rationales
Monitor neurological status every hour until stable, then every 2 hr: orientation, weakness, confusion, lethargy, drowsiness, obtundation, and motor function.	Fluid imbalance, acidosis, and electrolyte imbalances can precipitate changes in neurological function in patients with DKA. The severity of these neurological derangements reflects the severity of the imbalances and should improve with treatment.
Minimize effects of environment on mental status: 1. Reorient patient as needed. 2. Maintain quiet environment, minimizing extraneous stimuli. 3. Provide simple, brief explanations of activities, procedures, or equipment. 4. Provide meaningful, relaxing stimuli to patient. 5. Provide consistent caregivers when possible.	The stresses of the critical care environment (sensory overload, sensory deprivation, and sleep deprivation) can aggravate mental status changes produced physiologically. Taking preventive measures may minimize these environmental effects.
Provide for safety and minimize hazards related to immobility and alterations in consciousness: 1. Oral and skin care every 2 hr 2. Reposition every 1–2 hr 3. Active/passive ROM 4. Provide for elimination 5. Siderails up, bed in low position, bed check 6. Special mattress	Patients with altered levels of consciousness and compromised mobility and ability to perform ADLs are at high risk for skin breakdown, oral infections/sores, and falls.

Nursing Interventions	Rationales
Keep head of bed elevated 30°–45°.	The patient with altered mental status is at risk for vomiting and aspiration.
Obtain an order for a nasogastric tube in patients with altered level of consciousness.	Inserting a nasogastric tube and keeping the stomach empty will minimize the risk for vomiting and aspiration.

DISCHARGE PLANNING/CONTINUITY OF CARE

- Assess need for/type of long-term care and follow-up.
- If the discharge destination is home, assess existing supports and the need for assistance.
- Determine coping deficits/support needs and institute assistance measures.
- Determine knowledge deficits/teaching needs and document and institute a teaching plan.
- Refer patient to social services as appropriate.
- Communicate coping deficits/support needs and knowledge deficits/teaching needs to unit accepting patient on transfer.

REFERENCES

Graves, L. (1990). Diabetic ketoacidosis and hyperosmolar hyperglycemic nonketotic coma. *Critical Care Nursing Quarterly, 13*(3), 49–61.

Sabo, C. E. & Michael, S. R. (1989). Diabetic ketoacidosis: Pathophysiology, nursing diagnosis and nursing interventions. *Focus on Critical Care, 16*(1), 21–28.

Sauve, D. O. & Kessler, C. A. (1992). Hyperglycemic emergencies. *AACN Clinical Issues in Critical Care Nursing, 3*(2), 350–360.

Silverberg, J. D. & Kreisberg, R. A. (1990). Hyperglycemic disorders. *Problems in Critical Care, 4*(3), 355–371.

Siperstein, M. D. (1992). Diabetic ketoacidosis and hyperosmolar coma. *Endocrinology and Metabolism Clinics of North America, 21*(2), 415–432.

Yeates, S. & Blaufuss, J. (1990). Managing the patient in diabetic ketoacidosis. *Focus on Critical Care, 17*(3), 240–248.

DISTURBANCES OF ANTIDIURETIC HORMONE (ADH)

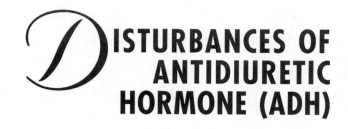

Produced in the supraoptic nuclei of the hypothalamus and released from the neurohypophysis (posterior pituitary) where it is stored, ADH acts on the renal distal and collecting tubules to cause reabsorption of water. In high concentrations, ADH also acts on smooth muscles of the arterioles to produce vasoconstriction. Release of ADH is mediated by both osmotic and nonosmotic factors: osmoreceptors in the hypothalamus respond to changes in extracellular osmolality; stretch receptors in the left atrium and baroreceptors in the carotid sinus and aortic arch respond to changes in circulating volume and blood pressure, respectively. Normally ADH is released in response to high serum osmolality, elevated serum sodium, decreased blood volume, decreased blood pressure, stress, trauma, hypoxia, pain, and anxiety. Certain drugs can also cause ADH release: barbiturates, morphine, vincristine, nicotine, general anesthetics, and carbamazepines. Other drugs inhibit ADH release: ethanol, glucocorticoids, phenytoin, adrenergic agents, and narcotic antagonists. Two common disturbances of ADH are diabetes insipidus (DI) and the syndrome of inappropriate antidiuretic hormone (SIADH).

DIABETES INSIPIDUS

Diabetes insipidus (DI) results from an ADH deficiency (neurogenic DI), ADH insensitivity (nephrogenic DI), or excessive water intake (secondary DI). The result is impaired renal conservation of water and profound diuresis. This defect may be permanent or transient.

ETIOLOGIES

- ADH deficiency (neurogenic DI)
  - idiopathic; familial/congenital
  - intracranial surgery especially in the region of the pituitary
  - tumors: craniopharyngioma, pituitary tumors, metastases

- infections: meningitis, encephalitis
- cranulomatous disease: tuberculosis, sarcoidosis
- severe head trauma or any disorder that causes increased intracranial pressure
- vascular disorders: aneurysms, Sheehan's syndrome
• ADH insensitivity (nephrogenic DI)
    - hereditary
    - renal disease: pyelonephritis, polycystic kidney disease, obstructive uropathy, transplant
    - multisystem disorders affecting kidneys: multiple myeloma, sickle cell disease, cystic fibrosis
    - metabolic disturbances: chronic hypokalemia or hypercalemia
    - drugs: ethanol, phenytoin, lithium carbonate, demeclocycline, amphotericin, methoxyflurane
• Excessive water intake (secondary DI)
    - osmoreceptors reset
    - psychogenic polydipsia
    - excessive intravenous fluid administration

CLINICAL MANIFESTATIONS

- Cardiovascular: Water loss produces
    - hypotension
    - PCWP < 8 mmHg
    - decreased skin turgor
    - dry mucous membranes
    - CVP < 2 mmHg
    - tachycardia
    - weight loss
- Renal: ADH suppression produces
    - pale, dilute urine
    - polyuria (5–40 L possible in 24 hr)
- Neurological: Decreased cerebral perfusion, cerebral dehydration, and hypernatremia produce
    - confusion
    - restlessness
    - coma
    - irritability
    - seizures
    - lethargy

CLINICAL/DIAGNOSTIC FINDINGS

- Urine osmolality inappropriately low in the face of high serum osmolality
- Urine specific gravity decreased
- Serum sodium > 145 mEq/L
- Serum osmolality > 295 mOsm/kg
- Plasma ADH < 1 pg/mL
- BUN and creatinine increased (hemoconcentration)

NURSING DIAGNOSIS: FLUID VOLUME DEFICIT

Related To
- Deficient ADH
- Renal cells insensitive to ADH
- Polyuria and inability to respond to thirst

Defining Characteristics

Hypotension
Tachycardia
Poor skin turgor
Hypernatremia (Na > 145 mEq/L)
Decreased urine specific gravity
Low urine osmolality in face of serum hyperosmolality (inappropriate)

Orthostatic changes
Weak pulses
CVP < 2 mmHg; PCWP < 8 mmHg

Patient Outcomes

Adequate fluid balance is maintained/restored, as evidenced by
- blood pressure within 10 mmHg patient baseline
- urine osmolality appropriate for serum osmolality
- heart rate 60–100 bpm
- normal skin turgor
- peripheral pulses return to baseline
- serum osmolality 275–295 mOsm/kg
- serum sodium 135–145 mEq/L
- CVP 2–10 mmHg; PCWP 8–12 mmHg

Nursing Interventions	Rationales
Monitor/document fluid status: intake and output, daily weight, and urine specific gravity.	Specific gravity reflects the concentration of the urine and helps to indirectly evaluate osmolality of the urine.
Monitor serum osmolarity and serum sodium.	Hyperosmolality and hypernatremia reflect excess water loss in relation to solutes (dilutional imbalance). Return of these values to normal range reflects a return of fluid balance.
Monitor for signs of continuing fluid deficit: hypotension, tachycardia, tachypnea, orthostatic changes, altered hemodynamics (decreased CVP/PCWP and CO/CI), weak peripheral pulses, poor skin turgor, and dry mucous membranes.	These parameters are utilized to evaluate the presence and severity of the fluid deficit.

Nursing Interventions	Rationales
Provide adequate fluids. If patient is able to drink, keep water pitcher full and within reach of patient. If patient is unable to drink, administer fluids to replace fluid loss milliliter for milliliter on an hourly basis.	If losses are not replaced immediately, the patient will rapidly develop hypovolemia and shock.
For central diabetes insipidus administer vasopressin and carbamazepine as prescribed and monitor for water overload.	Vasopressin replaces the absent or reduced ADH, causing water retention. Carbamazepine enhances the release of ADH and augments the renal response to ADH.
For nephrogenic diabetes insipidus administer chlorpropamide (Diabinese) as prescribed monitoring for hypoglycemia and thiazide diuretics and sodium restriction as prescribed.	Chlorpropamide is an antidiabetic agent that also stimulates ADH release and augments renal response to ADH. Because of its antidiabetic properties, the patient must be monitored for hypoglycemia. Thiazide diuretics combined with sodium restriction enhance water reabsorption.

SYNDROME OF INAPPROPRIATE ANTIDIURETIC HORMONE

The syndrome of inappropriate antidiuretic hormone (SIADH) is a syndrome characterized by release of ADH unrelated to plasma osmolality. In SIADH, normal feedback mechanisms no longer control ADH secretion. Because ADH acts on the renal tubules to cause water reabsorption, the patient develops water intoxication and dilutional hyponatremia.

ETIOLOGIES

- Ectopic ADH production
  - bronchogenic cancer most common (oat cell)
  - cancer of prostate, pancreas, or duodenum
  - Hodgkin's disease
  - nonmalignant pulmonary disease: viral pneumonia, tuberculosis, COPD, lung abscess
- Central nervous system disorders
  - head trauma
  - infections: meningitis, encephalitis, brain abscess
  - intracranial surgery, cerebral aneurysms, brain tumors, cerebral atrophy, CVA
  - Guillain-Barré syndrome, lupus erythematosus

- Drugs:
  - chlorpropamide (Diabinese)
  - antineoplastics (vincristine, cyclophosphamide)
  - anesthesia
  - acetaminophen
  - amitriptyline
  - thiazide diuretics
  - carbamazepine (Tegretol)
  - isoproterenol
  - pentamidine
  - tricyclic antidepressants
  - nicotine
- Positive pressure ventilation

CLINICAL MANIFESTATIONS

- Neurological: Brain cell swelling and resulting increased intracranial pressure produce
  - weakness
  - lethargy
  - mental confusion
  - seizures
  - difficulty concentrating
  - restlessness
  - headache
  - coma
- Gastrointestinal: Extracellular fluid congestion and hypernatremia produce
  - nausea
  - vomiting
  - decreased bowel sounds
  - anorexia
  - muscle cramps
- Cardiovascular: Water retention produces
  - weight gain
  - increased blood pressure
  - CVP > 10 mmHg
  - PCWP > 12 mmHg
- Renal: ADH oversecretion produces decreased urine output
- Pulmonary: Water retention produces
  - adventitious lung sounds
  - frothy, pink sputum
  - increased respirations
  - dyspnea

CLINICAL/DIAGNOSTIC FINDINGS

- Urine osmolality inappropriately concentrated in the presence of low serum osmolality
- Urine specific gravity increased
- Serum sodium < 135 mEq/L
- Serum osmolality < 275 mOsm/kg
- Plasma ADH > 5 pg/mL
- BUN and creatinine decreased (hemodilution)
- Urine sodium increased

▼

NURSING DIAGNOSIS: FLUID VOLUME EXCESS

Related To excess water retention from excess ADH

Defining Characteristics
Weight gain
Nausea
Hyponatremia (< 135 mEq/L)
BUN < 5 mg/dL
CVP > 10 mmHg; PCWP > 8 mmHg
Anorexia
Hypo-osmolality (< 275 mOsm/L)
Increased blood pressure
Creatinine < 0.6 mg/dL

Patient Outcomes
Adequate fluid balance is maintained/restored, as evidenced by:
- serum sodium 135–145 mEq/L
- serum osmolality 275–295 mOsm/kg
- weight return to patient baseline
- CVP 2–10 mmHg; PCWP 8–12 mmHg
- blood pressure return to patient baseline
- BUN and creatinine within normal limits

Nursing Interventions	Rationales
Monitor/record fluid balance: intake and output, daily weight, and urine specific gravity.	
Monitor serum sodium and osmolality levels.	Serum sodium and osmolality are low due to water retention and can produce neurological signs and symptoms. Return of these values to normal will reflect the success of therapeutic measures.

Nursing Interventions	Rationales
Monitor/record cardiovascular function: vital signs, hemodynamics, peripheral pulses, neck veins, and presence of peripheral edema.	Blood pressure, heart rate, and respiratory rate can all increase as the body attempts to cope with excess volume. Central venous pressure will increase with increased right ventricular volume. Pulmonary capillary wedge pressure may increase if the patient's left ventricle is unable to cope with the increased volume and begins to fail. If hypervolemia is severe, PCWP may increase with normal left ventricular function. If heart failure occurs, CO/CI will decrease. Full bounding pulses, neck vein distention, and peripheral edema are all indicators of fluid overload. Weak, thready pulses and flat neck veins may indicate fluid deficit.
Monitor/record respiratory function: respiratory rate and pattern, presence of adventitious lung sounds, and ability to mobilize pulmonary secretions.	These parameters can indicate whether fluid overload is compromising pulmonary status. Tachypnea, labored respirations, c/o SOB, or fine crackles are indicators of fluid overload and impending heart failure. The severely dehydrated patient may have difficulty mobilizing secretions.
Maintain fluid restriction.	A fluid restriction will prevent further fluid overload.
Administer hypertonic saline as prescribed and monitor closely for signs of hypernatremia, worsening fluid overload, and heart failure.	Hypertonic saline is used to replace serum sodium in patients with severe symptomatic hyponatremia but can in turn produce hypernatremia, fluid overload, and heart failure.
Administer diuretics as prescribed and document patient response.	Diuretics decrease the effectiveness of ADH and promote diuresis and free water clearance.

Nursing Interventions	Rationales
Administer lithium or demeclocyline as prescribed and monitor their effects.	Lithium and demeclocyline inhibit the action of ADH and promote water excretion.
Explain rationale for therapeutic measures to patient.	Fluid restrictions require the cooperation of the patient. The patient's understanding of therapeutic measures is an essential element of this cooperation.

▼

DISCHARGE PLANNING/CONTINUITY OF CARE

- Assess need for/type of long-term care and follow-up.
- If the discharge destination is home, assess existing supports and the need for assistance.
- Determine coping deficits/support needs and institute assistance measures.
- Determine knowledge deficits/teaching needs and document and institute a teaching plan.
- Refer patient to social services as appropriate
- Communicate coping deficits/support needs and knowledge deficits/learning needs to unit accepting the patient on transfer.

REFERENCES

Batcheller, J. (1992). Disorders of antidiuretic hormone secretion. *AACN Clinical Issues in Critical Care Nursing*, 3(2), 370–378.

Gotch, P. M. (1991). The endocrine system. In J. G. Alspach (Ed.), *Core curriculum for critical care nursing*, (4th ed., pp. 629–637). Philadelphia, PA: Saunders.

Hall, J. & Robertson, G. (1990). Diabetes insipidus. *Problems in Critical Care*, 4(3), 342–354.

Lindaman, C. (1992). SIADH: Is your patient at risk? *Nursing*, 22(6), 60–63.

Patterson, L. M. & Noroian, E. L. (1989). Diabetes insipidus versus syndrome of inappropriate antidiuretic hormone. *Dimensions of Critical Care Nursing*, 8(4), 226–234.

▼

Hyperglycemic Hyperosmotic Nonketotic Coma

Hyperglycemic hyperosmotic nonketotic coma (HHNC) is a hyperglycemic emergency caused by decreased utilization and increased production of glucose. It generally occurs in patients with non-insulin-dependent diabetes mellitus (NIDDM) or Type II diabetes, which means these patients have some endogenous supply of insulin. When a patient with NIDDM is continuously stressed, this supply of insulin may not be adequate to control serum glucose levels but is enough to prevent the production of the ketones seen in DKA. Without the ketoacidosis seen in DKA, these patients develop signs and symptoms later, producing a more severe hyperglycemia, hyperosmolality, and osmotic diuresis. The severe hyperosmolality impairs the thirst center in the hypothalamus, preventing these patients from responding to the significant water losses and producing a severe dehydration. This is compounded by the fact that HHNC develops more slowly (over days to weeks) allowing fluid and electrolyte derangements to become profound. The mortality rate in HHNC is high (14–63%) and results from the underlying illness, cardiovascular collapse, depression of CNS functions, emboli, renal failure, or electrolyte imbalance.

ETIOLOGIES

- Hyperglycemic hyperosmotic nonketotic coma occurs most frequently in middle-aged or elderly patients with NIDDM (40% not previously diagnosed) who are exposed to some continuous diabetogenic stress such as
  - infection: pneumonia, sepsis, urinary tract, cellulitis
  - acute illness: pancreatitis, cerebrovascular insult
  - chronic illness: renal disease, hypertension, heart disease, peripheral vascular disease
  - drugs that alter glucose metabolism: steroids, thiazide diuretics, phenytoin, chlorpromazine, mannitol, diazoxide, propranolol, cimetadine, calcium channel blockers, sympathomimetics
  - excessive parenteral glucose

- Iatrogenic stress (nondiabetics)
  - hyperalimentation
  - high-protein gastric tube feedings
  - hyperosmolar peritoneal dialysis

CLINICAL MANIFESTATIONS

- Early symptoms: weakness, lethargy, polyuria, polydipsia
- Cardiovascular: Dehydration from hyperglycemic osmotic diuresis produces
  - tachycardia
  - dry, warm skin
  - CVP < 2 mmHg
  - CO < 4 L/min
  - weak peripheral pulses
  - hypotension
  - dry mucous membranes
  - PCWP < 8 mmHg
  - CI < 2.5 L/min/m^2
  - shock
- Neurological: Brain cell dehydration produces
  - weakness
  - confusion
  - absent deep-tendon reflexes
  - positive Babinski
  - lethargy
  - seizures
  - paresis
  - coma
- Renal: Elevated glucose produces polyuria.
- Gastrointestinal: Diuresis produces
  - polydipsia
  - vomiting
  - weight loss

CLINICAL/DIAGNOSTIC FINDINGS

- Uncontrolled glucose levels produce
  - glycosuria
  - extreme hyperglycemia > 800 mg/dL
  - serum osmolality > 295 mOsm/L
- Osmotic diuresis produces
  - hypernatremia (>145 mEq/L)
  - hemoconcentration: increased BUN, hematocrit, albumin
  - normal to increased potassium initially; then decreased
  - hypophosphatemia (<2.5 mg/dL)
  - initial hypermagnesemia, then hypomagnesemia
- Absence of ketoacidosis produces
  - serum/urine ketones absent
  - pH > 7.35
  - HCO_3 > 21 mEq/L

NURSING DIAGNOSIS: FLUID VOLUME DEFICIT

Related To
- Osmotic diuresis
- Vomiting
- Total body water loss

Defining Characteristics
Tachycardia
CVP < 2 mmHg
CO < 4 L/min
Dry mucous membranes
Weak peripheral pulses
Shock

Hypotension
PCWP < 8 mmHg
CI < 2.5 L/min/m^2
Poor skin turgor
Weight loss

Patient Outcomes
Adequate fluid balance is maintained/restored, as evidenced by
- blood pressure within 10 mmHg patient baseline
- heart rate 60–100 bpm
- CVP 2–10 mmHg; PCWP 8–12 mmHg
- CO 4–8 L/min; CI 2.5–4 L/min/m^2
- normal skin turgor
- moist mucous membranes
- weight return to patient baseline

Nursing Interventions	Rationales
Monitor vital signs for hypotension, reflex tachycardia, and increased respiratory rate.	Fluid deficit produces hypotension, tachycardia, and increased respiratory rate. Hypotension, if prolonged, can produce other complications such as acute renal failure and must be corrected rapidly.
Monitor hemodynamic measurements for low CVP/PCWP and low CO/CI	Fluid volume deficit produces low CVP, PCWP, CO and CI. Low CO/CI, if prolonged, can produce other complications such as acute renal failure.
Monitor peripheral indicators of fluid deficits: peripheral pulses, skin turgor, and mucous membranes.	Weak, thready pulses, poor skin turgor, and dry mucous membranes indicate fluid volume deficit. Increased blood viscosity can lead to vascular thrombi.

Nursing Interventions

Monitor/record fluid balance: intake and output, hourly urine output, and daily weights.
Administer intravenous fluids as ordered, monitoring for signs and symptoms of fluid overload: increased heart rate, increased blood pressure, jugular venous distension, fine crackles, shortness of breath, increased CVP/PCWP, and increased weight over baseline.

Rationales

Fluid loss in HHNC averages 8–12 L or 20–25% of total body water. Generally, half of the fluid deficit is replaced in the first 12 hr using hypotonic crystalloid solutions, but since these patients are often elderly, they need to be monitored closely for fluid overload.

NURSING DIAGNOSIS: ELECTROLYTE IMBALANCE

Related To
- Decreased insulin
- Fluid shifts
- Vomiting

Defining Characteristics
Hyperglycemia (>800 mg/dL)
Hyponatremia (<135 mEq/L)
Hypokalemia (<3.5 mEq/L
Hypophosphatemia (<2.5 mg/dL)
Hypomagnesemia (<1.5 mg/dL)

Patient Outcomes
Serum glucose and electrolytes will return to normal range.

Nursing Interventions

Same as for diabetic ketoacidosis.

NURSING DIAGNOSIS: ALTERED THOUGHT PROCESSES

Related To
- Dehydration
- Electrolyte imbalance

Defining Characteristics
Confusion
Drowsiness
Lethargy
Convulsions

Patient Outcomes
The patient will return to baseline mentation.

Nursing Interventions
Same as for diabetic ketoacidosis.

DISCHARGE PLANNING/CONTINUITY OF CARE

- Assess need for/type of long-term care and follow up.
- If the discharge destination is home, assess existing supports and the need for assistance.
- Determine coping deficits/support needs and institute assistance measures.
- Determine knowledge deficit/teaching needs and document and institute a teaching plan.
- Refer patient to social services as appropriate.
- Communicate coping deficits/support needs and knowledge deficits/learning needs to unit accepting the patient on transfer.

REFERENCES

Graves, L. (1990). Diabetic ketoacidosis and hyperosmolar hyperglycemic nonketotic coma. *Critical Care Nursing Quarterly, 13*(3), 50–61.
Pope, D. W. & Dnasky, D. (1989). Hyperosmolar hyperglycemic nonketotic coma. *Emergency Medical Clinics of North America, 7,* 849–856.
Sauve, D. O. & Kessler, C. A. (1992). Hyperglycemic emergencies. *AACN Clinical Issues in Critical Care Nursing, 3*(2), 350–360.
Silverberg, J. D. & Kreisberg, R. A. (1990). Hyperglycemic disorders. *Problems in Critical Care, 4*(3), 355–371.
Siperstein, M. D. (1992). Diabetic ketoacidosis and hyperosmolar coma. *Endocrinology and Metabolism Clinics of North America, 21*(2), 415–432.

▼

HYPOGLYCEMIC CRISIS

Hypoglycemic crisis is defined as a decrease in plasma glucose levels to 50 mg/dL or below. Glucose levels are normally maintained by a balance between glucose release from the liver and insulin secretion. During the fasting state, glucagon stimulates hepatic glucose production and insulin is secreted in small amounts to maintain a relatively constant blood glucose level. During the postprandial state release of insulin increases to facilitate storage of glucose for future use. Hypoglycemia can occur during either of these states.

Hypoglycemic crisis occurs with rapid glucose uptake or utilization, with release of excess insulin, or when inadequate glucose is available for tissue needs. Since glucose is the preferred fuel of the brain and the brain is unable to store glucose, changes in the level of consciousness will occur. Prolonged lack of glucose to the brain can produce permanent damage. In an attempt to increase serum glucose levels, the body releases glucagon, cortisol, growth hormone, and epinephrine. The epinephrine release is responsible for the adrenergic signs and symptoms seen with hypoglycemia. These signs and symptoms are particularly prominent if the serum glucose falls rapidly.

ETIOLOGIES

Fasting Hypoglycemia
- Excess insulin
  - insulin or oral hypoglycemic agent dose greater than body's requirements
  - pancreatic islet cell tumors
- Factors that potentiate hypoglycemic medications
  - certain drugs: propranolol, oxytetracycline
  - chronic renal disease
  - liver disease that impairs drug degradation process
  - elderly patients on long-acting sulfonylureas
  - autoimmune phenomenon

- Underproduction of glucose
  - insufficient caloric consumption
  - heavy alcohol consumption with inadequate dietary intake
  - insufficient glucocorticoids
  - drugs: aspirin, disopyramide (Norpace), haloperidol (Haldol), propoxyphene HCl (Darvon), phenylbutazone
  - strenuous exercise/severe stress with inadequate dietary intake or decrease in insulin
  - Addison's disease, hypopituitarism
  - severe liver disease (loss of >80% function)

Postprandial Hypoglycemia
Too rapid glucose uptake and utilization:
- Gastrointestinal disease: subtotal gastrectomy, vagotomy, pyloroplasty, gastroenterostomy
- Extrapancreatic tumors
- Fructose intolerance
- Galactosemia
- Reactive hypoglycemia

CLINICAL MANIFESTATIONS

- Neurological: Decreased glucose supply to brain cells can produce
  - headache
  - irritability
  - inability to concentrate
  - nerve paresthesias
  - lethargy
  - weakness
  - slurred speech
  - confusion
  - dizziness
  - visual disturbances
  - fatigue
  - seizures
  - incoordination
  - unconsciousness
- Cardiovascular: Activation of the sympathetic nervous system and release of epinephrine can produce
  - cool, clammy skin
  - palpitations
  - tremors
  - anxiety
  - pallor
  - tachycardia
  - sweating
  - hunger

NOTE: Signs and symptoms as the result of epinephrine release usually occur when the glucose falls rapidly and can occur even if the glucose value is above 50 mg/dL. Neurological signs and symptoms are more closely related to actual glucose levels.

CLINICAL/DIAGNOSTIC FINDINGS

- Serum glucose < 50 mg/dL

▼

NURSING DIAGNOSIS: ALTERED NUTRITION—LESS THAN BODY REQUIREMENTS
Related To lack of glucose supply to cells

Defining Characteristics
Hypoglycemia (<50 mg/dL)
Palpitations
Pallor
Headache
Irritability
Fatigue
Cool, clammy skin
Tachycardia
Sweating
Confusion
Dizziness
Weakness

Patient Outcomes
The nutritional supply of glucose will be adequate, as evidenced by
- serum glucose 60–115 mg/dL
- absence of neurological signs of decreased glucose supply to brain
- absence of sympathetic effects of decreased glucose on the heart

Nursing Interventions	Rationales
Identify if patient is at risk for hypoglycemia: past experience with hypoglycemia (causes and symptoms), stability of serum glucose levels, and recent changes in insulin dose or diet.	It is difficult to identify a hypoglycemic crisis based on symptoms alone because many other conditions can produce similar symptomatology. Thus, any history you are able to obtain from the patient can provide valuable clues. It will also assist in development of an appropriate long-term treatment regimen for the patient.
Assess for cause of episode.	Determining what precipitated the hypoglycemic episode, for example, too much insulin, will enable the development of a patient-specific treatment regimen, reveal patient teaching needs, and assist in preventing future episodes.

Endocrine Care

Nursing Interventions	Rationales
Assess neurological and cardiovascular signs and symptoms during and after the episode.	Release of epinephrine is responsible for the palpitations, pallor, tachycardia, sweating, and cool, clammy skin seen with hypoglycemia. Lack of glucose to the brain is responsible for the neurological signs and symptoms (see Altered Thought Processes). These signs and symptoms should resolve when serum glucose levels are adequate.
Obtain serum glucose or glucose meter glucose if patient is exhibiting symptomatology.	This provides verification of the diagnosis.
Administer carbohydrate orally if patient is able: sweetened carbonated beverage or fruit juice, honey, skim milk, or glucose tablets.	All of these are quick sources of glucose and should raise serum glucose levels adequately.
Administer parenteral glucose (50% dextrose) as prescribed if patient is unable to take orally.	If a diabetic patient is comatose or has an altered level of consciousness, it is essential to increase the serum glucose immediately with 50% dextrose IV push to prevent permanent brain damage. This is so important that dextrose is frequently given prior to confirmation of the diagnosis with a serum glucose level.
Institute preventive interventions: 1. Monitor serum glucose trends. 2. Ensure bedtime snacks are given. 3. Monitor and record appetite and nutritional intake. 4. Consult with dietitian/nutritionist as needed. 5. Assess activity/exercise levels, particularly at home.	In diabetics, there must be a balance between nutritional, exercise, and insulin/oral hypoglycemic regimens to prevent either hypo- or hyperglycemic emergencies.

▼

NURSING DIAGNOSIS: ALTERED THOUGHT PROCESSES
Related To lack of glucose to the brain

Defining Characteristics
Impaired mentation
Irritability
Inability to concentrate
Unconsciousness
Dizziness
Lethargy
Seizures

Patient Outcomes
The patient will return to baseline mentation.

Nursing Interventions	Rationales
Assess for degree of physiological/psychological dysfunction: orientation, confusion, irritability, inability to concentrate, fatigue, weakness, lethargy, visual disturbances (blurred vision, diplopia), slurred speech, nerve paresthesias, and incoordination.	Decreased glucose supplies to the brain produce these neurological signs and symptoms. These signs and symptoms should resolve with adequate serum glucose levels.
Institute seizure precautions as appropriate: siderails up and padded and oral airway and oxygen at bedside.	Decreased glucose supplies to the brain can precipitate seizures. Precautions to prevent injury should be taken until the patient's level of consciousness has returned to patient baseline.
Provide for safety: siderails up and bed in low position; bed check, posey if confused; and call light, urinal, water, and so on, within reach.	Patients with altered levels of consciousness are at risk for injury and falls. Preventive measures to minimize such risks should be instituted.

Nursing Interventions	Rationales
Monitor glucose levels via lab or glucose meter.	
Minimize effects of environment on mental status: 1. Reorient patient as needed. 2. Maintain quiet environment, minimizing extraneous stimuli. 3. Provide simple, brief explanations of activities, procedures, or equipment. 4. Provide meaningful, relaxing stimuli to patient.	The stresses of the critical care environment (sensory overload, sensory deprivation, and sleep deprivation) can aggravate mental status changes produced physiologically. Taking preventive measures may minimize these environmental effects.

DISCHARGE PLANNING/CONTINUITY OF CARE

- Assess need for/type of long-term care and follow-up.
- If the discharge destination is home, assess existing supports and the need for assistance.
- Determine coping deficits/support needs and institute assistance measures.
- Determine knowledge deficits/teaching needs and document and institute a teaching plan.
- Refer patient to social services as appropriate.
- Communicate coping deficits/support needs and knowledge deficits/learning needs to unit accepting the patient on transfer.

REFERENCES

Bacchus, H. (1989). Heading off a diabetic crisis. *Emergency Medicine*, 21(20), 20–24, 26, 31–32.

Gotch, P. M. (1991). The endocrine system. In J. G. Alspach (Ed.), *Core curriculum for critical care nursing*, (4th ed., pp. 667–672). Philadelphia, PA: Saunders.

Gray, D. P. & Ludwig-Beymer, P. (1990). Alterations in hormonal regulation. In K. L. McCance & S. E. Huether (Eds.), *Pathophysiology: The biologic basis for disease in adults and children* (pp. 618–619). St. Louis, MO: Mosby.

Mulcahy, K. (1992). Hypoglycemic emergencies. *AACN Clinical Issues in Critical Care Nursing*, 3(2), 361–369.

MYXEDEMA COMA

Myxedema coma is the life-threatening end stage of improperly treated, neglected, or undiagnosed hypothyroidism. Most cases are elderly females, occur in winter months, and are associated with physiological or psychological stress or underlying illness. The addition of stress to an already hypothyroid patient accelerates the metabolism and clearance of whatever thyroid hormone is present. This creates a situation of increased hormone utilization but decreased production, precipitating a crisis state.

ETIOLOGIES

- Most cases
  - longstanding autoimmune disease of the thyroid (Hashimoto's thyroiditis)
  - surgical or radioactive iodine treatment for Graves' disease (hyperthyroidism) with inadequate hormone replacement
- Known precipitating factors
  - administration of central nervous system depressants (narcotics, barbiturates, or anesthesia)
  - critical illness
  - exposure to cold
  - infection, trauma
- Common underlying illnesses
  - anemia
  - aspiration
  - infections
  - pleural and pericardial effusions
  - ascites
  - heart failure
  - seizures

CLINICAL MANIFESTATIONS

- The earliest signs may be fatigue, weakness, muscle cramps, and intolerance to cold, but the clinical picture varies with rate of onset and severity.

- Neurological: Decreased metabolic rate and decreased cerebration produce
  - coarse, raspy, hoarse voice
  - delusions, paranoia
  - hearing loss
  - slow deliberate speech
  - vertigo
  - coma
  - depression
  - seizures
  - lethargy
  - slowed mentation
- Temperature: Decreased metabolic rate and thermal energy production produce
  - intolerance to cold
  - hypothermia
- Cardiovascular: Depressed cardiac function produces
  - LVSWI < 35 g/mL
  - bradycardia
  - CO < 4 L/min
  - distant heart tones
  - low-voltage EKG
  - RVSWI < 8.5 g/mL
  - pericardial effusions
  - CI < 2.5 L/min/m^2
  - hypotension
  - shock
- Pulmonary: Respirations are depressed, producing
  - decreased respirations
  - dyspnea on exertion
  - hypoventilation

  Fluid retention produces
  - pleural effusions
  - upper airway edema
- Gastrointestinal: Decreased metabolism produces
  - decreased appetite
  - constipation
  - decreased bowel sounds
  - paralytic ileus

  Fluid retention produces
  - weight gain
  - ascites
- Skeletal muscle: Slowed motor conduction produces
  - decreased tendon reflexes
  - sluggish movements

  Decreased calcium metabolism produces increased bone density.
- Integumentary: Decreased thyroid hormone produces
  - dry, flaky, cool, coarse skin
  - dry, coarse hair
  - yellow tint to skin
  - brittle nails
  - ecchymoses

  Water retention and decreased protein produce
  - interstitial edema
  - mucinous edema of eyelids, periorbital tissue, and dorsa of hands and feet

CLINICAL/DIAGNOSTIC FINDINGS

- Serum T_4 < 5 μg/dL
- Serum T_3 < 110 ng/100 mL
- Resin T_3 uptake < 25%
- TSH high (primary); normal or low (secondary)
- Serum sodium < 135 mEq/L
- Hypoglycemia (uncommon) (<60 mg/dL)
- Anemia (Hgb < 13 g/dL)

- Leukocytosis absent despite stress
- Elevated CPK, SGOT, LDH, cholesterol, triglycerides
- Respiratory acidosis: pH < 7.35, $PaCO_2$ > 45 torr
- Decreased platelets (<150,000/mm^3)

NURSING DIAGNOSIS: FLUID VOLUME EXCESS

Related To impaired water excretion

Defining Characteristics

Weight gain
Pericardial effusion
Ascites
CVP > 10 mmHg

Hyponatremia (<135 mEq/L)
Pleural effusion
Mucinous edema
PCWP > 12 mmHg

Patient Outcomes

Fluid balance is maintained/restored, as evidenced by
- absence of pericardial or pleural effusions
- serum sodium 135–145 mEq/L
- weight return to patient baseline
- absence of edema
- CVP 2–10 mmHg; PCWP 8–12 mmHg

Nursing Interventions	Rationales
Assess, monitor, and document cardiovascular status: vital signs, hemodynamic parameters, and peripheral pulses. Monitor for signs and symptoms of cardiac failure: increased CVP/PCWP, jugular venous distention, peripheral edema, c/o SOB, and fine crackles in lungs.	Fluid volume excess can produce cardiac failure, especially if the patient has decreased metabolism and/or underlying cardiac disease.
Monitor/maintain fluid balance: intake and output, hourly urine output, and daily weight. Maintain fluid restriction.	Patients with a fluid volume excess are commonly placed on fluid restrictions to restore fluid balance. Daily weights and intake and output provide an objective means of measuring progress toward getting rid of excess fluid.

Nursing Interventions	Rationales
Monitor serum sodium and watch for signs and symptoms of hyponatremia: changes in mental status and seizures.	Hyponatremia is caused by water retention in excess of sodium and can produce significant neurological changes and seizures.
Administer thyroid drugs (usually levothyroxine sodium) as prescribed and monitor for side effects such as angina, myocardial irritability, allergic skin reactions, and signs and symptoms of hyperthyroidism.	

NURSING DIAGNOSIS: DECREASED CARDIAC OUTPUT

Related To
- Decreased contractility
- Decreased heart rate
- Decreased stroke volume
- Pericardial effusions
- Dysrhythmias

Defining Characteristics
Bradycardia
PCWP > 12 mmHg
Distant heart sounds
LVSWI < 35 g/mL
Urine output < 30 mL/hr

CO < 4 L/min; CI < 2.5 L/min/m^2
CVP > 10 mmHg
Hypotension
RVSWI < 8.5 g/mL

Patient Outcomes
Hemodynamics and metabolic rate will be normal, as evidenced by
- CO 4–8 L/min; CI 2.5–4 L/min/m^2
- CVP 2–10 mmHg; PCWP 8–12 mmHg
- LVSWI 35–85 g/mL; RVSWI 8.5–12 g/mL
- blood pressure within 10 mmHg of patient baseline
- urine output > 30 mL/hr
- control of dysrhythmias
- no pericardial effusion

Nursing Interventions	Rationales
Assess/monitor cardiac output, cardiac index, pulmonary artery pressures (PAP, CVP, PCWP), and SVR. Assess/monitor heart sounds: diminished, murmur, and gallop. Assess/monitor blood pressure, heart rate, and rhythm Monitor for subjective complaints of chest pain or objective signs of ischemia (ST-segment changes on EKG). Institute treatment to control dysrhythmias according to protocols.	Decreased thyroid hormone levels depress cardiac function (decreased cardiac contractility, decreased heart rate, decreased stroke volume) and may cause pericardial effusions and dysrhythmias. Patients may also have severe atherosclerotic heart disease from high levels of cholesterol and triglycerides. These effects combine to place this patient at risk for cardiovascular collapse.
Administer volume or pressors cautiously to maintain blood pressure.	Patients in myxedema coma will be unable to respond to vasopressors until they have adequate levels of thyroid hormone available. Simultaneous administration of vasopressors and thyroid hormone is associated with myocardial irritability.

NURSING DIAGNOSIS: HYPOTHERMIA

Related To inability of body to retain heat

Defining Characteristics
Hypothermia   Intolerance to cold

Patient Outcomes
The patient will have a normal temperature.

Nursing Interventions	Rationales
Warm patient passively with blankets (no active warming).	More active rewarming with a heating blanket can result in peripheral vasodilatation, circulatory collapse, and death.
Monitor temperature every 1–2 hr or continuously with a probe. Control room temperature; avoid exposure to cold.	

NURSING DIAGNOSIS: ALTERED THOUGHT PROCESSES

Related To
- Slowed metabolism and cerebration
- Hyponatremia

Defining Characteristics

Delusions
Depression
Paranoia
Seizures
Slow speech, hoarse voice

Slowed mentation
Lethargy
Coma
Vertigo
Hearing loss

Patient Outcomes
The patient will return to baseline mentation and normal personality pattern (per significant other).

Nursing Interventions	Rationales
Assess for degree of physiological/psychological dysfunction: orientation; difficulty concentrating, slowed mentation; depression, lethargy; seizures, coma; vertigo, hearing loss; slow speech, and hoarse voice.	Low circulating thyroid levels produce a decreased metabolic rate and decreased cerebration resulting in neurological symptoms.
Minimize effects of environment on mental status: 1. Reorient patient as needed. 2. Provide simple, clear explanations of all activities, procedures, and equipment. 3. Minimize extraneous, meaningless stimuli. 4. Maintain quiet environment. 5. Provide for consistent caregivers when possible. 6. Encourage a significant other to stay with patient. 7. Promote sleep and rest.	The stresses of the critical care environment (sensory overload, sensory deprivation, and sleep deprivation) can aggravate mental status changes produced physiologically.

Nursing Interventions	Rationales
Monitor serum sodium and signs of hyponatremia (confusion, weakness, muscle twitching, nausea and vomiting, seizures).	Hyponatremia can alter mental status and produce seizures. Hyponatremia usually responds to thyroid replacement and water restriction.

NURSING DIAGNOSIS: INEFFECTIVE BREATHING PATTERN

Related To
- Hypoventilation
- Pleural effusions
- Decreased respiratory rate
- Muscle weakness
- Ascites

Defining Characteristics
Dyspnea on exertion
Decreased respiratory rate
Decreased breath sounds
Shallow respirations

Elevated $PaCO_2$ (>45 torr)
pH < 7.35

Patient Outcomes
An effective breathing pattern will be maintained/restored, as evidenced by
- normal rate and depth of ventilation
- $PaCO_2$ 35–45 torr, pH 7.35–7.45
- patient reports no dyspnea with activity

Nursing Interventions	Rationales
Assess hypometabolism's effect on breathing: rate, depth, and rhythm of respiration; airway and breathing effort, use of accessory muscles; breath sounds. Obtain ABG's, and pulse oximetry as prescribed and prn respiratory distress. Obtain pulmonary function parameters: tidal volume and vital capacity. Assess for subjective complaints of shortness of breath and dyspnea on exertion.	Hypothyroidism depresses respiratory function and produces fluid retention, both of which can cause problems with ventilation and oxygenation.
Monitor for anemia: Hgb < 13 g/dL, fatigue, weakness, and pale skin.	Hypothyroidism can cause anemia. Since red blood cells are responsible for oxygen transport to tissues, anemia can interfere with tissue oxygenation.
Monitor respiratory effort during activity. Support airway as appropriate: airway, supplementary oxygen, suctioning, intubation equipment/ventilator. Position patient for ease of respiratory effort, that is, head of bed is elevated. Provide quiet, restful environment. Allow frequent rest periods during activity. Minimize activity to decrease oxygen need. Send sputum for culture and sensitivity and administer antibiotics if prescribed.	
Minimize water retention by adhering to fluid restriction.	The water retention caused by hypothyroidism can cause fluid to accumulate within the lungs or in the pleural space. This can interfere with respiratory effort.

NURSING DIAGNOSIS: ACTIVITY INTOLERANCE
Related To muscle weakness

Defining Characteristics
Dyspnea on exertion
Fatigue
Unsteadiness on feet

Patient Outcomes
The patient's activity level will return to baseline.

Nursing Interventions	Rationales
During acute crisis, minimize physical activity. Provide all daily cares for patient. Maintain on bedrest.	Until thyroid levels are normalized, the patient needs to conserve energy for vital cardiac and respiratory function.
Allow for adequate rest/sleep periods: Minimize or group interruptions; assess patient's normal sleep patterns/habits and try to accommodate them; and maintain quiet, calm environment.	
Provide adequate nutrition	Decreased appetite and inadequate nutrition can contribute to muscle weakness and fatigue.
Increase activity gradually when patient is able. Monitor physical response to activity: blood pressure, heart rate and rhythm, and respiratory rate before, during, and after activity. Note tachycardia, dysrhythmias, dyspnea, pallor, diaphoresis, and dizziness or fatigue.	Heart rate, blood pressure, and respiratory rate should return to baseline within 4 min after activity.
Schedule activities to decrease energy expenditure spacing with rest periods. Assess strength and need for assistance as activity increases.	

DISCHARGE PLANNING/CONTINUITY OF CARE

- Assess need for/type of long-term care and follow-up.
- If the discharge destination is home, assess existing supports and the need for assistance.
- Determine coping deficits/support needs and institute assistance measures.
- Determine knowledge deficits/teaching needs and document and institute teaching plan.
- Refer patient to social services as appropriate.
- Communicate coping deficits/support needs and knowledge deficits/learning needs to unit accepting the patient on transfer.

REFERENCES

Gavin, L. A. (1991). Thyroid crises. *Medical Clinics of North America, 75*(1), 179–192.

Gotch, P. M. (1991). The endocrine system. In J. G. Alspach (Ed.), *Core curriculum for critical care nursing* (4th ed., pp. 644–650). Philadelphia, PA: Saunders.

Hays, J. H. (1990). Thyroid disease. *Problems in Critical Care, 4*(3), 325–341.

Isley, W. L. (1990). Thyroid disorders. *Critical Care Nursing Quarterly, 13*(3), 39–49.

Spittle, L. (1992). Diagnoses in opposition: Thyroid storm and myxedema coma. *AACN Clinical Issues in Critical Care Nursing, 3*(2), 300–308.

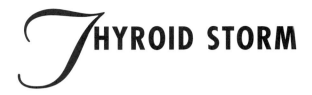HYROID STORM

Thyroid storm is a hyperdynamic, hypermetabolic state that results in life-threatening disruption of most body systems. It usually occurs in untreated or inadequately treated patients with hyperthyroidism. Thyroid hormone levels in these patients are no higher than those with uncomplicated hyperthyroidism; however, it appears that when hyperthyroid patients are stressed either physiologically or psychologically, this can trigger exaggerated responses to thyroid hormone. Elevation of thyroid hormone results in an increased rate of chemical reactions, increased metabolism, increased release of catecholamines, increased nutrient and oxygen consumption, increased heat production, alterations in fluid and electrolyte balance, and a catabolic state.

ETIOLOGIES

- The most common types of hyperthyroidism seen with thyroid storm
  - toxic diffuse goiter (Graves' disease)
  - unusually large toxic multinodular goiter
- The types listed above combined with stress
  - burns
  - general anesthesia
  - surgery
  - trauma
  - diabetic ketoacidosis
  - infection
  - severe emotional stress
- Mortality is usually related to the underlying illness.

CLINICAL MANIFESTATIONS

- Abrupt onset/most prominent: severe fever, marked tachycardia, tremors, delirium, stupor, coma
- Cardiovascular: Increased metabolism and increased catecholamines produce
  - dysrhythmias (PACs, atrial fibrillation, atrial flutter)

- $SvO_2 < 70\%$
- CO > 8 L/min
- CI > 4 L/min/m^2
- CVP > 10 mmHg
- PCWP > 12 mmHg
- palpitations
- pericardial rub, systolic murmur, third heart sound (S_3)
- elderly: angina and congestive heart failure

Enhanced oxygen and nutrient delivery to tissue produces warm, moist, pink skin.
- Gastrointestinal: Increased intestinal motility produces
  - abdominal pain
  - increased frequency of stools
  - nausea and vomiting

Increased metabolism and protein/fat degradation produce
  - weight loss
  - increased appetite
- Skin: Inadequate protein synthesis produces
  - petechiae
  - soft friable nails and thin skin
  - thin, fine, silky fragile hair
- Neurological: Hypermetabolism and increased cerebration produce
  - agitation
  - seizures
  - fear
  - mood swings
  - stupor
  - decreased attention span
  - increased irritability
  - delirium
  - overt psychoses
  - coma
- Ophthalmic: exopthalmos
- Pulmonary: Increased need for oxygen produces
  - dyspnea
  - tachypnea

Increased protein catabolism reduces protein in respiratory muscles, producing
  - muscle weakness
  - hypoventilation
  - respiratory failure
  - decreased lung capacity
  - CO_2 retention
- Skeletomuscular: Muscle protein degradation produces
  - fatigue
  - muscle weakness
  - tremors of tongue, eyelids, or eyeballs
  - muscle wasting
  - peripheral tremors
- Temperature: Loss of temperature regulation produces
  - excessive sweating
  - increased temperature
  - heat intolerance

CLINICAL/DIAGNOSTIC FINDINGS

- Abnormal liver function tests
- Anemia (Hgb < 13 g/dL)

- Hypokalemia (<3.5 mEq/L)
- Hyperglycemia (>115 mg/dL)
- Hypercalcemia (>10.5 mg/dL)
- Hyponatremia or hypernatremia
- BUN > 20 mg/dL
- Resin T_3 uptake > 35%
- T_3 > 230 ng/100 mL; T_4 > 12.5 μg/dL
- Leukocytosis (WBC > 10,000/mm^3)

NURSING DIAGNOSIS: DECREASED CARDIAC OUTPUT

Related To
- Dysrhythmias
- Extreme tachycardia
- Increased metabolic demands on heart
- Congestive heart failure

Defining Characteristics
Angina
CO < 4 L/min
CVP > 10 mmHg
MAP < 60 mmHg
Urine output < 30 mL/hr
Tachycardia
Decreased peripheral pulses
Signs of left- or right-sided failure

Dysrhythmias
CI < 2.5 L/min/m^2
PCWP > 12 mmHg
Hypotension
Systolic murmmur
Third heart sound (S_3)
SvO_2 < 70%

Patient Outcomes
Cardiac output will be maintained/restored, as evidenced by
- CO 4–8 L/min; CI 2.5–4 L/min/m^2
- PCWP 8–12 mmHg; CVP 2–10 mmHg
- blood pressure within 10 mmHg patient baseline
- MAP > 60 mmHg
- heart rate 60–100 bpm
- dysrhythmias controlled
- urine output > 30 mL/hr

54 Endocrine Care

Nursing Interventions	Rationales
Assess for identification of precipitating cause of thyroid storm, that is, underlying stressor.	
Assess/record blood pressure, MAP, respiratory rate, and heart rate (especially sleeping) Assess/record hemodynamics: PAP, PCWP, CVP, CO, CI, SvO_2, and SVR. Assess/record cardiac rhythm and dysrhythmias. Assess/record heart sounds: S_1, S_2, gallop, and murmur. Assess/record presence and strength of peripheral pulses. Assess for subjective c/o chest pain, palpitations, and SOB. Assess for objective signs of ischemia: cool, clammy skin; capillary refill time > 3 s; and decreased urine output.	Increased circulating thyroid hormone increases metabolism and catecholamine production. This hyperdynamic circulation puts tremendous stress on the heart and can lead to cardiovascular collapse. Baseline assessment and continuous/frequent monitoring are necessary to detect early signs of cardiovascular stress.
Identify patients at risk for failure and shock.	Patients who are elderly or have preexisting coronary artery disease or other cardiac risk factors are more likely to develop heart failure and shock.
Assess for previous history of chronic lung disease, heart block, and pulmonary edema.	Propranolol is contraindicated in these patients because it blocks stimulation of both $beta_1$ and $beta_2$ receptors producing decreased contractility, decreased heart rate, decreased AV conduction, and bronchoconstriction.
Monitor serum electrolyte status: potassium and calcium levels, and signs/symptoms of hypokalemia or hypercalcemia.	Increased thyroid hormone can produce hypokalemia and hypercalcemia, which in turn cause dysrhythmias and a further decrease in cardiac output.
Control temperature (see Hyperthermia).	
Provide adequate hydration.	Insensible losses will be much greater than normal due to hypermetabolism.

Nursing Interventions	Rationales
Administer digoxin as prescribed and monitor response.	Digoxin is given to patients in congestive heart failure or with tachyarrhythmias to slow heart rate and improve cardiac function.
Minimize demand on heart by controlling activity.	
Administer propranolol or calcium blockers as prescribed and monitor effects (blood pressure, heart rate, cardiac output, pulmonary artery pressures, pulmonary capillary wedge pressure, and central venous pressure).	Propranolol is the beta blocker of choice to antagonize the peripheral effects of thyroid hormone because of its ability to inhibit the peripheral conversion of T_4 to T_3 and the cardiac effects of excessive hormone. Recent research also indicates that calcium blockers can be effective in controlling heart rate and rhythm.
Administer drugs used to inhibit thyroid hormone biosynthesis (propylthiouracil) as prescribed and monitor for side effects.	Propylthiouracil (PTU) given orally is the drug of choice because it inhibits conversion of T_4 to T_3. Potential side effects include agranulocytosis, bleeding tendency, vertigo, drowsiness, nausea, and headaches.
Administer Lugol's solution or sodium iodide as prescribed and assess response.	Iodide agents inhibit release of hormone from the thyroid gland and may also inhibit production of thyroid hormones in high doses. These drugs must be given 1–2 hr after antithyroid drugs to prevent the iodide from being used to synthesize more thyroid hormone.

NURSING DIAGNOSIS: HYPERTHERMIA
Related To
- Increased heat production
- Increased metabolism
- Loss of temperature regulation

Defining Characteristics
Cold intolerance
Heat intolerance
Excessive sweating
Increased temperature

Patient Outcomes
The patient's temperature will return to normal range.

Nursing Interventions	Rationales
Monitor patient's temperature every hour; continuously with probe if possible.	
Assess fluid status: hourly urine output; intake and output; daily weight; diaphoresis, skin turgor, and mucous membranes.	The high body temperatures produced by thyroid storm can significantly increase insensible fluid loss.
Utilize cooling measures to decrease temperature: ice packs to axillae and groins, cooling mattress, minimal covers, and controlled room temperature. Administer acetaminophen (no aspirin) as prescribed.	Aspirin increases the level of free thyroxine.
Administer antibiotics as prescribed if infection is a precipitator.	

NURSING DIAGNOSIS: INEFFECTIVE BREATHING PATTERN

Related To
- Decreased vital capacity
- Hypoventilation
- Increased oxygen need from hypermetabolism
- Muscle weakness
- CO_2 retention

Defining Characteristics
PaO_2 < 60 torr
Shallow respirations
$PaCO_2$ > 45 torr
Lung vital capacity < 10 mL/kg
SvO_2 < 60%
Tachypnea

Patient Outcomes
An effective breathing pattern is maintained/restored, as evidenced by:
- normal respiratory rate, depth, and pattern

- normal $PaCO_2$ (35–45 torr) and pH (7.35–7.45) or return to patient baseline
- PaO_2 > 60 torr
- vital capacity > 10 mL/kg, tidal volume 5–7 mL/kg
- resolution of muscle weakness
- patient reports breathing easier
- SvO_2 > 60%

Nursing Interventions	Rationales
Assess respiratory status: airway and breathing effort and use of accessory muscles; rate and depth of respiration; breath sounds; ABGs/pulse oximetry; pulmonary function parameters (tidal volume, vital capacity); and subjective complaints of shortness of breath and dyspnea on exertion.	Increased thyroid levels increase the respiratory rate because of increased oxygen need related to increased metabolism. At the same time increased catabolism can weaken respiratory muscles, making it more difficult for the patient to maintain adequate oxygenation.
Support airway as appropriate: airway, supplementary oxygen, suctioning, and intubation equipment/ventilator.	Supportive measures may be required to ensure an adequate breathing pattern.
Position patient for ease of respiratory effort, that is, head of bed elevated.	
Provide quiet, restful environment. Allow frequent rest periods and minimize activity	Adequate rest and decreased activity decrease oxygen need.
Send sputum for culture and sensitivity and administer antibiotics as prescribed.	Hypoventilation, muscle weakness, and decreased vital capacity can cause retention of secretions and development of pulmonary infection. Untreated pulmonary infection will aggravate the already impaired breathing pattern.

NURSING DIAGNOSIS: ACTIVITY INTOLERANCE

Related To
- Extreme energy expenditure
- Muscle protein degradation in skeletal muscles that exceeds protein synthesis

Defining Characteristics

Dyspnea
Peripheral tremors
Generalized muscle wasting
Tremors of tongue, eyelids, or eyeballs
Weakness especially in proximal limbs

Fatigue
Weight loss

Patient Outcomes

The patient's activity level will return to baseline.

Nursing Interventions	Rationales
Assess for causes of fatigue, that is, treatments, medications, inadequate nutrition, and inadequate sleep. During acute crisis, minimize physical activity: Provide all daily cares for patient and maintain on bedrest. Allow for adequate rest/sleep periods: 1. Minimize or group interruptions. 2. Assess patient's normal sleep patterns/habits and try to accommodate them. 3. Maintain a quiet, calm environment. 4. Administer sedatives if prescribed and assess effectiveness. 5. Assess for and provide patient with calming diversional activities.	
Provide adequate nutrition.	
After acute crisis is resolved, monitor physical response to activity: blood pressure, heart rate and rhythm, and respiratory rate before, during, and after activity. Note tachycardia, dysrhythmias, dyspnea, pallor, diaphoresis, dizziness, or fatigue.	Heart rate, blood pressure, and respiratory rate should return to baseline within 4 min after activity.
Schedule activities to decrease energy expenditure spacing with rest periods.	
Assess muscle strength and need for assistance as activity increases.	

Nursing Interventions	Rationales
Administer oxygen during activity.	Oxygen administration can increase activity tolerance.

NURSING DIAGNOSIS: ALTERED THOUGHT PROCESSES

Related To
- Hypermetabolism
- Increased cerebration

Defining Characteristics
Agitation
Decreased attention
Mood swings
Paranoia
Stupor
Elderly: depression and apathy
Delirium
Increased irritability
Nervousness
Psychosis

Patient Outcomes
- The patient's mentation and behavior will return to baseline.
- The patient's personality (per significant others) will return to baseline.

Nursing Interventions	Rationales
Assess for degree of physiological/psychological dysfunction: orientation, irritability, nervousness, agitation; memory, attention span, mood swings, fear, paranoia, level of consciousness, and tremors (tongue, eyes, peripheral).	
Minimize effects of environment on mental status: 1. Reorient patient as needed. 2. Maintain quiet environment, minimizing extraneous stimuli. 3. Provide simple, brief explanations of activities, procedures, or equipment. 4. Provide meaningful, relaxing stimuli to patient. 5. Provide for consistent caregivers when possible. 6. Encourage family/significant other to stay with patient.	The stressors of the critical care environment (sensory overload, sensory deprivation, and sleep deprivation) can aggravate mental status changes produced physiologically.

Nursing Interventions	Rationales
Initiate protective measures for patient with convulsions/agitation/delusions: padded siderails, soft restraints, and close supervision. Assist patient with daily cares as needed. Provide all cares if level of consciousness is decreased.	

DISCHARGE PLANNING/CONTINUITY OF CARE

- Assess need for/type of long-term care and follow-up.
- If the discharge destination is home, assess existing supports and the need for assistance.
- Determine coping deficits/support needs and institute assistance measures.
- Determine knowledge deficits/teaching needs and document and institute teaching plan.
- Refer patient to social services as appropriate.
- Communicate coping deficits/support needs and knowledge deficits/learning needs to unit accepting the patient on transfer.

REFERENCES

Gavin, L. A. (1991). Thyroid crises. *Medical Clinics of North America*, *75*(1), 179–192.

Gotch, P. M. (1991). The endocrine system. In J. G. Alspach (Ed.), *Core curriculum for critical care nurses* (4th ed., pp. 637–644). Philadelphia, PA: Saunders.

Hays, J. H. (1990). Thyroid disease. *Problems in Critical Care*, *4*(3), 325–341.

Isley, W. L. (1990). Thyroid disorders. *Critical Care Nursing Quarterly*, *13*(3), 39–49.

Spittle, L. (1992). Diagnoses in opposition: Thyroid storm and myxedema coma. *AACN Clinical Issues in Critical Care Nursing*, *3*(2), 300–308.

Gastrointestinal Care

ABDOMINAL AORTIC ANEURYSM

Traditionally, abdominal aortic aneurysms (AAAs) are thought to be the result of atherosclerotic changes in the wall of the vessel. Specifically, the media layer of the vessel wall which is normally elastic is replaced by a thin collagenous layer. This thinned wall is brittle and easily disrupted. The lumen of the aneurysmal vessel wall is also lined with thrombus. As the aneurysm grows in diameter, it may also lengthen, causing the vessel to become tortuous. Aneurysms can enlarge and usually do so over years. If pressure waves in the artery overcome the strength of the stiffened aneurysmal wall, the vessel can rupture or dissect, causing a life-threatening emergency. In dissection, a tear in the tunica intima of the aorta, with a surge of blood into the media, separates the intima from the adventitia. Abdominal aortic aneurysms are common and rank as the thirteenth leading cause of death in the United States. Most aortic aneurysms arise below the renal arteries and involve the lower abdominal aorta. Elective surgery is generally considered in patients with aneurysms larger than 4 or 5 cm.

ETIOLOGIES

- Hypertension
- Smoking
- Genetic
- Aging of the aorta
- Increased proteolysis

CLINICAL MANIFESTATIONS

- Gastrointestinal: A ruptured abdominal aorta produces
  - sudden onset of abdominal discomfort or back pain
  - abdominal distention
  - pulsatile abdominal mass
  - abdominal tenderness and guarding

- Cardiovascular: Hypovolemia associated with intra-abdominal hemorrhage produces
  - hypotension
  - cardiac dysrhythmias
  - tachycardia
  - CO < 4 L/min; CI < 2.5 L/min/m^2
  - weak rapid pulse
  - cold, pale skin
  - CVP < 2 mmHg; PCWP < 8 mmHg
- Renal: Renal artery stenosis with infrarenal abdominal aortic aneurysm produces
  - hypertension   – creatinine > 1.2 mg/dL

  Expanding or rupturing AAA produces
  - renal colic-type pain   – gross hematuria
  - pulsating urination   – flank or testicular pain
  - suprapubic pain
- Vascular: Iliac occlusive disease produces
  - unilateral buttock or thigh claudication
  - diminished femoral pulsations
  - impotence

  Atheroemboli to the lower extremities produce
  - painful and cyanotic toes   – palpable pulses
  - tingling/numbness in legs
- Neurological:
  - CVA   – paraplegia

CLINICAL/DIAGNOSTIC FINDINGS

- Aneurysm on computerized tomography (CT) scan

NURSING DIAGNOSIS: ALTERED TISSUE PERFUSION—CENTRAL AND PERIPHERAL

Related To intra-abdominal hemorrhage

Defining Characteristics
CO < 4 L/min   CI < 2.5 L/min/m^2
CVP < 2 mmHg   PCWP 8 mmHg
Hypotension   Tachycardia
Skin cool, pale, and dry

Patient Outcomes
Central and peripheral perfusion and hemodynamics are supported, as evidenced by

- MAP > 70 mmHg
- CO 4–8 L/min; CI 2.5–4 L/min/m^2
- CVP 2–10 mmHg; PCWP 8–12 mmHg
- heart rate 60–100 bpm
- warm, pink skin

Nursing Interventions	Rationales
Monitor cardiovascular status: respiratory rate, heart rate and blood pressure, including orthostatic changes, hemodynamics (CVP, PCWP, CO, CI, MAP), and peripheral pulses.	Increased respiratory rate, increased heart rate, decreased blood pressure and/or orthostatic changes, low CVP, PCWP, CO/CI, and MAP, and weak peripheral pulses indicate persistent decreased perfusion. Early in the process, the blood pressure may be elevated due to activation of the sympathetic nervous system.
Monitor peripheral circulation: skin color and temperature, quality of peripheral pulses, and capillary refill time (CRT).	Cool, clammy, pale skin, weak peripheral pulses or increased CRT indicate decreased circulating volume and peripheral perfusion.
Administer colloids and crystalloids as prescribed to maintain perfusion pressure. Administer blood products as prescribed. Monitor for patient response.	Replacement of blood and fluid lost can reestablish perfusion to core organs until surgery can be performed.

NOTE: Patients with ruptured abdominal aortic aneurysm usually require immediate surgical repair after medical stabilization. Interventions to maintain perfusion are initiated and continued throughout the surgical procedure.

Administer positive inotropic agents as prescribed and monitor patient response.	Inotropic agents may be required to maintain blood pressure if unable to do so with fluids.

NURSING DIAGNOSIS: HIGH RISK FOR INJURY— ANEURYSMAL RUPTURE

Risk Factors
- Hypertensive crisis
- Increased ventricular contraction velocity related to aortic dissection

Patient Outcomes

Injury is prevented, as evidenced by
- blood pressure return to patient baseline
- heart rate 60–100 bpm
- prevention of progression of dissection

Nursing Interventions	Rationales
Monitor for signs of aneurysm rupture, including abdominal distention, increased abdominal girth, sudden decrease in blood pressure, sudden change in level of consciousness, loss of peripheral pulses, and tachycardia.	Aneurysm rupture requires immediate surgical intervention.
Administer antihypertensives to maintain blood pressure within prescribed parameters: nitroprusside, beta blockers, and ace inhibitors.	Lowering the blood presssure decreases contraction velocity in the aorta and may prevent/halt progression of the dissection.
Administer calcium channel blockers and/or beta blockers as prescribed and monitor patient response.	Calcium channel blockers and beta blockers decrease ventricular conduction velocity.

NURSING DIAGNOSIS: HIGH RISK FOR INJURY—EMBOLIC

Risk Factors
- Stasis of blood
- Irregular blood flow
- Irregularity in vessel wall

Patient Outcomes

The patient will have an absence of or early detection of emboli.

Nursing Interventions	Rationales
Monitor peripheral circulation: pulses, capillary refill time, pain, and color.	Emboli may travel to feet causing pain in toes and feet, pallor of toes, or blue toes.

Nursing Interventions	Rationales
Monitor renal function: urine output every hour, serum BUN, and creatinine.	Microemboli to kidneys can produce diuresis of dilute urine and increased serum BUN and creatinine. Macroemboli can produce oliguria (urine output < 30 mL/hr).
Monitor for abdominal pain or tenderness.	Emboli may occlude the superior or inferior mesenteric artery, causing pain or tenderness.

NURSING DIAGNOSIS: ACUTE PAIN

Related To
- Aortic vessel expansion
- Aortic dissection

Defining Characteristics
Back pain
Flank pain
Abdominal tenderness
Renal/colic-type pain

Patient Outcomes
Pain is controlled, as evidenced by the patient's subjective report of tolerable pain.

Nursing Interventions	Rationales
Assess complaints of pain, noting location, character, and intensity. Use pain-rating scale for objective measure of reported pain.	Changes in location or intensity of pain may indicate complications such as an expanding dissection or rupture.
Assess factors which increase or decrease pain (e.g., position).	

NOTE: Analgesia may not be ordered, as increasing pain is an important diagnostic cue. Surgical intervention is usually indicated when the patient experiences increased pain.

NURSING DIAGNOSIS: KNOWLEDGE DEFICIT
Related To new diagnosis

Defining Characteristics
Patient expresses lack of understanding regarding diagnosis.

Patient Outcomes
The patient will be able to
- describe the pathophysiology of abdominal aortic aneurysm.
- list health practices which may contribute to expansion of the aneurysm.
- identify signs and symptoms of a rupturing aneurysm.

Nursing Interventions	Rationales
Assess patient knowledge base of disease process. Provide medication instructions: name, action, dose, and schedule for antihypertensives. Explain relationship to aneurysm. Instruct patient about hazards of smoking if appropriate. Teach patient signs and symptoms of aortic aneurysm dissection/rupture.	
Discuss with patient need and rationale for continued follow-up of the aneurysm (size).	Aneurysms generally expand at a rate of 0.4 cm/year. Surgical repair is considered with aneurysms over 4–5 cm.
Discuss with patient reasons for absence of symptoms/plan of care.	

DISCHARGE PLANNING/CONTINUITY OF CARE

- Assess need for/type of long-term care and follow-up.
- If the discharge destination is home, assess existing supports and the need for assistance.
- Determine coping deficits/support needs and institute assistance measures.
- Determine knowledge deficits/teaching needs and document and institute a teaching plan.
- Refer patient to social services as appropriate.
- Communicate coping deficits/support needs and knowledge deficits/teaching needs to unit accepting the patient on transfer.

REFERENCES

Asfoura, J. Y. & Vidt, D. G. (1991). Acute aortic dissection. *Chest*, *99*(3), 724–729.

Dobrin, P. B. (1989). Pathophysiology and pathogenesis of aortic aneurysms. *Surgical Clinics of North America*, *69*(4), 687–701.

Fann, J. I., Sarris, G. E., Mitchell, R. S., Shumway, N. E., Stinson, E. B., Oyer, P. E., & Miller, D. C. (1990). Treatment of patients with aortic dissection presenting with peripheral vascular complications. *Annals of Surgery*, *12*(1), 705–713.

Neerukonda, S. K., Vijay, N. R., Jantz, R. D., Schoonmaker, F. W., & Saxena, A. K. (1991). Aortic dissection: Diagnosis and management. *Hospital Practice*, *26*(2), 66–75.

Reuler, J. B. & Kumar, K. L. (1991). Abdominal aortic aneurysm. *Journal, of General Internal Medicine*, *4*(6), 360–366.

Rutherford, R. B. & McCroskey, B. L. (1989). Ruptured abdominal aortic aneurysms. *Surgical Clinics of North America*, *69*(4), 859–868.

Schulze, C. (1990). Aortic dissection: An ICU crisis. *RN*, *8*, 42–46.

▼

ABDOMINAL SURGERY

Gastrointestinal surgery may be used to treat ulcer disease, gastrointestinal perforation or obstruction, tumors or lesions which result in ischemic bowel, or inflammation of any portion of the bowel. Abdominal surgery is also indicated with pathology of accessory organs of the gastrointestinal tract, including the gallbladder, pancreas, and liver. Abdominal trauma may also require surgical intervention.

Postoperatively, the bowel is decompressed until gastrointestinal function is restored. Drains are often placed in abdominal wounds to facilitate drainage of secretions. Pain related to the incision, fluid and electrolyte balance, and wound care management are priorities. Respiratory complications related to splinting of the abdomen due to pain are also a potential hazard. Nursing care is focused on monitoring and interventions to prevent postoperative complications.

ETIOLOGIES

- Esophageal disorders secondary to
  - gastroesophageal reflux
  - cancer
  - varices
- Gastric or duodenal ulcer disease
  - perforation
  - hemorrhage
  - gastric outlet obstruction
- Tumors
  - malignant
  - benign tumors with bleeding, obstruction, or intussusception
- Gastrointestinal obstruction
  - simple mechanical obstruction
  - strangulation obstruction
  - vascular obstruction

- Inflammation of the bowel
  - regional ileitis
  - regional enterocolitis
  - Crohn's disease
  - diverticulitis with perforation, obstruction, or fistula formation
- Disorders of accessory organs of the gastrointestinal system
  - cholecystitis
  - pancreatic cancer/pancreatitis
  - liver tumor
- Abdominal trauma

CLINICAL MANIFESTATIONS

- Gastrointestinal: Intestinal obstruction, paralytic ileus, and inflammation may produce
  - pain
  - abdominal rigidity
  - abdominal tenderness, rebound tenderness
  - abdominal distention
  - nausea and vomiting
  - abnormal bowel sounds (hyperactive, diminished, or absent)
  - loss of appetite
  - constipation, obstipation
  - diarrhea

  Bleeding may produce
  - hematemesis
  - bloody mucus
  - bloody diarrhea
  - maroon stools
  - melena
- Cardiovascular: Hypovolemia from third spacing of fluid may produce
  - hypotension
  - tachycardia
  - CO < 4 L/min
  - CI < 2.5 L/min/m^2
- Pulmonary: Atelectasis from surgery, anesthesia, and splinting of painful abdominal incision may produce
  - decreasing Pao$_2$
  - Paco$_2$ > 45 torr
  - inability to move secretions
  - confusion/somnolence/restlessness/irritability
  - increased respiratory rate
  - fever
  - adventitious breath sounds
  - decreased breath sounds
  - unequal chest excursion

CLINICAL/DIAGNOSTIC FINDINGS

- WBC count > 10,000/mm^3
- Potassium < 3.5 mEq/L
- Sodium imbalance (increased or decreased)
- Hematocrit < 35
- Hemoglobin < 13 g/dL
- Abnormal liver function tests (with GI bleeding)
  - PT > 13 s

- PTT > 45 s
- alkaline phosphate > 100 IU/L
- albumin < 3.5 g/dL
- ammonia > 45 µg/dL

NURSING DIAGNOSIS: ACUTE PAIN

Related To
- Abdominal incision
- Intestinal distention, obstruction, strangulation
- Wound infection

Defining Characteristics
Patient reports of severe abdominal pain
Splinting of abdomen/respirations
Abdominal guarding
Direct and rebound tenderness

Patient Outcomes
The patient reports alleviation of pain or reduction in pain using a pain-rating scale.

Nursing Interventions	Rationales
Perform a complete asssessment of pain to include location, characteristics, and precipitating factors. Observe for nonverbal cues: grimacing and guarding.	
Assess integrity of nasogastric suction.	Intestinal distention or secretion accumulation increases patient discomfort.
Assess wound status: inflammation, drainage, and redness	Wound infection may be a source of discomfort.
Implement measures (pharmacologic, nonpharmacologic, interpersonal) to facilitate pain relief before pain becomes severe. Implement prior to painful procedures.	Early intervention will prevent the pain response from escalating. Pharmacologic agents and other strategies are less effective when the patient is experiencing severe pain.

Nursing Interventions | Rationales

Nursing Interventions	Rationales
Utilize a multidisciplinary approach to pain management.	
Teach patient pain-rating scale and document pain rating.	
Teach patient splinting of incision.	
Provide information to promote patient knowledge of pain experience.	

NURSING DIAGNOSIS: HIGH RISK FOR FLUID VOLUME DEFICIT

Risk Factors
- Blood loss
- Fluid sequestration in abdominal cavity (third spacing)
- Nasogastric suction

Patient Outcomes
Adequate fluid balance is maintained/restored, as evidenced by
- blood pressure return to patient baseline
- CO 4–8 L/min; CI 2.5–4 L/min/m^2
- CVP 2–10 mmHg; PCWP 8–12 mmHg
- heart rate 60–100 bpm
- pink, moist mucous membranes
- warm, pink skin
- urine output > 30 mL/hr

Nursing Interventions	Rationales
Assess peripheral indicators of fluid balance: mucous membranes and skin turgor.	
Monitor cardiovascular status for signs of fluid depletion: heart rate, blood pressure including orthostatic changes, hemodynamics (CVP, PCWP, CO, CI, MAP), and peripheral pulses.	Increased heart rate, decreased blood pressure and/or orthostatic changes, low CVP, PCWP, CO/CI, and MAP, and weak peripheral pulses indicate persistent hypovolemia. Normalization of these measurements will reflect adequate fluid volume replacement.

Abdominal Surgery 73

74 Gastrointestinal Care

Nursing Interventions	Rationales
Monitor and record fluid status: intake and output and daily weight.	Hypovolemia can occur due to fluid sequestration in the abdominal cavity or gastrointestinal losses from surgery/nasogastric tube (NG) suction.
Monitor cardiac rhythm (EKG) and document changes.	Loss of electrolytes, especially potassium and calcium, can cause heart rhythm abnormalities
Monitor renal function: BUN, creatinine, specific gravity, and hourly urine output.	These measures indicate the adequacy of fluid volume replacement. A low urine output indicates decreased renal perfusion and inadequate fluid replacement.
Administer hypotonic solutions (D_5W, D_5 ½NS) as prescribed and monitor patient response.	Hypotonic solutions correct intracellular dehydration by causing water to move from the vascular space into the cells.
Administer isotonic solutions (normal saline, lactated Ringer's) as prescribed and monitor patient response.	Isotonic solutions are indicated for extracellular hydration.
Combine crystalloid (normal saline, lactated Ringer's) and colloid (Hespan, plasmanate) solutions as prescribed and monitor patient response.	Crystalloid and colloid solutions replace intravascular volume.
Administer electrolytes as prescribed and monitor effects.	
Instruct patient to avoid rapid position changes.	During hypovolemia, orthostatic changes can produce dizziness and syncope.

NURSING DIAGNOSIS: IMPAIRED GAS EXCHANGE
Related To
- Effect of anesthesia and surgery
- Splinting of respirations from abdominal incision

Defining Characteristics

Decreasing PaO$_2$
PaCO$_2$ > 45 torr
Inability to move secretions
Confusion, somnolence, irritability, restlessness
Decreased breath sounds/adventitious sounds

SaO$_2$ < 90%
pH < 7.35

Patient Outcomes

The patient will demonstrate effective gas exchange, as evidenced by
- PaO$_2$ > 60 torr
- SaO$_2$ > 90%
- PaCO$_2$ 35–45 torr or return to baseline
- clear, equal breath sounds
- alert/oriented or mental status return to baseline

Nursing Interventions	Rationales
Auscultate breath sounds, noting areas of decreased or absent ventilation and presence of adventitious sounds.	Ineffective gas exchange and retention of secretions results in areas of atelectasis, changing the character of breath sounds.
Monitor respiratory laboratory data: PaO$_2$, PaCO$_2$, SaO$_2$.	PaO$_2$, and SaO$_2$ will indicate the adequacy of gas exchange. The PaCO$_2$ measures the adequacy of ventilation.
Perform therapies to remove secretions: 1. Do physiotherapy. 2. Encourage slow deep breathing, turning, and coughing. 3. Teach how to cough effectively. 4. Teach how to splint respirations. 5. Remove secretions by suctioning if required. 6. Assist with incentive spirometer as appropriate.	Retained secretions cause ventilation/perfusion mismatch.
Administer analgesia as prescribed to maintain optimal comfort.	Splinting of respirations due to pain may contribute to impaired gas exchange.
Administer aerosol/nebulizer treatments as prescribed and monitor patient response.	Breathing treatments humidify secretions and facilitate their removal.

Nursing Interventions	Rationales
Administer humidified oxygen as prescribed and monitor patient response (pulse oximetry).	

NURSING DIAGNOSIS: HIGH RISK FOR INFECTION

Risk Factors
- Wound
- Immunosuppression

Patient Outcomes
Infection in abdominal wound is absent, as evidenced by
- clean granulation tissue
- absence of drainage
- WBC count 5,000–10,000/mm^3
- afebrile

Nursing Interventions	Rationales
Monitor appearance of incision line and surrounding tissue.	Redness, warmth, swelling, or complaints of pain or tenderness indicate infection.
Monitor for wound drainage: color, amount, and odor. Culture if appropriate.	Purulent wound drainage indicates infection.
Monitor for systemic effects of infection: temperature and vital signs.	Fever, tachycardia, and tachypnea are systemic signs of infection.
Monitor WBCs and differential count.	An elevated WBC count with a differential shift to the left (more bands than segs) indicates acute infection.
Use aseptic technique for dressing changes.	
Promote nutritional intake.	Adequate intake of calories and nutrients, especially protein, is essential for wound healing and prevention of infection.
If wound infection occurs, administer antibiotics as prescribed.	

NURSING DIAGNOSIS: ALTERED NUTRITION — LESS THAN BODY REQUIREMENTS

Related To
- Nasogastric suction
  See Appendix A
- Paralytic ileus

DISCHARGE PLANNING/CONTINUITY OF CARE

- Assess need for/type of long-term care and follow-up (ostomy/wound care).
- If the discharge destination is home, assess existing supports and the need for assistance.
- Determine coping deficits/support needs and institute assistance measures.
- Determine knowledge deficits/teaching needs and document and institute a teaching plan (wound care, activity limitations).
- Refer patient to social services as appropriate.
- Communicate coping deficits/support needs and knowledge deficits/teaching needs to unit accepting the patient on transfer.

REFERENCES

Hall, L., Wood, D. H., & Schmidt, G. A. (1991). *Principles of critical care* New York, NY: McGraw-Hill.

Herr, K. A. & Mobily, P. R. (1992). Interventions related to pain. In G. M. Bulechek & J. C. McCloskey (Eds.), Symposium on Nursing Interventions. *Nursing Clinics of North America*, 27(2), 347–369.

Kinney, M. R., Packa, D. R., & Dunbar, S. B. (1993). *AACN'S clinical reference for critical care nursing* (3rd ed.) New York, NY: McGraw-Hill.

Sleisenger, M. H. & Fordtran, J. S. (1989). *Gastrointestinal Disease: Pathophysiology, Diagnosis, Management* (4th ed.). Philadelphia, PA: Saunders.

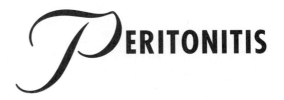Peritonitis

The most common cause of an acute abdomen is peritonitis, which is an inflammation of the peritoneum with an infective or irritating agent. Primary peritonitis results from a primary infection of the peritoneum. The bacterial agent is thought to gain access to the peritoneum through the vascular system or the fallopian tubes. Secondary peritonitis results from contamination of the peritoneal cavity from an altered or defective visceral wall. Contamination from the stomach, pancreas, and upper small bowel causes a chemical reaction from the spillage of digestive enzymes. Contamination from the lower small bowel and colon results in inflammation from the entry of bacterial content into the peritoneal cavity.

The attempt of the peritoneum to localize the contamination is the peritoneal defense mechanism and explains the presenting signs and symptoms of acute abdomen. The local reactions of the peritoneum involve vascular dilatation and increased capillary permeability. This allows large numbers of polymorphonuclear leukocytes to pour into the peritoneal cavity to phagocytize foreign material. The contaminated peritoneum is "walled off" by fibroplastic exudate which is deposited and seals off the adjacent bowel, mesentery, and omentum from the inflamed area. Diffuse peritonitis will result if this peritoneal defense mechanism is overwhelmed.

Vascular dilatation and increased capillary permeability also increase the absorptive capacity of the peritoneum, allowing for absorption of bacteria and toxins into the bloodstream. These vascular changes also lead to fluid shifts from the extracellular fluid compartment into the peritoneum, which depletes circulating blood volume.

Postoperative peritonitis can occur after any abdominal surgery, particularly in patients with preexisting nutritional depletion and electrolyte imbalances.

The treatment of primary peritonitis is supportive therapies, including intravenous fluid replacement, monitoring, and antibiotics. Surgery is usually indicated with secondary causes of peritonitis after the patient's cardiovascular and respiratory statuses have been stabilized.

ETIOLOGIES

- Primary peritonitis
  - cirrhosis
  - nephrosis
  - ascites
  - tuberculous invasion
  - altered host immune response
- Secondary peritonitis
  - perforated peptic ulcer
  - ruptured appendix
  - ischemic bowel disease
  - rupture of a viscus (trauma)
  - gangrenous bowel
  - bowel obstruction
  - pancreatitis
  - perforated colon
  - peritoneal dialysis
  - surgery of the abdomen

CLINICAL MANIFESTATIONS

- Gastrointestinal: Chemical irritation of the peritoneum produces
  - abdominal pain
  - rebound tenderness
  - abdominal muscle rigidity
  - abdominal distention
  - nausea and vomiting
  - decreased or absent bowel sounds
- Cardiovascular: Hypovolemia from third spacing of fluids, prolonged vomiting, and activation of catecholamines produce
  - decreased CO/CI
  - hypotension
  - weak rapid pulse
  - diaphoresis
  - weakness
  - fever
  - water and sodium retention
  - potassium loss
- Pulmonary: Chemical irritation with resultant pain, abdominal distention, and increased metabolic requirements for oxygen produce
  - shallow respirations
  - rapid respirations
- Renal: Hypovolemia and presence of circulating toxins, pigments, and necrotic tissue products produce
  - decreased urinary output
  - concentrated urine

CLINICAL/DIAGNOSTIC FINDINGS

- Spread of infectious organisms produces
  - elevated leukocyte level (polymorphonuclear cells)
  - positive peritoneal lavage (WBC > 500/mm^3, RBC > 50,000/mm^2)
  - positive culture and sensitivity of peritoneal aspirate

- positive systemic culture and sensitivity
- A perforated viscus produces
  - free air on abdominal radiograph
  - signs of fluid in abdomen or edema of the intestinal wall on abdominal radiograph

NURSING DIAGNOSIS: ACUTE PAIN

Related To
- Chemical irritation of the parietal peritoneum (containing somatic nerves)
- Abdominal distention

Defining Characteristics
Patient complaint of acute abdominal pain
Fetal position
Abdominal guarding
Direct and rebound tenderness

Patient Outcomes
The patient will report abdominal pain is relieved or tolerable (0–3 on pain-rating scale of 0–10).

Nursing Interventions	Rationales
Assess patient anxiety. Administer sedatives with analgesics as required.	Anxiety may heighten pain perception.
Assess pain based on pain-rating scale and document.	A scale allows for objective assessment of subjective perception of pain.
Administer analgesic as prescribed and monitor patient response.	Note: Physician may limit pain medication to monitor progression of peritoneal irritation.
Encourage bedrest. Minimize activities. Assist patient to most comfortable position. Splint painful area.	Bedrest decreases peritoneal irritation. Knee to chest position decreases intensity of pain. Semi-Fowler's position allows for fluid drainage by gravity, reducing abdominal tension and decreasing pain. Careful movement and splinting reduces muscle tension, which may promote comfort.

Nursing Interventions	Rationales
Provide alternate comfort measures, that is, massage, back rubs, and relaxation techniques.	Alternate comfort measures can promote relaxation and may refocus attention from pain.

NURSING DIAGNOSIS: FLUID VOLUME DEFICIT

Related To
- Fluid shift from extracellular, intravascular, and interstitial compartments into the peritoneal cavity (third spacing)
- Prolonged vomiting

Defining Characteristics

Hypotension
Tachycardia
Mental status changes
Cool, clammy skin
Sodium > 145 mEq/L
BUN > 20 mg/dL

CVP < 2 mmHg
PCWP < 8 mmHg
Hyperventilation
Urine output < 30 mL/hr
Increased urinary sodium

Patient Outcomes
Fluid volume will be restored, as evidenced by
- blood pressure return to baseline (MAP > 60 mmHg)
- heart rate 60–100 bpm
- urine output > 30 ml/hr
- CVP 2–10 mmHg
- PCWP 8–12 mmHg
- warm, dry skin
- mentation return to baseline
- absence of hemoconcentration

Nursing Interventions	Rationales
Assess for peripheral indicators of fluid balance: mucous membranes, skin turgor, and thirst.	
Monitor and record fluid balance: intake and output and daily weight.	Daily weights and intake and output provide a means to trend and evaluate fluid balance over a 24-hr period.

Nursing Interventions	Rationales
Monitor indicators of intravascular volume, including vital signs, pulmonary artery pressure readings, CO, CI, urine output, peripheral circulation, and mentation.	Normalization of these measurements will reflect adequate fluid volume replacement.
Monitor serum electrolytes and urinary electrolytes.	Electrolyte levels may be increased if fluid volume deficit results in hemoconcentration. Electrolyte levels may be decreased if large amounts of fluid are lost into the peritoneal cavity or in the vomitus.
Monitor renal function: BUN, creatinine, and hourly urine output	BUN and creatinine reflect renal function and their increase forewarns of prolonged decreased renal perfusion and hypovolemia. A low urine output and high specific gravity show decreased renal perfusion and inadequate fluid replacement.
Restore fluid volume with colloids and crystalloids as prescribed and according to fluid assessments.	
Monitor patient response.	
Measure abdominal girth every shift.	Increasing abdominal girth indicates increased third spacing of fluid into the peritoneum.
Avoid abrupt changes in position until fluid balance is restored.	During hypovolemia, orthostatic changes can produce dizziness and syncope.

NURSING DIAGNOSIS: HIGH RISK FOR INFECTION

Risk Factors
- Peritonitis
- Sepsis/septic shock
- Abscess formation
- Wound evisceration

Patient Outcomes
Patient will remain infection free, as evidenced by
- absence or resolution of fever

- WBC 5,000–10,000/mm^3
- negative culture and sensitivity reports
- clear chest x-ray

Nursing Interventions	Rationales
Assess bowel sounds.	Decreased/absent bowel sounds may indicate an ileus which in turn may be an indication of an abdominal source of infection.
Monitor for fever, hypotension, and tachycardia in patients at high risk for infection.	
Monitor quality of all drainage. Culture as appropriate.	A change in the characteristics of drainage indicates infection.
Monitor results of laboratory and diagnostic tests: WBC count and serial blood and sputum, urine, and wound cultures.	
Monitor abdominal girth and tenderness and rigidity of the abdomen.	Increased abdominal girth, tenderness, and/or rigidity of the abdomen indicates third spacing of fluid and possible bacterial contamination.
Use aseptic technique.	
Provide frequent oral care.	Colonization of the oral mucosa is a source of infection.
Administer fluid replacement as prescribed and monitor patient response.	
Administer antibiotics as prescribed.	
Administer peritoneal dialysis with antibiotics as prescribed.	Direct instillation of antibiotics into the abdomen may be used to treat inflammation of the peritoneum.
Prepare patient for surgery.	Most patients with secondary peritonitis require surgical intervention.

▼

NURSING DIAGNOSIS: INEFFECTIVE BREATHING PATTERN/ IMPAIRED GAS EXCHANGE

Related To
- Abdominal distention
- Pleural effusion
- Pain

Defining Characteristics
Increased respiratory rate
$SaO_2 < 90\%$
Atelectasis on chest x-ray
Subjective complaint of dyspnea
Pleural effusion on chest x-ray
Decreasing PaO_2
$PaCO_2 > 45$ torr
pH < 7.35
Decreased breath sounds
Presence of crackles

Patient Outcomes
Breathing patterns and gas exchange are effective, as evidenced by
- respiratory rate 10–20
- $PaO_2 > 60$ torr
- $SaO_2 > 90\%$
- $PaCO_2$ 35–45 torr or return to baseline
- pH 7.35–7.45
- clear breath sounds
- chest x-ray return to baseline
- no reports of dyspnea

Nursing Interventions	Rationales
Monitor respiratory status: respiratory rate, arterial blood gases, pulse oximetry, breath sounds, and chest x-rays.	
Position patient in semi-Fowler's position.	This allows for free movement of diaphragm.
Administer pain medication as prescribed and monitor effects.	Judicious use of pain medication decreases splinting of respirations due to pain, without respiratory compromise.
Administer chest physiotherapy. Turn and reposition.	Chest physiotherapy and turning promotes gas exchange.
Encourage deep breathing and coughing and use of incentive spirometer. Administer oxygen as prescribed and monitor patient response (pulse oximetry). Assist with aspiration of pleural effusion as needed.	

DISCHARGE PLANNING/CONTINUITY OF CARE

- Assess need for/type of long-term care and follow-up
- If the discharge destination is home, assess existing supports and the need for assistance
- Determine coping deficits/support needs and institute assistance measures.
- Determine knowledge deficits/teaching needs and document and institute a teaching plan.
- Refer patient to social services as appropriate.
- Communicate coping deficits/support needs and knowledge deficits/teaching needs to unit accepting the patient on transfer.

REFERENCES

Berk, J. E., Haubrich, W. S., Kalser, M. H., Roth, J. L., & Schaffner, F. (1985). *Gastroenterology* (4th ed.) Philadelphia, PA: Saunders.

Hall, L., Wood, D. H., Schmidt, G. A. (1991). *Principles of critical care.* New York, NY: McGraw-Hill.

Kinney, M. R., Packa, D. R., & Dunbar, S. B. (1993). *AACN'S clinical reference for critical-care nursing* (3rd ed.) New York, NY: McGraw-Hill.

Sleisenger, M. H. & Fordtran, J. S. (1989). *Gastrointestinal disease: Pathophysiology, diagnosis, management* (4th ed.) Philadelphia, PA: Saunders.

Stabile, B. E. (1992). Current surgical management of duodenal ulcers. *Surgical Clinics of North America*, 72(2), 335–353.

ACUTE GASTROINTESTINAL BLEED

Life-threatening gastrointestinal bleeding most often originates in the upper tract and is caused primarily by gastric ulcers from peptic ulcer disease or disease of the esophagus. Peptic ulcer disease is the most common cause of upper gastrointestinal tract bleeding. These ulcers are characterized by a break in the mucosa extending through the muscularis mucosae. Excess secretion of acid is important to the pathogenesis of the ulcer development coupled with impaired ability of the mucosa to secrete the quantity and quality of mucus for protection. Esophageal bleeding can be the result of varices that develop from increased portal venous pressure or from a linear tear of the esophagel and/or gastric mucosa (Mallory Weiss tear).

Bleeding from the lower gastrointestinal tract rarely causes hemodynamic compromise. The patient, however, may present with orthostatic vital signs from slower blood loss.

The clinical manifestations of the patient presenting with gastrointestinal tract bleeding varies considerably, depending on the amount and the rapidity of blood loss. In addition to signs of blood loss from the tract, signs of cardiovascular compensatory mechanisms or decreased perfusion to core body organs predominate.

Most gastrointestinal bleeding is self-limiting and requires medical intervention only. Surgical therapy is considered if the bleed is massive and conventional medical therapies are unsuccessful.

ETIOLOGIES

- Peptic ulcer disease
  - gastric ulcer
  - duodenal ulcer
  - Zollinger-Ellison syndrome
- Portal hypertension with development of varices
  - esophageal
  - gastric
  - hemorrhoids

- Pathology of the esophagus
  - cancer
  - Mallory Weiss tear
- Pathology of the stomach
  - cancer
  - erosive gastritis
- Pathology of the intestine
  - ulcerative colitis
  - polyps
  - diverticula
  - hemorrhoids
  - aortointestinal fistula
  - Crohn's disease
  - neoplasms
  - arteriovenous malformation
- Coagulation disorders: disseminated intravascular coagulation (DIC)
- Medications
  - aspirin
  - corticosteroids
  - nonsteroidal anti-inflammatory drugs
  - anticoagulants

CLINICAL MANIFESTATIONS

- Gastrointestinal: Bleeding above the ligament of Treitz (at the duodenal-jejunal junction) can produce
  - hematemesis (bright red or coffee ground)
  - melena (tarry or maroon stools)

  Blood in the gastrointestinal tract can produce
  - hyperactive bowel sounds
  - vomiting
- Cardiovascular: Hypovolemia can produce
  - tachycardia
  - hypotension
  - orthostatic hypotension
  - cool, clammy skin
  - CO < 4 L/min
  - CI < 2.5 L/min/m^2
  - decreased preload indicators (CVP/PCWP)
  - dysrhythmias
- Neurological: Hypovolemia and decreased perfusion produce
  - anxiety
  - restlessness
  - change in mental state
- Pulmonary: Hypovolemia and decreased perfusion produce
  - hyperventilation
  - respiratory alkalosis
- Renal: Hypovolemia and hypotension produce
  - decreased urine output

CLINICAL/DIAGNOSTIC FINDINGS

- Loss of blood volume produces
  - hemoglobin < 13 g/dL
  - hematocrit < 35% (women); < 42% (men)
  - decreasing PaO_2
  - BUN > 20 mg/dL
  - creatinine > 1.2 mg/dL
  - sodium > 145 mEq/L
  - PT > 13 s
  - PTT > 45 s
  - platelet count < 150,000/mm^3
- Body stress response activation of sympathetic nervous system produces
  - glucose > 115 mg/dL
  - white blood cell count > 10,000/mm^3
  - respiratory alkalosis ($PaCO_2$ < 35 torr; pH > 7.45)
  - temperature elevation
- Loss of gastric contents associated with hematemesis and vomiting produce a potassium level below 3.5 mEq/L.
- Decreased tissue perfusion produces
  - metabolic acidosis (HCO_3 < 21 mEq/L; pH < 7.35)
  - ammonia > 45 µg/dL

NURSING DIAGNOSIS: FLUID VOLUME DEFICIT

Related To active loss of blood from gastrointestinal tract

Defining Characteristics

Hypotension
CO < 4 L/min
CVP < 2 mmHg
Tachycardia
Skin and mucous membranes are cool, pale, and dry
Urine output < 30 mL/hr
CI < 2.5 L/min/m^2
PCWP < 8 mmHg

Patient Outcomes

Adequate fluid balance is maintained/restored, as evidenced by
- MAP > 70 mmHg
- CO 4–8 L/min; CI 2.5–4 L/min/m^2
- CVP 2–10 mmHg; PCWP 8–12 mmHg
- heart rate 60–100 bpm
- pink, moist mucous membranes
- warm, pink skin
- urine output > 30 mL/hr

Nursing Interventions	Rationales
Monitor/record cardiovascular status: blood pressure, heart rate including orthostatic changes; hemodynamics (CVP, PCWP, CO, CI, MAP), and peripheral pulses.	Increased heart rate, decreased blood pressure, and/or orthostatic changes; low CVP, PCWP, CO, CI, and MAP; and weak peripheral pulses indicate persistent hypovolemia. Normalization of these measurements will reflect adequate fluid replacement. Prevent fluid overload through continuous assessment during fluid administration.
Monitor/record fluid balance: intake and output and daily weight.	Intake and output and daily weight provide a means to trend and evaluate fluid balance.
Monitor renal function: BUN, creatinine, and hourly urine output.	BUN and creatinine reflect renal function, and their increase indicates prolonged decreased renal perfusion. Decreased urine output is an early sign of decreased perfusion and inadequate fluid replacement.
Monitor coagulation studies and complete blood count.	This enables monitoring of the patient's response to treatments and enables prevention of complications related to coagulation defects.
Administer intravenous colloids, crystalloids, or blood products as prescribed until signs and symptoms of hypovolemia decrease and the patient stabilizes. Monitor for signs of fluid overload such as increased CVP/PCWP, adventitious lung sounds, jugular venous distension, increased peripheral edema, and respiratory distress. Inform patient of need for blood replacement as necessary.	Initially colloids or crystalloids are used for fluid resuscitation. Blood losses greater than 1500 mL require blood replacement in addition to fluids.

Nursing Interventions	Rationales
Perform nasogastric lavage as appropriate.	Lavage is a controversial intervention. It may disturb blood clots over bleeding sites. It may be used to remove blood from the stomach to prepare the patient for endoscopy. Room temperature solution should be used. Iced solutions, however, may decrease the ability of blood to form clots.
Administer electrolyte replacements as ordered until signs and symptoms of electrolyte imbalance are corrected.	With gastrointestinal blood loss and associated vomiting, sodium and potassium may be lost.
Hematest all excretions and observe for blood in emesis, sputum, feces, urine, and nasogastric and wound drainage. Document color, amount, and character of gastrointestinal secretions (emesis, stools).	Monitoring of blood loss is important to evaluate the outcomes of treatment.
Administer medications (vasopressin) as prescribed and monitor response.	Vasopressin or pitressin lowers portal hypertension and decreases the flow of blood at the site of bleeding by producing splanchnic vasoconstriction.
Avoid extremes in gastric pH by administration of medications, for example, antacids and histamine-2 blocking agent.	Antacids are a direct alkaline buffer used to control gastric pH. Histamine H_2 antagonistic drugs decrease the production of gastric acid by inhibiting the action of histamine.
Maintain pressure in cuffed/balloon nasogastric tube (Sengstaken Blakemore).	With bleeding esophageal varices, special nasogastric tubes with a balloon in the esophagus and/or stomach are used to tamponade bleeding vessels.
Instruct patient on procedures (e.g., endoscopy, sclerotherapy) if appropriate.	Anticipatory teaching immediately prior to the procedure assists the patient in understanding and preparing mentally for the prescribed procedure or treatment.

Clinical Clip

The most accurate assessment parameters for the amount of blood loss in gastrointestinal bleeding are the vital signs.

NURSING DIAGNOSIS: HIGH RISK FOR IMPAIRED GAS EXCHANGE

Risk Factors
- Decreased oxygen-carrying capacity (decreased hemoglobin)
- Aspiration

Patient Outcomes
Gas exchange between the alveoli of the lungs and the vascular system is adequate, as evidenced by
- $PaO_2 > 80$ torr
- $PaCO_2$ return to baseline
- normal pH
- $SaO_2 > 90\%$
- absence of gastric contents in lung secretions
- absence of restlessness, confusion, irritability, dizziness
- heart rate 60–100 bpm
- airways clear of mucus
- breath sounds clear

Nursing Interventions	Rationales
Assess oxygenation status (PaO_2, pulse oximetry).	
Monitor hemoglobin.	Hemoglobin carries oxygen in the blood stream.
Auscultate breath sounds, noting areas of decreased or absent ventilation and the presence of adventitious sounds.	
Administer oxygen as prescribed. Remove secretions by coughing or suctioning. Note characteristics.	
Alleviate fear and/or anxiety. Promote activities to provide rest.	Activity or inadequate rest can increase oxygen demand.

Nursing Interventions

Prevent aspiration: Monitor for abdominal distention; position patient with head of bed up if possible; and treat nausea and vomiting promptly.

Rationales

Blood accumulated in the stomach may precipitate vomiting and possible aspiration.

NURSING DIAGNOSIS: ALTERED TISSUE PERFUSION— CENTRAL AND PERIPHERAL

Related To
- Decreased circulating volume
- Hypotension

Defining Characteristics
Confusion or change in level of consciousness
CO < 4 L/min; CI < 2.5 L/min/m^2
SVR > 1200 dyn/s/cm^{-5}
Hypotension
Cool, clammy skin
CVP < 2 mmHg; PCWP < 8 mmHg
Urine output < 30 mL/hr
Tachycardia
Weak, thready peripheral pulses

Patient Outcomes
Central and peripheral perfusion are stable, as evidenced by
- MAP > 60 mmHg
- CO 4–8 L/min; CI 2.5–4 L/min/m^2
- CVP 2–10 mmHg; PCWP 8–12 mmHg
- SVR 800–1200 dyn/s/cm^{-5}
- Svo_2 > 70%
- mental status returning to patient baseline
- warm, dry skin
- urine output > 30 mL/hr

Nursing Interventions	Rationales
Monitor heart rate, respiratory rate, and blood pressure.	Blood pressure will remain low until low volume is corrected by administration of colloids and crystalloids. Heart rate and respiratory rate will be elevated as long as tissue perfusion is inadequate.
Monitor CO/CI and SVR.	Cardiac output is a major determinant of tissue perfusion. Increased SVR, resulting from vasoconstriction, decreases tissue perfusion.
Monitor CVP, PCWP, and Svo_2.	Low CVP and PCWP indicate hypovolemia. A low Svo_2 indicates inadequate tissue perfusion.
Monitor for changes in patient's mental status.	Hypovolemia may produce changes in mental status due to decreased cerebral perfusion.
Monitor urine output hourly.	Decreased urine output is an early sign of decreased perfusion to the kidney.
Monitor peripheral circulation: Inspect skin, noting color and temperature; check quality of peripheral pulses and capillary refill time (CRT).	Cool, clammy, pale skin, weak peripheral pulses, or increased CRT indicate decreased circulating volume and decreased peripheral perfusion.
Provide preventive skin care: 1. Changes position regularly. 2. Keep skin clean and dry. 3. Inspect skin for erythema/blanching with position change. 4. Gently massage vulnerable areas with position change. 5. Utilize specialized mattress or bed in patients on bedrest and/or with decreased spontaneous movement. 6. Provide range-of-motion exercises. Consult physical therapy.	Decreased tissue perfusion puts the patient at risk for skin breakdown. The frequency of nursing interventions should be increased if any reddened areas do not resolve within 1 hr.

NURSING DIAGNOSIS: KNOWLEDGE DEFICIT

Related To discharge regimen

Defining Characteristics
Patient expresses lack of understanding of diagnosis and/or discharge regimen.

Patient Outcomes
The patient will be able to
- verbalize dietary, medication, and activity regimens.
- describe signs and symptoms that require medical interventions.

Nursing Interventions	Rationales
Assess patient's level of understanding and ability to comprehend.	
Describe discharge dietary regimen: Avoid caffeine, alcohol, and food known to patient to cause dyspepsia. The patient should be encouraged to eat nutritional meals at regular intervals.	
Describe discharge medication regimen, including names of drug and purpose, specific dosage schedule in hours, expected adverse side effects and how to deal with them, avoidance of medications that will irritate the gastric or esophageal mucosa (i.e., nonsteroidal anti-inflammatory drug), and stopping smoking.	
Identify signs and symptoms of early bleeding: dizziness and change in vision, sudden or gradual weakness, coffee ground emesis, or melena. See Appendix B.	

DISCHARGE PLANNING/CONTINUITY OF CARE

- Assess need for/type of long term-care and follow-up.
- If the discharge destination is home, assess existing supports and the need for assistance.
- Determine coping deficits/support needs and institute assistance measures.
- Determine knowledge deficits/teaching needs and document and institute a teaching plan.
- Refer patient to social services as appropriate.
- Communicate coping deficits/support needs and knowledge deficits/teaching needs to unit accepting patient on transfer.

REFERENCES

Burns, S. M. & Martin, M. J. (1990). Vasopressin/nitroglycerin therapy in the patient with variceal bleeding. *Critical Care Nurse*, 10(9), 42–49.

Dudnick, R., Martin, P., & Friedman, L. S. (1991). Management of bleeding ulcers. *Medical Clinics of North America*, 75(4), 947–965.

Eisenberg, P. (1990). Monitoring gastric pH to prevent stress ulcer syndrome. *Focus on Critical Care*, 17(4), 316–322.

Jacoby, A. G. & Wiegman, M. V. (1990). Cardiovascular complications of intravenous vasopressin therapy. *Focus on Critical Care*, 17(1), 63–66.

Mertz, H. R. & Walsh, J. H. (1991). Peptic ulcer pathophysiology. *Medical Clinics of North America*, 75(4), 799–814.

Pierce, J. D., Vilkerson, E., & Griffiths, S. A. (1990). Acute esophageal bleeding and endoscopic injection sclerotherapy. *Critical Care Nurse*, 10(9), 67–72.

Rubin, W. (1991). Medical treatment of peptic ulcer disease. *Medical Clinics of North America*, 74(4), 981–998.

▼

ACUTE PANCREATITIS

Acute pancreatitis is characterized by an inflammatory response and potential necrosis of pancreatic cells resulting from premature activation of pancreatic enzymes within the pancreas. The disease ranges in severity from a mild self-limiting form to a severe necrotizing process. In the mild form, edema of glandular and interstitial tissue predominates. In the severe form, the initial damage of pancreatic cells is thought to cause a cycle where release and activation of digestive enzymes lead to generalized pancreatic necrosis with disruption and thrombotic occlusion of vessels in and around the pancreas. The substrates released not only cause a local inflammation and pathology in and around the pancreas but also can trigger systemic complications when released into the circulation. Multisystem failure can predominate in this fulminant form.

Significant clinical symptoms include abdominal pain, nausea, and vomiting. The patient may also present with signs of hypovolemic shock with associated sequestration of fluid in the peritoneum as a result of inflammation of pancreatic cells. Respiratory failure and pancreatic septic processes are the most common complications of acute pancreatitis and most significantly impact morbidity and mortality in this patient population.

ETIOLOGIES

- Biliary tract disease
- Alcoholic disease
- Pancreatic disease
- Posttraumatic (abdominal)
- Pregnancy
- Retrograde pancreatography
- Hyperlipoproteinemia
- Drugs
    - acetaminophen
    - cimetidine
    - estrogens
    - clonidine
    - corticosteroids
    - furosemide

- lipids
- procainamide
- sulfa antibiotics
- opiates
- rifampin
- thiazides
- Hepatitis B
- Coxsackie virus
- Atheroembolism
- Lupus erythematosus
- Posttransplantation
- Shock

CLINICAL MANIFESTATIONS

- Gastrointestinal: Pancreatic inflammation and/or necrosis can produce:
  - pain
  - nausea
  - abdominal distention
  - abdominal tympany
  - vomiting
  - low-grade fever
  - abdominal guarding
  - hypoactive bowel sounds
- Severe disease: above signs and
  - ascites
  - palpable abdominal mass
  - jaundice
  - hypovolemic shock
  - Grey Turner's sign (bluish discoloration around flank)
  - Cullen's sign (bluish discoloration around umbilicus)

CLINICAL/DIAGNOSTIC FINDINGS

- Pancreatic inflammation/necrosis can produce
  - serum amylase > 85 IU/L
  - serum pancreatic isoamylase > 50%
  - urine amylase > 15 IU/hr
  - serum lipase > 24 IU/dL
  - serum triglycerides > 150 mg/dL
  - pancreatic/parapancreatic abscess or pseudocyst per abdominal computed tomography, ultrasound, magnetic resonance imaging

NURSING DIAGNOSIS: FLUID VOLUME DEFICIT

Related To
- Fluid sequestration in abdominal cavity
- Vomiting
- Pancreatic vascular interruption by inflammatory process

Defining Characteristics

Signs of hypovolemic shock: hypotension, tachycardia, mental status changes, hyperventilation, cool clammy skin, decreased urine output
Precipitous vomiting
Increased serum electrolytes (hemoconcentration)
Hypernatremia (sodium > 145 mEq/L)
Increased urinary sodium
BUN > 20 mg/dL
With vascular interruption: hematocrit < 35% (female); < 42% (male)
With hemoconcentration: hematocrit > 47% (female); > 52% (men)

Patient Outcomes

Fluid volume will be restored, as evidenced by
- blood pressure return to baseline (MAP > 60 mmHg)
- heart rate 60–100 bpm
- urine output > 30 mL/hr
- CVP 2–10 mmHg
- PCWP 8–12 mmHg
- potassium 3.5–5.0 mEq/L
- hematocrit 30%

Nursing Interventions	Rationales
Monitor for signs and symptoms of hemorrhage: low hematocrit and hemoglobin, Cullen or Grey Turner's sign, and increasing abdominal girth	
Monitor outcomes of fluid replacement therapy, including blood pressure and heart rate, intake and output, preload indicators (CVP, PCWP), skin turgor, capillary refill, mucous membranes, and thirst.	Blood pressure (decreased) and heart rate (increased) are the most sensitive clinical signs of volume status. The PCWP is the most sensitive measure of the adequacy of volume status and left ventricular filling pressure.
Restore fluid volume with colloids, crystalloids, or blood products as prescribed and monitor effects.	Colloids or crystalloids may be used to restore volume. There is theoretical support for the use of fresh frozen plasma because it contains components of plasma antiprotease and plasma fibronectin which are depleted in acute pancreatitis. Packed red blood cells may be required with vascular interruption of the pancreas.

Nursing Interventions / Rationales

Nursing Interventions	Rationales
Maintain patent intravenous access (central line preferred).	
Maintain on bedrest until fluid volume status is restored.	The patient is at risk for orthostatic hypotension.

NURSING DIAGNOSIS: ACUTE PAIN

Related To
- Interruption of blood supply to the pancreas
- Peritoneal irritation from activated pancreatic exocrine enzymes
- Edema or distention of the pancreas

Defining Characteristics
Patient reports acute abdominal pain (severe, relentless, knifelike; midepigastrium or periumbilical region): fetal position, abdominal guarding, and direct and rebound tenderness.

Patient Outcomes
The patient will report abdominal pain is relieved or tolerable (0–3 on pain-rating scale of 0–10).

Nursing Interventions	Rationales
Assess degree of pain by having patient use pain-rating scale and document pain rating.	A scale allows for objective assessment of the subjective perception of pain.
Assess patient anxiety. Administer sedatives with analgesics as required.	Anxiety may heighten pain perception.
Administer nonopiate analgesics. Schedule pain medications initially to prevent severe pain episodes.	Morphine may cause spasm of the sphincter of Oddi, which may worsen pain. Scheduled doses of pain medication are more effective with severe pain.
Maintain NPO as long as patient reports abdominal pain and NG to intermittent suction.	Fluids in the gastrointestinal tract stimulate pancreatic exocrine secretion and will promote the cycle of pancreatic inflammation.

Nursing Interventions

Encourage bedrest. Minimize activities. Assist patient to most comfortable position.

Rationales

Bedrest decreases pancreatic exocrine secretion, an etiology of pain. Knee-to-chest position decreases the intensity of the pain.

NURSING DIAGNOSIS: ALTERED NUTRITION—LESS THAN BODY REQUIREMENTS

Related To
- Prolonged NPO status and hypomotility of the intestines
- Nausea and vomiting
- Impaired nutrient metabolism
- Altered production of digestive exocrine enzymes

Defining Characteristics
Negative nitrogen balance
Albumin < 3.5 g/dL
Total protein < 6 g/dL
Serum bicarbonate < 18 mEq/L

Patient Outcomes
Nutritional balance will be restored, as evidenced by
- positive nitrogen balance
- serum albumin 3.5–5 g/dL
- total protein 6–8 g/dL
- absence of muscle wasting
- absence of metabolic acidosis

Nursing Interventions

Assess nutritional status through laboratory analysis of nitrogen balance, albumin, and total protein

Rationales

These are the most accurate indicators of nutritional balance in the critically ill. Daily weights are more reflective of fluid balance.

Nursing Interventions	Rationales
Administer total parenteral nutrition as prescribed. Avoid lipid therapy. Monitor for signs and symptoms of complications of TPN therapy, including line sepsis, hyperglycemia, and electrolyte imbalance.	Total parenteral nutrition allows for complete rest of the pancreas and therefore inhibits pancreatic exocrine secretion. Hyperlipidemia is associated with severe pancreatitis, and thus lipids should be avoided, especially in patients with severe manifestations of the disease.
Maintain strict NPO. Administer elemental enteral feedings as prescribed into the jejunum.	Pancreatic stimulation is bypassed by infusing distal to the duodenum.
See Appendix A.	

NURSING DIAGNOSIS: ELECTROLYTE IMBALANCE

Related To
- Prolonged vomiting
- Fluid sequestration from activated pancreatic enzymes and inflammatory response

Defining Characteristics
Calcium < 8.5 mg/dL
Sodium < 135 mEq/L
Potassium < 3.5 mEq/L

Patient Outcomes
Electrolyte balance will be restored, as evidenced by
- serum calcium 8.5–10.5 mg/dL
- serum potassium 3.5–5.0 mEq/L
- serum sodium 135–145 mEq/L

Nursing Interventions	Rationales
Monitor serum calcium. Infuse replacements through central line and monitor response. With severe hypocalcemia, place patient in seizure precautions. Monitor for prolonged Q-T interval on EKG.	Hypocalemia is associated with severe manifestations of acute pancreatitis.

Nursing Interventions	Rationales
Monitor serum potassium and infuse 20 mEq KCl over 1 hr to replace until level is greater than 4.0 mEq/L. Monitor EKG for ventricular dysrhythmias.	Potassium may be lost from prolonged vomiting, NG suction, and fluid sequestration.
Monitor serum sodium and for signs of hyponatremia (weakness, confusion, muscle twitching, anorexia, nausea, and vomiting)	

NURSING DIAGNOSIS: IMPAIRED GAS EXCHANGE

Related To
- Pulmonary complications of pancreatic inflammation and mediated responses
- Fluid overload during intravascular rehydration
- Atelectasis from diaphragmatic splinting due to pain

Defining Characteristics
Decreasing PaO$_2$
Acute respiratory distress syndrome
Pleural effusion
Pulmonary emboli

Patient Outcomes
Gas exchange will be restored, as evidenced by
- PaO$_2$ > 60 torr
- SaO$_2$ > 90%
- respiratory rate 12–20
- absence of effusions, areas of consolidation, acute respiratory distress syndrome (ARDS) on chest x-ray

Nursing Interventions	Rationales
Perform respiratory assessment and correlate with arterial blood gas analysis, pulse oximetry, and chest x-ray results.	Hypoxemia is a common complication from acute pancreatitis from mechanisms which are not well understood. Acute respiratory distress syndrome is associated with fulminant forms of the disease.

Nursing Interventions	Rationales
Administer oxygen therapy to maintain arterial oxygen tension and oxygen saturation.	
Perform peritoneal lavage.	Peritoneal lavage is used to clear activated mediators and enzymes from the peritoneal cavity. These substances are associated with severe pulmonary and pancreatic septic complications of acute pancreatitis.

DISCHARGE PLANNING/CONTINUITY OF CARE

- Assess need for/type of long-term care and follow-up.
- If the discharge destination is home, assess existing supports and the need for assistance.
- Determine coping deficits/support needs and institute assistance measures.
- Determine knowledge deficits/teaching needs and document and institute a teaching plan.
- Refer patient to social services as appropriate.
- Communicate coping deficits/support needs and knowledge deficits/teaching needs to unit accepting patient on transfer.

REFERENCES

Brown, A. (1991). Acute pancreatitis. *Focus on Critical Care, 18*(2), 121–130.

Hadeley, S. & Fitzsimmons, L. (1990). Acute pancreatitis: A life-threatening emergency. *Topics in Emergency Medicine, 12*(2), 39–47.

Jones, M. L. & Neoptolemos, J. (1990). Recent advances in the treatment of acute pancreatitis. *Surgical Annual, 22*, 235–255.

Pitchumoni, C. S., Agarwal, J., & Jain, N. K. (1988). Systemic complications of acute pancreatitis. *American Journal of Gastroenterology, 83*(6), 597–608.

FULMINANT HEPATIC FAILURE

The liver is one of the most complex organs of the body performing over 400 functions. Some of these are filtration of blood in the gastrointestinal tract; secretion of bile; carbohydrate, fat, and protein metabolism; storage of blood, glucose, vitamins, and minerals; production and removal of blood-clotting components; and detoxification of drugs and other substances. Fulminant hepatic failure results when the liver is unable to perform its many functions.

Causes of liver failure are many and include both inflammatory and fibrotic processes. For example, in viral hepatitis, there is massive necrosis of liver cells. In alcoholic cirrhosis, liver cells are replaced by fibrous tissue. Fatty liver is the result of fat droplet deposits within liver cells.

ETIOLOGIES

- Inflammatory liver disease with liver necrosis secondary to
  - hepatitis A, B, non-A, non-B, C, D, and E
  - toxic ingestions of drugs (e.g., acetaminophen, halothane, methyldopa) and chemicals and poisons (e.g., chlorinated hydrocarbons, phosphorus, aflatoxin)
  - liver tumors
  - herpes
  - heat stroke
- Fibrotic liver disease secondary to cirrhosis of the liver
  - alcohol ingestion
  - biliary disease
  - cardiac disease
  - viral hepatitis
- Fatty liver deposits secondary to
  - alcohol ingestion
  - dietary influences
  - steatosis

CLINICAL MANIFESTATIONS

- Cardiovascular: Loss of filtration mechanisms in the liver and portal hypertension can produce
  - hyperdynamic circulation
  - dysrhythmias
  - portal hypertension
- Renal: Loss of liver filtration mechanisms, altered protein metabolism functions, and the inability to regulate sodium and fluid balance can produce
  - ascites
  - edema
  - decreased intravascular volume
  - hypokalemia
  - dilutional hyponatremia
  - hepatorenal syndrome
- Endocrine: Loss of liver detoxification of hormones can produce
  - increased aldosterone
  - increased antidiuretic hormone
- Gastrointestinal: Loss of liver secretory processes and altered substrate metabolism can produce
  - decreased appetite
  - diarrhea
  - bleeding disorders
  - malnutrition
  - nausea and vomiting
- Hematological: Loss of liver secretory processes, portal hypertension, and altered protein metabolism can produce
  - esophageal and/or gastric varices
  - anemia
  - impaired coagulation
  - DIC
- Neurological: Loss of liver metabolism of ammonia can produce
  - hepatic encephalopathy
  - cerebral edema
- Immunological: Loss of Kupffer cell phagocytic mechanisms can produce infection
- Skin: Portal hypertension, impaired bilirubin metabolism and loss of liver cell detoxification mechanisms can produce
  - jaundice
  - spider angiomas
  - pruritis

CLINICAL/DIAGNOSTIC FINDINGS

- Decreased liver secretory functions can produce
  - total bilirubin > 1 mg/dL; direct > 0.4 mg/dL
  - urine bilirubin positive or > 0.02 mg/dL
  - urobilinogen > 1 Ehrlich unit/dL (estimated)
  - PT > 13 s
  - PTT > 45 s
  - albumin < 3.5 g/dL
  - fibrinogen < 200 mg/dL
- Liver cell necrosis can produce
  - SGOT/AST > 36 IU/L

- SGPT/ALT > 24 IU/L
- alkaline phosphate > 100 IU/L
- Decreased liver detoxification functions can produce
  - ammonia > 45 µg/dL
  - cholesterol > 210 mg/dL

NURSING DIAGNOSIS: FLUID VOLUME: DEFICIT

Related To
- Portal hypertension and risk for variceal bleed
- Third spacing of peritoneal fluid
- Coagulation abnormalities

Defining Characteristics
Hypotension
CVP < 2 mmHg
Skin cool, pale, and dry
Urine output < 30 mL/h
Platelet count < 50,000/mm^3
PT > 13 s

Tachycardia
PCWP < 8 mmHg
Dry mucous membranes
Hemoglobin < 13 g/dL
Hematocrit < 25%
PTT > 45 s

Patient Outcomes
Adequate fluid balance is maintained/restored, as evidenced by
- MAP > 60 mmHg
- CVP 2–10 mmHg; PCWP 8–12 mmHg
- heart rate 60–100 bpm
- pink, moist mucous membranes
- warm, pink skin
- urine output > 30 ml/hour
- hematocrit > 25%
- hemoglobin 10–12 g/dL
- platelet count 50,000–80,000/mm^3
- absence of bleeding

Nursing Interventions	Rationales
Assess for peripheral indicators of fluid balance: mucous membranes, skin turgor, and thirst.	
Monitor cardiovascular status: vital signs, including orthostatic changes, hemodynamics, and peripheral pulses.	Increased respiratory rate, increased heart rate, decreased blood pressure and/or orthostatic changes, low CVP, PCWP, and MAP, and weak peripheral pulses indicate persistent hypovolemia. Normalization of these measurements will reflect adequate fluid volume replacement.
Monitor fluid balance: daily weight, intake, and output.	Daily weights and intake and output provide a means to trend and evaluate fluid balance.
Monitor renal function: hourly urine output, BUN, and creatinine. Notify the physician if urine output is less than 30 mL/hr.	In the absence of hepatorenal failure, a urine output below 30 mL/hr and a rising BUN and creatinine reflect inadequate renal perfusion due to inadequate fluid volume replacement.
Monitor complete blood count and coagulation functions.	Hepatic failure can produce abnormal coagulation function, resulting in occult and/or frank bleeding.
Administer intravenous fluid/blood products as prescribed until signs and symptoms of hypovolemia and blood loss stabilize. Monitor for signs and symptoms of cardiovascular overload with fluid replacement.	Colloids and cystalloids are used to replace blood loss if the volume is less than 800 mL and the hematocrit is greater than 25%. Packed red blood cells are usually given with moderate to severe blood loss (>800 mL). Monitoring should be done, especially in the presence of cardiac disease, to prevent fluid overload.
Avoid abrupt changes in position (to upright) until fluid balance is restored.	During hypovolemia, orthostatic changes can produce dizziness and syncope.

Nursing Interventions	Rationales
Administer vasopression as prescribed. Monitor for complications: hypertension, dysrhythmias, fluid retention, and hyponatremia.	Vasopression acts directly on the gastrointestinal smooth muscle and its ability to contract. It is used to attempt to lower portal venous pressure by vasoconstriction. Hypertension and dysrhythmias may result from vasoconstriction of coronary and systemic arteries. By altering the permeability of the renal collecting ducts, vasopression allows reabsorption of water, producing fluid retention and dilutional electrolyte imbalances (hyponatremia). Total body sodium is usually increased with liver failure; thus interpretation of sodium must be done with caution.
Maintain balloon tamponade according to protocol. Monitor for complications: pharyngeal obstruction (asphyxia) and mucosal erosion (bleeding).	Bleeding esophageal varices may require special NG tubes with a balloon in the esophagus and/or stomach to apply direct pressure (tamponade) to bleeding vessels (e.g., Sengstaken-Blakemore tube). Excessive/prolonged balloon pressure can cause mucosal erosion and worse bleeding. Displacement of the tube can cause pharyngeal obstruction and respiratory distress.
Assist with sclerotherapy. Monitor for complications: oozing, increased temperature, and ARDS.	Sclerotherapy involves injection of a sclerosing agent such as sodium tetradeclysulfate into the varix or surrounding tissue of the bleeding vessel, causing thrombosis and sclerosis of the vein. Acute respiratory distress syndrome may result if sodium morrhuate is used, as this drug contains fatty acids which have been associated with pulmonary toxicity.

NURSING DIAGNOSIS: ALTERED NUTRITION—LESS THAN BODY REQUIREMENTS

Related To
- Decreased hepatic fat
- Decreased carbohydrate and protein metabolism
- Decreased storage of vitamins and minerals
- Decreased intake

Defining Characteristics
Decreased weight
Decreased appetite
Nausea and vomiting
Serum albumin < 3.5 g/dL
Serum transferrin < 200 mg/dL

Patient Outcomes
Nutritional balance is restored, as evidenced by
- albumin 3.5–5 g/dL
- serum transferrin 200–360 mg/dL
- sufficient protein intake for liver regeneration
- positive nitrogen balance
- increased appetite
- stabilized weight/weight gain
- absence of nausea and vomiting

Nursing Interventions	Rationales
Assess nutritional status. Consult dietitian for basal energy expenditure calculations and calorie requirements.	Critically ill patients require 1.5–3 times their normal calories because of the stress response.
Assess gastrointestinal motility. Assess tolerance to enteral feedings: Note bowel sounds, complaints of nausea/vomiting, abdominal discomfort, and presence of altered elimination patterns. Check gastric residuals every 4 hr.	The gastrointestinal tract should be used to provide nutrients if at all possible.

Nursing Interventions	Rationales
Monitor laboratory studies: serum albumin, total lymphocyte count, serum transferrin, total protein, and serum glucose.	Serum albumin and total lymphocyte count reflect the adequacy of nutrition. Serum transferrin, a circulating protein involved with iron transport, may be decreased by liver disease. Serum proteins may be low due to impaired hepatic metabolism or losses due to ascites. Glucose may be decreased because of impaired gluconeogenesis, decreased glycogen stores, or inadequate intake. Glucose may be increased with the high glucose content of parenteral feedings.
Limit protein intake if ammonia levels are elevated.	A high protein diet can increase levels of serum ammonia due to the liver's inability to convert ammonia to urea for excretion. Elevated ammonia and urea produce changes in neurological functioning.
Weigh daily. Monitor intake and output. Compare changes in fluid status.	Weight is not a direct indicator of nutritional status because of fluid alterations with liver failure. The tricep skin fold test may be more useful.
Administer vitamin supplements as prescribed.	In liver failure, the liver loses the ability to store vitamins. The patient may have a poor tolerance to fat which decreases absorption of fat-soluble vitamins.
See Appendix A.	

NURSING DIAGNOSIS: ALTERED THOUGHT PROCESSES

Related To
- Impaired handling of ammonia
- Aggressive diuretic therapy
- Diet
- Medications which require liver metabolism
- Decreased perfusion states

Defining Characteristics
Behavioral changes
Mental status changes: confusion, lethargy, amnesia
Delirium
Seizures
Coma

Patient Outcomes
The patient's thought processes will return to baseline, as evidenced by
- mental function return to baseline
- arterial ammonia 15–45 μg/dL

Nursing Interventions	Rationales
Assess for changes in mentation.	Changes in level of consciousness may indicate progression of liver dysfunction.
Monitor serum electrolytes, pH, ammonia, and BUN.	Hypokalemia and metabolic alkalosis increase production and absorption of ammonia. Accumulation of nitrogenous products (BUN) potentiates the development of encephalopathy.
Limit factors which may precipitate or exacerbate encephalopathy with impaired hepatocellular function, including constipation, infections, oral protein load, electrolyte imbalance, acid-base imbalance, diuretic therapy, diarrhea, vomiting, hypoglycemia, hypotension, hemorrhage into the gastrointestinal tract, dehydration, azotemia, sedative-hypnotic drugs, barbiturates, and benzodiazepines.	
Protect from injury during altered states of consciousness. Reorient patient to environment.	Confusion and aggressive behavior may develop.
Administer neomycin sulfate as prescribed and monitor effects.	Neomycin suppresses urea-splitting bacteria, decreasing ammonia degradation and ammonia production.

Nursing Interventions	Rationales
Administer lactulose as prescribed and monitor effects.	The laxative effect of lactulose promotes excretion of blood and protein from the gut, decreasing the production of ammonia.
Restrict hepatotoxic drugs.	In liver failure, drug metabolism is decreased and may result in toxic doses.
Limit protein by mouth.	Protein, if broken down in the intestine, produces ammonia.

NURSING DIAGNOSIS: INEFFECTIVE BREATHING PATTERN

Related To
- Impairment of lung expansion due to ascites
- Impaired level of consciousness
- Immune system depression

Defining Characteristics
Dyspnea
Tachypnea
Decreased respiratory depth
$PaCO_2$ > 45 torr
Decreasing PaO_2
Use of accessory muscles
Altered chest excursion

Patient Outcomes
A normal breathing pattern is restored, as evidenced by
- absence of dyspnea
- $PaCO_2$ return to baseline
- PaO_2 > 80 torr or return to baseline
- respiratory rate 12–20
- chest excursion and depth return to baseline
- absence of lung infection

Nursing Interventions	Rationales
Monitor respiratory status: respiratory rate, breath sounds, depth of respirations, and lung excursion.	Ineffective breathing patterns are best assessed through assessment of respiratory rate and depth. Adventitious breath sounds may be an early sign of lung consolidation. Rapid, shallow respirations may be present due to ascites and hypoxia.
Monitor ABGs for increasing $PaCO_2$ and decreasing PaO_2	Increased $PaCO_2$ is associated with ineffective breathing (hypoventilation). Hypoxia may also result.
Monitor temperature and WBC count and note changes in characteristics of sputum or associated symptoms.	An increased temperature, increased WBC count, and thickened and/or foul smelling sputum may indicate development of a respiratory infection. Other associated symptoms include adventitious breath sounds, decreased breath sounds, or increased respiratory rate.
Encourage patient to cough and deep breathe. Perform chest physiotherapy as needed.	These measures assist in lung expansion and clearing of secretions.
Administer medications (diuretics/salt poor albumin) as prescribed and monitor effects. Assist with paracentesis.	Ascites may limit movement of the diaphragm and cause ineffective, shallow breathing. Medications and/or paracentesis may be used to decrease ascites.
Keep head of bed elevated. Reposition from side to side.	Head of bed elevation reduces pressure on the diaphragm, allowing for free movement.
Administer oxygen or ventilatory support as prescribed and monitor patient response.	An ineffective breathing pattern may require assistance with a ventilator or oxygen therapy to maintain respirations and oxygenation.

NURSING DIAGNOSIS: HIGH RISK FOR IMPAIRED SKIN INTEGRITY

Risk Factors
- Altered nutritional state
- Impaired liver metabolism of toxins and/or medications
- Altered circulation
- Edema
- Bile salt accumulation
- Decreased level of consciousness

Patient Outcomes
Skin integrity is maintained/restored, as evidenced by
- Intact skin surface
- Intact mucous membranes

Nursing Interventions	Rationales
Assess oral mucosa. Provide frequent mouth care.	
Provide preventive skin care: 1. Change position regularly. 2. Keep skin clean and dry. 3. Inspect skin for erythema/bleeding with position change. 4. Gently massage vulnerable areas with position change. 5. Utilize special mattress/bed in patients with limited mobility or bedrest restrictions. 6. Encourage range-of-motion exercises.	Preventive measures/ongoing intervention prevents skin breakdown.
Administer antipyretics as ordered. Use nondrying soap for bathing and apply lotion to dry skin area.	Dry skin and pruritus caused by hepatic failure can result in scratching and potential skin breakdown.

DISCHARGE PLANNING/CONTINUITY OF CARE

- Assess need for/type of long-term care and follow-up.
- If the discharge destination is home, assess existing supports and the need for assistance.
- Determine coping deficits/support needs and institute assistance measures.
- Determine knowledge deficits/teaching needs and document and institute a teaching plan.
- Refer patient to social services as appropriate.
- Communicate coping deficits/support needs and knowledge deficits/teaching needs to unit accepting patient on transfer.

REFERENCES

Bosche, J., Pizcueta, P., Feu, F., Fernández, M., & García-Pagán, J. C. (1992). Pathophysiology of portal hypertension. *Gastroenterology Clinics of North America, 21*(1), 1–14.

Burns, S. M. (1990). VP/NTG therapy in the patient with variceal bleeding. *Critical Care Nurse, 10*(9), 42–49.

Gammal, S. H. & Jones, A. (1989). Hepatic encephalopathy. *Medical Clinics of North America, 73*(4), 793–813.

Katelaris, P. H. & Jones, D. B. (1989). Fulminant hepatic failure. *Medical Clinics of North America, 10*(9), 955–970.

Matloff, D. S. (1992). Treatment of acute variceal bleeding. *Gastroenterology Clinics of North America, 21*(1), 103–118.

Pierce, J. D., Wilkerson, E., & Griffiths, S. A. (1990). Acute esophageal bleeding and endoscopic injection sclerotherapy. *Critical Care Nurse, 10*(9), 67–72.

▼

Hematological Care

▼

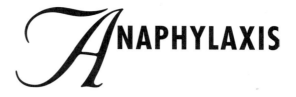

ANAPHYLAXIS

Anaphylaxis is a dramatic hypersensitivity reaction. It is a form of distributive shock where profound arterial vasodilation may result in cardiovascular collapse. This is a cell-mediated immunological response. Reactions are allergic, mediated via mast cell-bound, allergen-specific immunoglobulin E (IgE) antibodies. Cutaneomucous, cardiovascular, and bronchial signs, either isolated or associated, are the dominant clinical features. The initial treatment for this potentially life-threatening problem is to administer drug therapy to decrease the formation of mediators, decrease the release of mediators, or alter the effect of mediators.

ETIOLOGIES

- Food allergy
- Drug reaction
  - beta-lactam antibiotics
  - sulfonamides
  - sulfa diuretics
  - dilantin
  - aspirin
  - anesthetics
- Volume substitutes
- Insects
- Exercise induced
- Latex
- Chemotherapeutic agents
- Vaccines
- Contrast media
- Allergenic extract

CLINICAL MANIFESTATIONS

- The IgE-mediated response with release of proteases from the mast cell produces
  - fatigue
  - urticarial reaction: swelling, itching, burning
  - erhythematous eruption
- Vascular damage and changes in vascular permeability produce
  - swelling of eyelids, lips, tongue
  - hoarseness
  - wheezing
  - cough
  - tachypnea
  - syncope
  - palpitations
  - stridor
  - tachycardia
  - cold extremities
  - difficulty/noisy inspiration
  - tightness in chest
  - dyspnea
  - rhonchi
  - chest pain
  - cyanosis
  - hypotension
  - nausea
  - pelvic pain

CLINICAL/DIAGNOSTIC FINDINGS

There are no specific clinical/diagnostic findings used to diagnose anaphylaxis. Diagnosis is based on the clinical findings.

NURSING DIAGNOSIS: INEFFECTIVE BREATHING PATTERN

Related To
- Bronchospasm
- Edema of the tongue, larynx

Defining Characteristics
Noisy, difficult inspiration
Hoarseness
Tachypnea
Wheezing
Dyspnea
Cyanosis
Tightness in chest
Increased $PaCO_2$ with decreasing pH
Use of accessory muscles of ventilation

Patient Outcomes
Breathing pattern is restored/returned to baseline, as evidenced by
- respiratory rate 12–20 at rest
- $PaCO_2$ return to baseline
- pH 7.35–7.45

- absence of stridor
- absence of adventitious breath sounds

Nursing Interventions	Rationales
Assess level of consciousness.	Level of consciousness may decrease as the adequacy of alveolar ventilation decreases.
Assess breathing pattern.	A baseline assessment assists in guiding further intervention.
Pass oropharyngeal airway.	An airway may be needed to relieve upper airway obstruction.
Consider endotracheal intubation and mechanical ventilation.	Assisted ventilation will improve the ventilatory pattern returning pH and $PaCO_2$ to within normal limits.
Administer subcutaneous, intramuscular, or intravenous epinephrine as prescribed and monitor effects.	The alpha-adrenergic properties of epinephrine produce bronchodilation and increase inotropic and chronotropic cardiac activity.
Administer parenteral H_1 antihistamines as prescribed and monitor effects.	The H_1 antihistamines supplement the effect of epinephrine and help to reduce itching associated with urticaria.
Administer parenteral corticosteroids as prescribed and monitor effects.	Corticosteroids may help reverse shock or bronchospasm and correct urticaria or angioedema.
Administer oxygen as prescribed and monitor patient response (pulse oximetry).	Supplementary oxygen may be needed to improve oxygenation and prevent bronchoconstriction.
Position patient with head of bed elevated.	Elevating the head of the bed facilitates diaphragmatic descent for best use of ventilatory muscles.
Administer intravenous aminophylline as prescribed and monitor drug levels and effects.	Aminophylline is used for bronchodilation.
Administer nebulized bronchodilators as prescribed and monitor effects.	Nebulized bronchodilators are used as an adjunct therapy for bronchospasm.
Administer atropine sulfate as prescribed and monitor effects.	Atropine is used to treat refractory bradycardia associated with acute anaphylactic reactions.

NURSING DIAGNOSIS: DECREASED CARDIAC OUTPUT

Related To
- Release of histamine
- Secretion of endogenous catecholamines

Defining Characteristics

SVR < 800 dyn/s/cm^{-5}
Tachycardia
CI < 2.5 L/min/m^2
PCWP < 8 mmHg
Cardiovascular collapse

Hypotension
CO < 4 L/min
Urine output < 30 mL/hr
Dysrhythmias

Patient Outcomes
Cardiac output will be maintained/restored, as evidenced by
- MAP 60–90 mmHg
- heart rate 60–100 bpm
- PCWP 8–12 mmHg
- SVR 800–1200 dyn/s/cm^5
- urine output > 30 mL/hr
- absence of dysrhythmias
- absence of cardiovascular collapse

Nursing Interventions	Rationales
Assess and document cardiovascular status: blood pressure and heart rate, hemodynamics (MAP, PCWP, CO/CI), peripheral pulses, and cardiac rhythm. Assess signs of cardiovascular collapse (bradycardia, hypotension, decreased CO/CI, decreased MAP, weak peripheral pulses).	Arterial hypotension is caused by the direct effect of the peripheral vasodilation of histamine. Tachycardia results secondarily from the release of histamine as well as secretion of catecholamines.
Establish large venous access.	
Administer volume expanders as prescribed until MAP > 60 mmHg; PCWP 8–12 mmHg.	Anaphylaxis is a form of distributive shock. Fluids maintain preload with the associated vasodilation.

Nursing Interventions	Rationales
Administer epinephrine as prescribed and monitor effects.	The alpha effects of this drug correct arterial and venous vasodilation, restore systemic arterial pressure, and reduce capillary permeability. The beta effects increase cardiac contractility.
Administer glucagon as prescribed if unresponsive to epinephrine and monitor effects.	Patients with anaphylaxis who are receiving concurrent therapy with beta-blocking agents may be refractory to the usual doses of epinephrine. Glucagon increases intracellular cyclic adenosine monophosphate (AMP).
Elevate patient's legs.	Elevation of the legs increases venous return and therefore cardiac output.
Administer positive inotropic drugs as prescribed and monitor effects.	Inotropic drugs may be needed to increase myocardial contractility and cardiac output.

DISCHARGE PLANNING/CONTINUITY OF CARE

- Assess need for/type of long-term care and follow-up.
- If the discharge destination is home, assess existing supports and the need for assistance.
- Determine coping deficits/support needs and institute assistance measures.
- Determine knowledge deficits/teaching needs and document and institute a teaching plan.
- Refer patient to social services as appropriate.
- Communicate coping deficits/support needs and knowledge deficits/learning needs to unit accepting the patient on transfer.

REFERENCES

Banov, C. H. (1991). Current review of anaphylaxis and its relationship to asthma. *Allergie et Immunologie, 23*(10), 417–420.

Eon, B., Papazian, L., & Gouin, R. (1991). Management of anaphylactic and anaphylactoid reactions during anesthesia. *Clinical Reviews in Allergy, 9,* 415–429.

Leach, S. R. (1991). Cardiovascular collapse following infusion of 5% albumin. *Journal of the American Association of Nurse Anesthetists, 59*(6), 592–594.

Nocils, A. W. (1992). Exercise-induced anaphylaxis and urticaria. *Clinics in Sports Medicine, 11*(2), 303–312.
Sussman, G. L. & Dolovick, J. (1989). Prevention of anaphylaxis. *Seminars in Dermatology, 8*(3), 158–165.
Wiggins, C. A., Dykewicz, M. S., & Patterson, R. (1989). Idiopathic anaphylaxis: A review. *Annals Allergy, 62,* 1–5.
Yunginger, J. W. (1992). Anaphylaxis. *Current Problems in Pediatrics, 22*(5), 130–146.

▼

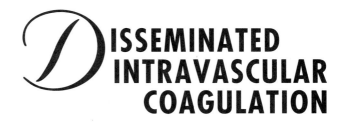ISSEMINATED INTRAVASCULAR COAGULATION

Disseminated intravascular coagulation (DIC) is a syndrome where hemorrhage and thrombosis occur simultaneously. This is a result of an overstimulation of normal coagulation/fibrinolysis processes. As a syndrome, DIC is triggered by another pathology. After the coagulation system has been activated, thrombin and plasmin circulate systemically, promoting both coagulation and fibrinolysis. Fibrin (clots) in the microcirculation lead to microvascular and macrovascular thrombosis. The clinical manifestations of DIC depend on the intensity and duration of the activation of blood coagulation, the rate of thrombi formation and dissolution, the rate of blood flow, and the function and status of the liver, bone marrow, and macrophage system.

ETIOLOGIES

- Obstetrical accidents
    - amniotic fluid embolism
    - eclampsia
    - abortion
    - retained fetus syndrome
- Septicemia
    - gram negative
    - gram positive
- Malignancy
- Burns
- Viremias
- Crush injuries
- Liver disease
    - obstructive jaundice
    - acute heptic failure
- Intravascular hemolysis
    - hemolytic transfusion reactions
    - massive transfusions

- Prosthetic devices
  - intra-aortic balloon
- Surgical procedures (postoperative damage)
- Heat stroke
- Snake bites
- Fat and other pulmonary emboli

CLINICAL MANIFESTATIONS

- Activation of thrombin produces
  - fever
  - hypoxemia
  - acidosis
- Bleeding and shift of fluid from the vascular to the interstitial space produce
  - hypotension
  - bleeding from invasive sites
  - hematomas
  - petechiae
  - invasive line oozing
  - subcutaneous hematomas
  - tachycardia
  - ecchymosis
  - decreased urine output
  - gangrene
  - surgical wound bleeding
- Thrombi deposition in the microcirculation produces
  - acral cyanosis (purple discoloration of the feet, hands, nose, and cheeks)
  - cold extremities
  - tachypnea
  - chest pain
  - dyspnea
  - hemoptysis

CLINICAL/DIAGNOSTIC FINDINGS

- D-dimer > 0.5 mg/L
- Platelet count < 50,000/mm^3
- Fibrin split products > 10 µg/mL
- Antithrombin III < 70% activity
- PT > 13 s
- PTT > 45 s
- Thrombin time > 15 s
- Fibrinogen level < 200 mg/dL
- Protamine sulfate strongly positive

NURSING DIAGNOSIS: ALTERED TISSUE PERFUSION—CENTRAL AND PERIPHERAL

Related To
- Decreased circulating volume

- Small- and large-vessel thrombosis
- Impaired blood flow to organs

Defining Characteristics

Confusion
CI < 2.5 L/min/m^2
Weak, thready peripheral pulses
Cool, clammy skin
PCWP < 8 mmHg

CO < 4 L/min
Hypotension
Tachycardia
CVP < 2 mmHg
Urine output < 30 mL/hr

Patient Outcomes

Central and peripheral tissue perfusion will be restored, as evidenced by
- blood pressure return to baseline
- MAP > 60 mmHg
- CO 4–8 L/min; CI 2.5–4 L/min/m^2
- CVP 2–10 mmHg; PCWP 8–12 mmHg
- peripheral pulses that are palpable to patient baseline
- sensorium that returns to patient baseline
- warm, dry skin
- urine output > 30 mL/hr

Nursing Interventions	Rationales
Assess for signs of neurovascular occlusion: hemiplegia, syncope, CVA-like symptoms, paresthesia, and confusion. Assess for signs of renal occlusion: progressive oliguria, hematuria, and renal failure. Assess for signs of mesenteric occlusion: abdominal pain, decreased bowel sounds, and abdominal distension. Assess for signs of pulmonary occlusion: shortness of breath, chest pain, and hemoptysis.	Microvascular thromboses of the brain, kidneys, GI tract, and lungs may occur as the result of DIC.
Monitor heart rate, respiratory rate, and blood pressure.	Heart rate and respiratory rate will be elevated as long as tissue perfusion is low. Blood pressure will be low until low volume is corrected by administration of intravenous fluids.

Nursing Interventions	Rationales
Monitor and record CO/CI.	Cardiac output is a major determinant of tissue perfusion. A low CO/CI indicates volume replacement is not yet adequate.
Monitor peripheral circulation: Inspect skin, noting color and temperature; check quality of peripheral pulses and capillary refill time (CRT).	Cool, clammy, pale skin, weak peripheral pulses, or increased CRT indicate decreased circulating volume and peripheral perfusion.
Collaboratively treat underlying clinical disorder.	The most important component of treatment is to control or reverse the process that initiated DIC.
Replace fluids with crystalloids as prescribed and monitor effects.	Fluids may be needed to correct hypovolemia.
Note hourly changes in urine output.	Urine output reflects kidney perfusion. A low urine output indicates inadequate volume.
Provide preventive skin care: 1. Regularly change position. 2. Keep skin clean and dry. 3. Inspect skin for erythema/blanching with each position change. 4. Utilize specialized mattress or bed in patients on bedrest and/or with decreased spontaneous movement.	Decreased tissue perfusion puts the patient at risk for skin breakdown. The frequency of position changes, skin care, and skin inspection should be increased if any reddened areas do not resolve within 1 hr.

NURSING DIAGNOSIS: HIGH RISK FOR INJURY

Risk Factors
- Thrombin activation
- Hemorrhage

Patient Outcomes
The patient will be free of injury related to hemorrhage, as evidenced by
- blood pressure return to baseline
- heart rate 60–100 bpm
- hemoglobin 13–18 g/dL

- hematocrit 35–47% in women; 42–52% in men
- no clinical signs of altered hemostasis

Nursing Interventions	Rationales
Assess for oral, nasal, scleral, rectal, or vaginal bleeding.	
Assess neurological status.	Intracerebral bleeding may occur and must be detected early.
Assess for hemoptysis, tachypnea, dyspnea, or orthopnea.	Thrombi and/or bleeding may occur in the pulmonary system.
Assess for bone and joint pain.	Bleeding may occur into joint spaces.
Assess hydration status: skin turgor, intake and output, daily weight, and mucous membranes.	
Monitor vital signs.	Blood pressure (decreased) and pulse (increased) are the most accurate indicators of the amount of bleeding.
Monitor laboratory values associated with hemostasis: hematocrit, platelets, fibrinogen levels, PT, and PTT.	
Monitor for clinical signs of altered hemostasis: petechiae, purpura, acral cyanosis, gangrene, surgical wound bleeding, bleeding from invasive lines, and subcutaneous hematomas.	These signs are suggestive of DIC.
Hematest urine, guaiac stool, and emesis.	Bleeding may occur in the kidneys or gastrointestinal tract.
Measure abdominal girth.	Abdominal girth increases with intra-abdominal bleeding.
Transfuse with blood component therapy as prescribed and monitor effects: packed red blood cells, whole blood, platelets, fresh frozen plasma, antithrombin concentrate, prothrombin complex, and cryoprecipitate.	Packed red blood cells and whole blood are used to replace blood loss and elevate hematocrit and protein levels. Platelets are used to restore the platelet count for hemostasis. Fresh frozen plasma is used to replace clotting factors. Antithrombin concentrate is used to stop the intravascular clotting process.

Nursing Interventions

Nursing Interventions	Rationales
Titrate heparin infusion as prescribed to maintain PTT at 1.5 times the control and monitor effects.	Heparin may inactivate thrombin or prevent the activation of thrombin and stop the intravascular clotting process.
Administer aminocaproic acid (Amicar) as prescribed and monitor patient response.	Aminocaproic acid inhibits fibrinolysis and therefore prevents the dissolution of clots (and bleeding).

NURSING DIAGNOSIS: HIGH RISK FOR IMPAIRED TISSUE INTEGRITY

Risk Factors
- Small- and large-vessel thrombosis
- Impaired blood flow
- Ischemia

Patient Outcomes
The patient's skin integrity will be restored/maintained.

Nursing Interventions	Rationales
Apply gentle, consistent pressure to bleeding sites.	
Provide for safety: Pad siderails and remove sharp objects from environment.	
Maintain central intravenous access.	
Limit injections and invasive procedures.	
Avoid rectal temperatures and tubes.	
Maintain clean, dry dressings.	
Provide for oral hygiene.	

NURSING DIAGNOSIS: HIGH RISK FOR DECREASED CARDIAC OUTPUT

Risk Factors
- Decreased preload
- Increased afterload

Patient Outcomes
Cardiac output will be maintained/restored, as evidenced by
- blood pressure at patient baseline
- CO 4–8 L/min; CI 2.5–4 L/min/m^2
- urine output > 30 mL/hr
- heart rate 60–100 bpm

Nursing Interventions	Rationales
Assess and document cardiovascular status: heart rate, respiratory rate, blood pressure, hemodynamics (CVP/PCWP, CO/CI, MAP), peripheral pulses, and signs of cardiovascular collapse (bradycardia, hypotension, decreased CO/CI, decreased MAP, weak peripheral pulses).	Decreased preload associated with hemorrhage causes decreased venous return to the heart and decreased CO. Increased afterload also decreases CO but does so by increasing the resistance against which the heart must work.
Identify causes of any dysrhythmias and treat according to protocol. Assess effect on cardiac output.	Dysrhythmias may further decrease CO.
Administer vasoactive drugs as prescribed and monitor patient response.	Postive inotropic agents may be needed to support CO.
Reduce myocardial oxygen consumption by providing a calm environment, administering sedatives and comfort measures.	
Administer fluids as prescribed to maintain MAP > 60 mmHg.	Maintaining MAP will optimize preload.

NURSING DIAGNOSIS: HIGH RISK FOR IMPAIRED GAS EXCHANGE

Risk Factors
- Decreased circulating hemoglobin
- Intrapulmonary shunting
- Failure of diffusion across alveolar-capillary membrane

Patient Outcomes
Gas exchange will be maintained/restored, as evidenced by
- PaO_2 within patient baseline
- $SaO_2 > 90\%$
- ABGs within normal limits
- normal hemoglobin (13–18 g/dL)

Nursing Interventions	Rationales
Monitor hemoglobin, PaO_2, and SaO_2	Hemoglobin is the major oxygen-carrying compound. The PaO_2 reflects how much of the oxygen is in the plasma. The saturation of hemoglobin is reflected by SaO_2. Oxygen transport is compromised with oxygen saturation below 90%.
Monitor arterial pH and blood lactate levels.	Arterial pH and blood lactate reflect overall acid-base balance.
Administer oxygen and make changes according to blood gas analysis or pulse oximeter changes.	Supplementary oxygen may be necessary to provide adequate gas exchange.
Consider application of continuous positive airway pressure (CPAP) or mechanical ventilation with positive end-expiratory pressure (PEEP).	The CPAP and PEEP cause alveolar hyperinflation, increasing surface area available for gas exchange.
Tracheal suction with red rubber catheters prn.	Endotracheal suctioning removes secretions and debris from the tracheobronchial tree and promotes airway patency. Using a red rubber catheter will minimize soft-tissue damage and prevent bleeding.

Nursing Interventions	Rationales
Limit patient activities. Provide an environment conducive to rest. Provide for rest periods.	Activity and inadequate rest can increase oxygen consumption.

DISCHARGE PLANNING/CONTINUITY OF CARE

- Based on underlying pathology/etiology, assess need for/type of long-term care and follow-up.
- If the discharge destination is home, assess existing supports and the need for assistance.
- Determine coping deficits/support needs and institute assistance measures.
- Determine knowledge deficits/teaching needs and document and institute a teaching plan.
- Refer patient to social services as appropriate.
- Communicate coping deficits/support needs and knowledge deficits/learning needs to unit accepting the patient on transfer.

REFERENCES

Bailes, B. K. (1992). Disseminated intravascular coagulation. *Association of Operating Room Nurses Journal, 55*(2), 517–528.

Bell, T. N. (1990). Disseminated intravascular coagulation in shock. *Critical Care Nursing Clinics of North America, 2*(2), 255–267.

Bick, R. L. & Kunkel, L. A. (1992). Disseminated intravascular coagulation syndromes. *International Journal of Hematology, 55,* 1–26.

Esparaz, B. & Green, D. (1990). Disseminated intravascular coagulation. *Critical Care Nursing Quarterly, 13*(2), 7–13.

Gibney, E. J. & Hayes, D. B. (1990). Coagulopathy and abdominal aortic aneurysm. *European Journal of Vascular Surgery, 4,* 557–562.

Meriney, D. K. (1990). Diagnosis and management of acute promyelocytic leukemia with disseminated intravascular coagulopathy: A case study. *Oncology Nursing Form, 17*(3), 379–383.

Suchak, B. A. & Corazon, B. B. (1989). Disseminated intravascular coagulation: A nursing challenge. *Orthopaedic Nursing, 8*(6), 61–69.

Turner, G. (1991). Disseminating intravascular coagulation (DIC): Nursing interventions. *Advancing Clinical Care, March/April,* 19–23.

HUMAN IMMUNODEFICIENCY VIRUS

Human immunodeficiency virus (HIV) is a cytopathic virus that can lead to impairment and lysis of cells of the immune system, in particular T_4 lymphocytes. Infected cells cannot proliferate, function, or communicate effectively, disrupting the body's normal immunological defense mechanisms. This dysfunction permits HIV to spread unrestrained, directly infecting cells throughout the body while its effects on the immune system permit opportunistic infections and tumors to occur. The result is acquired immunodeficiency syndrome (AIDS) or AIDS-related complex.

Human immunodeficiency virus is contracted via blood transmission, sexual contact, and perinatally. Clinical signs of infection may not appear for 5–7 years after exposure, but the ultimate mortality rate for AIDS is 100%. Clinical manifestations are the result of opportunistic infections, tumors, and/or direct infection of cells. Particularly devastating and potentially lethal to these patients are changes in the neurological, cardiovascular, pulmonary, renal, and gastrointestinal systems.

ETIOLOGIES

- Pulmonary changes
    - pneumocystis carnii pneumonia
    - cytomegalovirus pneumonia
    - bacterial pneumonia
    - nonspecific interstitial pneumonitis
    - tuberculosis
    - *Mycobacterium avium-intracellulare*
    - Kaposi's sarcoma
- Cardiovascular changes
    - bacterial endocarditis
    - nonbacterial thrombotic endocarditis
    - Kaposi's sarcoma of myocardium
    - tuberculosis pericarditis

- fungal pericarditis
- myocarditis
- Neurological changes
  - HIV encephalopathy
  - opportunistic infections: *Toxoplasma gondii*, *Cryptococcus neoformans*, progressive multifocal leukoencephalopathy (human papovavirus)
  - malignancy: lymphomas
  - HIV peripheral neuropathy
- Gastrointestinal changes
  - toxic megacolon
  - biliary tract disease
  - pancreatitis
  - obstruction/perforation of GI tract
  - Kaposi's sarcoma
  - infectious agents: *Cryptosporidium*, *Mycobacterium*, *Isospora*, cytomegalovirus, *Giardia*, *Salmonella*, herpes
  - AIDs enteropathy
- Renal changes
  - hemodynamic instability
  - nephrotoxic agents
  - AIDS-related glomerulopathy

CLINICAL MANIFESTATIONS

- Neurological: Demyelinization, neurotoxins, inflammation, cortical atrophy, vacuolar myelopathy, infection, and/or malignancy can produce
  - memory loss
  - disorientation
  - clumsiness
  - vision changes
  - coma
  - gait disturbances
  - hallucinations
  - confusion
  - psychotic behavior
  - spastic paraparesis
  - peripheral paresthesia
  - headache
  - aphasia
  - seizures
- Renal: Dehydration, hypovolemia, decreased glomerular filtration, tubular necrosis, altered renal circulation, and/or glomerulosclerosis can produce
  - oliguria
  - azotemia
- Cardiovascular: Accumulation of HIV proteins in cardiac tissue, myocyte necrosis, and release of lymphokines that depress cardiac function can produce
  - congestive heart failure
  - dysrhythmias
  - hypotension
- Gastrointestinal: Infectious agents, malignant lesions, enteropathy, and/or villous atrophy can produce

- diarrhea
- abdominal pain
- cachexia
- weight loss
- signs of dehydration
- upper GI bleed
- dysphasia
- steatorrhea
- nausea and vomiting
- Pulmonary: Infectious agents, malignant lesions, and interstitial disorders produce
  - dyspnea
  - adventitious lung sounds
  - tachypnea
  - decreased pulse oximetry
  - cough
  - decreased lung sounds
  - decreased PaO_2

CLINICAL/DIAGNOSTIC FINDINGS

- CSF fluid: mild mononuclear pleocytosis, increased protein, elevated $beta_2$–microglobulin, neopterin, and quinolinic acid
- CT scan: cerebral atrophy, lesions
- Lymphocyte count < $1000/mm^3$
- CD4 cell count < $200/mm^3$
- Erythrocyte sedimentation rate > 15–25 mm/hr
- LDH > 155 units (pneumocystis carinii pneumonia)
- Chest x-ray: infiltrates, pleural effusion, cavitation, cardiac effusions, dilated heart chambers
- Positive sputum gram stain/culture
- Positive stool cultures
- Serum albumin < 3.5 g/dL, transferrin < 250 mg/dL
- Vitamin B_{12} < 100 pg/mL; folic acid < 5.9 µg/mL
- Proteinuria, hematuria, leukocyturia
- BUN > 20 mg/dL; and creatinine > 1.2 mg/dL
- Electrolyte and acid/base disturbances
- Positive HIV

NURSING DIAGNOSIS: IMPAIRED GAS EXCHANGE

Related To
- Weakness
- Pneumonia

Defining Characteristics
Dyspnea
PaO_2 < 80 torr
Fever/chills
Tachypnea
SaO_2 < 90%
Adventitious lung sounds
Cough

Patient Outcomes
Adequate gas exchange will be maintained/restored, as evidenced by
- absence of dyspnea/tachypnea
- $SaO_2 > 90\%$
- clear lung sounds
- $PaO_2 > 80$ torr
- absence of cough

Nursing Interventions	Rationales
Assess and record respiratory function: rate, rhythm, and depth of respiration. Auscultate breath sounds. Assess ability to handle oral and pulmonary secretions. Assess for signs of respiratory distress: use of accessory muscles, tachypnea, and anxiety. Obtain ABGs, pulse oximetry as ordered and prn changes in respiratory function. Assess effects of activity on respiratory function.	Respiratory function may be altered by AIDS-related pneumonias, pneumonitis, tuberculosis, or Kaposi's sarcoma.
Support airway as appropriate: oral/nasal airway, supplementary oxygen, suctioning, intubation, and mechanical ventilation. Position patient for ease of respiratory effort, that is, head of bed (HOB) elevated. Reposition patient regularly.	
Monitor fluid balance closely	Too little fluid can interfere with mobilization of secretions

Nursing Interventions

Administer pentamidine as prescribed and monitor for side effects: hypotension, azotemia, dysrhythmias, pancreatitis, hypoglycemia, nausea, and vomiting.
Administer trimethoprim-sulfamethoxazole (TMP-SMX) as prescribed and monitor for side effects: rash, fever, leukopenia, thrombocytopenia, hyponatremia, and abnormal liver function tests.
Administer diaminodiphenylsulfone (Dapsone) as prescribed and monitor for side effects: nausea, vomiting, allergic dermatitis, hemolytic anemia, and peripheral neuropathy.
Administer clindamycin and primaquine as prescribed and monitor for side effects: skin rash.
Administer trimetrexate as prescribed and monitor for side effects: granulocytopenia, thrombocytopenia, and rash.

Rationales

The primary therapy for pneumocystis carinii pneumonia is pentamidine or TMP-SMX (Septra or Bactrim), but other drugs may also be used.

NURSING DIAGNOSIS: DECREASED CARDIAC OUTPUT

Related To
- Myocardial damage
- Pericardial effusions
- Congestive cardiomyopathy

Defining Characteristics
CVP > 10 mmHg
CO < 4 L/min
Hypotension
Dysrhythmias
Signs of congestive heart failure

PCWP > 12 mmHg
CI < 2.5 L/min/m^2
Tachycardia

Patient Outcomes
Cardiac output will be maintained/restored as evidenced by
- CO 4–8 L/min; CI 2.5–4 L/min/m^2
- CVP 2–10 mmHg; PCWP 8–12 mmHg
- blood pressure within 10 mmHg of patient baseline
- absence of signs of heart failure
- absence of dysrhythmias

Nursing Interventions	Rationales
Monitor/document hemodynamic status: blood pressure, heart rate, respiratory rate, hemodynamics (CO, CI), and signs of congestive heart failure (peripheral edema, neck vein distention, shortness of breath, adventitious lung sounds).	Human immunodeficiency virus can directly depress/alter cardiac function via accumulation of HIV proteins in cardiac tissue, myocyte necrosis, and release of lymphokines.
Monitor/document fluid balance: intake and output and daily weight	Hypovolemia or hypervolemia can further compromise cardiac function.
Institute treatment to control dysrhythmias according to protocols.	
Administer medications as prescribed for stabilization of blood pressure.	Hypotension may occur due to autonomic neuropathy. Fludrocortisone may be used.

NURSING DIAGNOSIS: HIGH RISK FOR INFECTION

Risk Factors
- Immunosuppression
- Debilitated state

Patient Outcomes
The patient will not contract further infections while hospitalized.

140 Hematological Care

Nursing Interventions	Rationales
Assess for/minimize potential sites of infection: intravenous access, Foley catheter, and oral cavity. Monitor temperature, white blood cell (WBC) count and WBC differential. Maintain protective precautions.	
Administer antibiotics as prescribed and monitor effects/complications. Provide intravenous site care every 24 hr. Change intravenous site every 72 hr.	
Provide frequent oral care.	The AIDS patient is particularly prone to gingivitis and *Candida* infections.

NURSING DIAGNOSIS: ALTERED SENSORY PERCEPTION
Related To neurological involvement

Defining Characteristics
Confusion
Psychomotor slowing
Spasticity
Ataxia
Visual loss
Slowed verbal response
Weakness: arms > legs
Hyperreflexia
Seizures
Headache

Patient Outcomes
Sensory-perceptual alterations will be minimized during hospitalization.

Nursing Interventions	Rationales
Assess/monitor/record neurological deficits: level of consciousness, orientation/memory, clarity of speech, muscle strength/movement, and vision loss.	Human immunodeficiency virus can produce neurological deficits via demyelinization, neurotoxins, inflammation, cortical atrophy, vacuolar myelopathy infection, or malignancy.
Assess need for medications for anxiety or psychosis. Administer as prescribed and monitor/record patient response.	Benzodiazepines may be prescribed for anxiety. Haloperidol or chlorpromazine may be used for acute psychosis.

Nursing Interventions	Rationales
Provide orientation with each contact. Provide orienting clues in room, that is, clocks and calendars. Protect from injury: siderails up; bed in low position; leave night light on; and needed items placed within easy reach. Offer meaningful stimulation (radio, TV). Keep verbal instructions simple and concrete; give only one instruction at a time. Provide continuity of caregivers as much as possible. Allow verbalization of frustrations/concerns and provide support and encouragment.	
Provide adequate rest periods.	
Administer medications for headache as prescribed and monitor response.	Low-dose amitriptyline is used to manage headaches. Headaches are believed to be related to disturbed serotonin metabolism caused by systemic/local production of cytokines.
Administer medications for dementia and monitor response.	Zidovudine may improve AIDS dementia.

NURSING DIAGNOSIS: IMPAIRED SKIN INTEGRITY

Related To
- Bacterial/fungal infections
- Kaposi's sarcoma
- Decreased level of activity

Defining Characteristics
Pruritis
Lesions
Impetigo

Dryness
Skin breakdown
Dermatitis

Nursing Interventions | Rationales

Nursing Interventions	Rationales
Inspect skin regularly, documenting changes: appearance, location, and size of lesions, signs of infection/skin breakdown, pain, and location/amount of edema.	The AIDS patient is prone to skin breakdown due to Kaposi's sarcoma, infections (candidiasis, varicella zoster, herpes simplex virus) and drug reactions.
Apply nonperfumed, alcohol-free skin moisturizers.	Dry skin is frequently an ongoing problem.
Turn and reposition at least every 2 hr. Utilize specialized mattress or bed. Encourage ambulation as early as possible. Keep edematous extremities elevated.	
Provide meticulous oral care: mouth rinse, lip moisturizer, and oral irrigation and suction if unable to rinse on own. Administer oral antifungal/antiviral medications as prescribed.	
Avoid use of tape as much as possible.	Tape can cause breakdown of skin and/or pain
Keep skin clean and dry. Prevent/protect from friction or rubbing. Administer medications to prevent itching as prescribed and monitor response	

NURSING DIAGNOSIS: ALTERED NUTRITION—LESS THAN BODY REQUIREMENTS

Related To
- Villous atrophy of intestine
- Gingivitis
- Massive proteinuria
- Chronic diarrhea
- Esophagitis

Defining Characteristics
Weight loss   Diarrhea
Dysphagia   Sore mouth

Nausea and vomiting
Fatigue
Transferrin < 200 mg/dL
Vitamin B$_{12}$ < 100 pg/mL

Weakness
Albumin < 3.5 g/dL
Folic acid < 5.9 μg/mL

Nursing Interventions	Rationales
Monitor fluid balance.	Poor oral intake, nausea and vomiting, and diarrhea can cause hypovolemia.
Administer drugs to correct gingivitis/esophagitis as prescribed and record results: 1. gingivitis: Nystatin swish and swallow; clotrimazole (mycelex troches) 2. *Candida* esophagitis: above plus miconazole, ketoconazole, fluconazole 3. cytomegalovirus esophagitis: ganciclovir 4. herpes simplex virus esophagitis: acyclovir, foscarnet 5. amphotericin Provide high-protein, high-calorie diet. Schedule medications that may cause nausea away from meal times. Medicate for nausea and vomiting and monitor response. See Appendix A	

NURSING DIAGNOSIS: DIARRHEA

Related To
- Infectious agents
- Enteropathy
- Villous atrophy

Patient Outcomes
The patient will have normal bowel elimination as evidenced by absence of diarrhea.

Nursing Interventions	Rationales
Assess/monitor effects of diarrhea on fluid balance: intake and output and daily weights; measure stools if possible and include in intake and output.	
Monitor serum electrolytes and acid-base balance.	Diarrhea can cause hypokalemia and metabolic acidosis (loss of HCO_3).
Monitor for signs of dehydration: decreased blood pressure, orthostatic changes, tachycardia, decreased urine output, and decreased CVP/PCWP. Monitor/record frequency and consistency of bowel movements. Administer adequate fluids and electrolytes to replace losses. Provide low-residue, high-protein, high-calorie diet Administer antidiarrheal medications as prescribed and monitor/record response.	
Administer medications to combat infection as prescribed and monitor response.	Most cases of diarrhea are caused by opportunistic infection by parasites, bacteria, viruses, or fungi.

NURSING DIAGNOSIS: ACTIVITY INTOLERANCE

Related To
- Malnutrition
- Weight loss
- Fever

Defining Characteristics
Dyspnea on exertion
Clumsiness
Muscle weakness

Fatigue
Gait disturbance

Patient Outcomes
The patient will be able to tolerate the prescribed activity level.

Nursing Interventions	Rationales
Assess muscle strength and need for assistance with ADLs.	
Assess/monitor physical response to activity: blood pressure, heart rate and rhythm, and respiratory rate before, during, and after activity. Note tachycardia, dysrhythmias, dyspnea, pallor, diaphoresis, dizziness, or fatigue.	Blood pressure, heart rate, and respiratory rate should return to baseline within 4 min after activity.
Assess/monitor tolerance to visitors, limiting visits as necessary. Assist with activity as needed, increasing activity gradually. Allow for adequate rest/sleep periods: Minimize or group interruptions, assess normal sleep patterns/habits and try to accommodate them, and maintain a quiet, calm environment.	
Provide adequate nutrition.	Inadequate nutrition will contribute to muscle weakness and fatigue.

NURSING DIAGNOSIS: INEFFECTIVE INDIVIDUAL COPING

Related To
- Stigma attached to AIDS
- Anxiety/depression related to possible death

Patient Outcomes
The patient will utilize effective coping strategies.

Nursing Interventions	Rationales
Assess past and current coping mechanisms.	This provides data to enable assistance of patient in developing effective coping mechanisms.
Assess effect of diagnosis on social relationships/ support systems.	
Assess/record and carry out patient's wishes concerning life-sustaining treatment. Reassure they will not be abandoned.	Patients may feel that a decision not to resuscitate may mean they will no longer be cared for.

Nursing Interventions	Rationales
Assess need for/administer antidepressants as prescribed and monitor response.	
Allow patient to express feelings/frustrations. Spend time with patient.	This helps establish a trusting and supportive relationship between the patient and nurse.
Explain use of isolation precautions to patient.	Isolation precautions may increase anxiety and feelings of social isolation.
Encourage contact with significant others.	Significant others are an important source of support and encouragement.
Assist in development of effective coping strategies based on personal strengths and experiences. Refer to support groups/counseling/community resources as appropriate. Provide accurate medical information concerning treatment rationales, alternatives, benefits, and risks. Support the patient's capacity for hope and autonomy.	

DISCHARGE PLANNING/CONTINUITY OF CARE

- Assess need for/type of long-term care and follow-up.
- If the discharge destination is home, assess existing supports and the need for assistance.
- Determine coping deficits/support needs and institute assistance measures.
- Determine knowledge deficits/teaching needs and document and institute a teaching plan.
- Refer patient to social services as appropriate.
- Communicate coping deficits/support needs and knowledge deficits/learning needs to unit accepting the patient on transfer.

REFERENCES

Brew, B. J. (1992). Central and peripheral nervous system abnormalities. *Medical Clinics of North America, 76*(1), 63–81.

Cuff, P. A. (1990). Acquired immunodeficiency syndrome and malnutrition, Role of gastrointestinal pathology. *Nutrition in Clinical Practice, 5*(2), 43–53.

Gee, G., Wong, R., & Moran, R. (1989). Current treatment strategies for HIV infection. *Seminars in Oncology Nursing, 5*(4), 249–254.

Henry, S. B. & Holzemer, W. L. (1992). Critical care management of the patient with HIV infection who has *Pneumocystis carinii* pneumonia. *Heart & Lung, 21*(3), 243–249

Lovejoy, N. C. & Rumley, R. (1992). AIDS epidemiology and pathology, Implications for intensive care units. *Critical Care Nursing Clinics of North America, 4*(3), 383–394.

McMahon, K. M. & Coyne, N. (1989). Symptom management in patients with AIDS. *Seminars in Oncology Nursing, 5*(4), 289–301.

Nyamathi, A. & Servellen, G. (1989). Maladaptive coping in the critically ill population with acquired immunodeficiency syndrome, Nursing assessment and treatment. *Heart & Lung, 18*(2), 113–120.

Pearlstein, G. (1990). Renal system complications in HIV infection. *Critical Care Nursing Clinics of North America, 2*(1), 79–88.

Singer, P., Askanazi, J., Akiva, L., Bursztein, S., & Kvetan, V. (1990). Reassessing intensive care for patients with the acquired immunodeficiency syndrome. *Heart & Lung, 19*(4), 387–394.

Tanowitz, H. B., Simon, D., & Wittner, M. (1992). Gastrointestinal manifestations. *Medical Clinics of North America, 76*(1), 45–62.

Timby, B. K. (1992). Pneumocystosis in patients with acquired immunodeficiency syndrome. *Critical Care Nurse, 12*(7), 64–71

Tribett, D. (1989). *Pneumocystis carinii* pneumonia in the patient with acquired immune deficiency syndrome. In K. T. Von Rueden & C. A. Walleck (Eds.), *Advanced critical care nursing*, (pp. 309–324). Rockville, MD: Aspen.

White, D. A. & Zaman, M. K. (1992). Pulmonary disease. *Medical Clinics of North America, 76*(1), 19–44.

▼

Neurological Care

ACUTE SPINAL CORD INJURY

Trauma to the spinal cord can produce impairment of blood supply, laceration, contusion, or hemorrhage. Spinal cord injuries usually occur as the result of (1) flexion rotation, dislocation, or fracture dislocation; (2) hyperextension; or (3) compression of the spinal column. The result is varying degrees of temporary and/or permanent deficits. Factors which determine the degree of deficit include (1) level of injury (see Table 17.1), (2) type/mechanism of injury, (3) complete damage (permanent motor and sensory loss below the level of the lesion) or incomplete damage (varying motor and sensory loss) (see Table 17.2), and (4) upper motor neuron damage (muscle spasticity, increased tendon reflexes) or lower motor neuron damage (muscle flaccidity, loss of muscle tone, muscle atrophy and loss of reflexes).

Spinal shock may occur immediately (30–60 min) after the injury. This is a state of transient reflex depression resulting in complete loss of motor, sensory, reflex, and autonomic function below the level of injury. Recovery usually begins within 3 weeks and may take as long as 4 months. The return of reflexes indicates the end of spinal shock.

Autonomic dysreflexia is a syndrome that reflects an excessive autonomic response to stimuli and is a medical emergency. It may occur with injuries at T6 or above and does not occur until spinal shock subsides. Stimuli that precipitate it may include bladder distention, distended bowel or digital stimulation, skin stimulation, and exposure to hot or cold. If not treated immediately, it can produce fatal seizures, subarachnoid hemorrhage, and/or CVA.

ETIOLOGIES

- Auto/motorcycle accidents
- Sports injuries (gymnastics, football)
- Falls or jumps
- Gunshot wounds/stab wounds
- Diving accidents

Table 17.1 • Levels and Consequent Results of Spinal Injury

Level	Result
C1–C4	Quadriplegia with intercostal and diaphragm paralysis
C4–5	Quadriplegia with possible phrenic nerve involvement
C5–6	Quadriplegia with gross arm movement; diaphragm spared
C6–7	Quadriplegia with biceps intact
C7–8	Quadriplegia with triceps/biceps intact; no intrinsic hand muscles
T1–T5	Paraplegia with some impairment of intercostal muscles (diaphragmatic breathing)
T6–L1	Spastic paralysis in legs; at T6 no abdominal reflexes
L1–L5	Independent motor abilities; sensation impaired in legs and saddle region
S1–S5	No paralysis of legs below S3; sensation impaired in saddle area, scrotum, glans penis, perineum, upper 3rd posterior thigh and anal area

Note: C = cervical, T = thoracic, L = lumbar, S = sacral.

CLINICAL MANIFESTATIONS

- Spinal Shock
  - hypotension
  - urinary retention
  - flaccid paralysis
  - poikilothermism
  - absence of reflexes
  - bradycardia
  - bowel paralysis (ileus)
  - vasovagal reflex
  - hypoventilation
- Autonomic dysreflexia
  - paroxysmal hypertension
  - blurred vision
  - profuse sweating above level of injury
  - pounding headache
  - bradycardia

Table 17.2 • Types of Incomplete Cord Transection

Type	Result
Brown-Séquard syndrome	Unilateral motor paralysis; contralateral loss of pain, temperature and touch sensation
Anterior cord syndrome	Complete motor paralysis; loss of pain and temperature; some preservation touch, pressure, position and vibration
Central cord syndrome	Arms greater motor loss than legs; some sensory impairment in upper extremities

▼

- flushing/splotching face and neck
- nasal congestion
- piloerection
- nausea
- pupil dilatation

CLINICAL/DIAGNOSTIC FINDINGS

- Spinal x-rays: fractures, dislocation, degeneration
- Tomography: bony lesions difficult to visualize on x-ray
- Myelogram: occlusion of spinal subarachnoid space
- CT scan: bony lesions or other spinal cord pathology
- Magnetic resonance imaging (MRI): bony deformities, spinal cord pathology

NURSING DIAGNOSIS: DECREASED CARDIAC OUTPUT

Related To
- Interruption of sympathetic nervous system (spinal shock)
- Stimulation of sympathetic nervous system (autonomic dysreflexia)

Defining Characteristics

Spinal shock
Hypotension
Bradycardia
SVR < 800 dyn/s/cm^{-5}
CVP < 2 mmHg; PCWP < 8 mmHg
CO < 4 L/min
CI < 2.5 L/min/m^2
Urine output < 30 mL/hr

Autonomic dysreflexia
Hypertension
Bradycardia

Patient Outcomes
Cardiac output will be maintained/restored, as evidenced by
- blood pressure return to baseline
- heart rate 60–100 bpm
- CO 4–8 L/min; CI 2.5–4 L/min/m^2
- CVP 8–10 mmHg; PCWP 8–12 mmHg
- urine output > 30 mL/hr

Nursing Interventions	Rationales
Assess for cause of autonomic dysreflexia: bladder distention, bowel distention, urinary tract infection, pressure sores, noxious stimuli, discomfort	Remedying the cause will reverse the responses seen with autonomic dysreflexia.
Monitor/record cardiovascular status: vital signs, hemodynamic parameters, and peripheral pulses.	Loss of sympathetic tone with spinal shock produces vasodilation, decreased SVR, and hypotension. Bradycardia occurs secondary to loss of sympathetic influence on the heart. Autonomic dysreflexia can cause paroxysmal hypertension and bradycadia.
Monitor/record fluid balance: daily weight and intake and output.	
Monitor for signs of pulmonary edema: PCWP > 20 mmHg, decreased CO, fine crackles in lungs, decreased pulse oximetry, decreased PaO_2, shortness of breath, and tachypnea.	Pulmonary edema can occur due to massive sympathetic discharge from mechanical injury to the spinal cord producing increased afterload, hypertension, bradycardia, and dysrhythmias. These changes can produce left ventricular strain and failure and disruption of pulmonary capillary endothelium.
Monitor for signs of autonomic dysreflexia: headache, blurred vision, profuse sweating and flushing above level of injury, nausea, pupil dilatation and piloerection, and chills and pallor below the level of injury.	The spinal cord lesion prevents transmission of sympathetic discharges elicited by noxious stimuli below the lesion.
Administer fluids as ordered to maintain adequate circulating volume. Monitor for signs of fluid overload.	Fluids may pool in the periphery due to vasodilatation causing a decrease in circulating volume.
Apply thigh-high elastic hose.	An elastic hose will decrease venous dilation and pooling of blood in the lower extremities.
Apply abdominal binder.	This helps prevent fluid shifts when the patient is placed upright.

Nursing Interventions	Rationales
Monitor for blood pressure changes after position change.	The patient with spinal cord injury loses the ability to compensate for postural changes.
Administer medications to maintain blood pressure as prescribed and monitor patient response.	
Administer atropine for symptomatic bradycardia per protocol.	
Institute measures to control hypertension caused by autonomic dysreflexia. Elevate the head of the bed. Administer antihypertensives if necessary and monitor patient response.	
Administer steroids if prescribed and monitor for side effects (GI bleeding, infection, hyperglycemia).	Steroid use is controversial but is believed to decrease spinal cord edema.
Administer diuretics as prescribed and monitor response.	Mannitol decreases spinal cord interstitial pressure. Furosemide decreases spinal cord venous pressure.

NURSING DIAGNOSIS: INEFFECTIVE BREATHING PATTERN

Related To loss of intercostal muscle, abdominal muscle, and/or diaphragmatic muscle innervation

Defining Characteristics
Hypoventilation
$PaCO_2$ > 45 torr
Tidal volume < 5 mL/kg
Vital capacity < 10 mL/kg
PaO_2 < 80 torr
SaO_2 < 90%
Retention of secretions

Patient Outcomes
The patient's breathing pattern will be maintained/restored, as evidenced by
- tidal volume 5–7 mL/kg
- PaO_2 > 80 torr
- SaO_2 > 90%
- vital capacity > 10 mL/kg
- $PaCO_2$ 35–45 torr

Nursing Interventions	Rationales
Assess/record respiratory function: rate, rhythm, and depth of respiration; breath sounds; ABGs and pulse oximetry as ordered and prn respiratory distress. Assess for signs of respiratory distress: use of accessory muscles.	High-level injuries can affect the diaphragm and sensorimotor function necessary to breathe and/or take deep breaths.
Measure tidal volume and vital capacity at regular intervals.	A vital capacity of under 10mL/kg may indicate the need for intubation.
Support airway as appropriate: oral/nasal airway, supplementary oxygen, suctioning, intubation, and mechanical ventilation. Position patient for ease of respiratory effort, that is, head of bed elevated.	
Assist patient with coughing and deep breathing using quad coughing technique (press with heel of hand between umbilicus and xiphoid during coughing).	This maneuver generates positive airway pressure and assists removal of secretions.
Induce cough with suctioning if necessary.	
Monitor for bradycardia during suctioning.	Due to lack of inhibition of vagal impulses, the patient may experience bradycardia during suctioning.

NURSING DIAGNOSIS: IMPAIRED PHYSICAL MOBILITY

Related To
- Compression of the spinal cord
- Vertebral column instability
- Forced immobilization by traction

Defining Characteristics
Muscle flaccidity/spasticity
Paresis of one or more extremities

Patient Outcomes

The patient will
- maintain full joint range of motion.
- exhibit no signs of complications.
- have no further damage to the spinal cord.

Nursing Interventions	Rationales
Assess leg/arm movement: 1. finger flexion, extension, and spreading 2. wrist flexion/extension 3. forearm pronation/supination 4. elbow flexion/extension 5. arm abduction/adduction 6. shoulder shrugging 7. hip flexion/extension 8. knee flexion/extension 9. foot dorsal/plantar flexion 10. toe flexion/extension	This provides baseline data to monitor improvement or worsening of the patient's deficit.
Assess leg/arm strength: against resistance, against gravity, and contraction present/not present. Assess ability for purposeful movement.	
Perform active/passive range-of-motion exercises.	
Support extremities with pillows to prevent or reduce swelling and maintain proper alignment.	
Utilize measures to maintain normal alignment and positioning of extremities: hand splints, boots, or high tops.	
Get patient out of bed (OOB) when spine is stabilized. Change position slowly.	
Utilize specialized bed such as rotating bed to provide pressure relief. Inspect skin every 2 hr for signs of reddening or breakdown. Keep off reddened areas as much as possible.	
Avoid neck movement (upper spinal injury) or hip movement (lower spinal injury) until approved by physician.	These movements may cause further spine injury by increasing pressure on the spinal cord.

Nursing Interventions | Rationales

Nursing Interventions	Rationales
Maintain correct alignment of spinal column at all times. If patient is in traction, ensure pulley weights hang freely.	
Monitor for signs of deep-vein thrombosis: measure and record calf and thigh circumference and assess legs for redness, increased temperature, or edema.	Prolonged bedrest and lack of normal muscle contraction increase the risk for thrombophlebitis.
Monitor for signs of pulmonary embolus: decreased breath sounds, decreased pulse oximetry, shortness of breath, and tachypnea.	
Apply/maintain elastic hose and/or intermittent pneumatic compression devices to lower extremities.	These prevent venous stasis and decrease the risk of thrombus formation.
Administer low-dose heparin as prescribed and monitor for side effects.	Low-dose heparin can prevent the formation of thrombi.
Maintain skin integrity. Turn and reposition frequently. Assess pressure points for redness, blanching, or breakdown with every position change. Keep skin clean, avoiding hot water and overdrying. Provide frequent mouth care.	

NURSING DIAGNOSIS: ALTERED SENSORY PERCEPTION— TACTILE

Related To
- Altered sensory reception
- Altered sensory transmission
- Altered sensory integration

Defining Characteristics
Decreased sensation in affected limbs

Patient Outcomes
The patient will remain free from injury.

Nursing Interventions	Rationales
Assess and record sensory deficit: deep touch, pain, temperature, and proprioception.	Deep touch and proprioception test the posterior column tract. Pain and temperature test the spinothalamic tract.
Provide safe environment: siderails up, bed in low position, protect from thermal injury, and place objects where patient can see them. Assist patient with ADLs as needed.	
Provide oral suctioning with oral hygiene if needed.	The patient may have difficulty swallowing secondary to altered sensation.
Assist patient in positioning/maintaining spinal alignment as prescribed.	The patient will be totally dependent in relation to position changes. Proper body alignment is essential to preventing further injury.
Institute measures to promote relaxation: radio, TV, visitors, and relaxation tapes. Encourage significant others to talk to and touch patient. Explain procedures and cares. Explain environment and reorient frequently. Provide meaningful tactile stimuli to area where sensation intact.	This helps reduce anxiety for both the patient and significant others.

NURSING DIAGNOSIS: INEFFECTIVE THERMOREGULATION
Related To autonomic dysfunction

Defining Characteristics
Hypothermia/hyperthermia depending on environmental temperature

Patient Outcomes
Patient will maintain normal core temperature.

Nursing Interventions

Monitor temperature every 2 hr until stable.
Provide warming measures if hypothermic.
Ensure cool environment if hyperthermic.

Rationales

Injuries above T6 cause interruption of sympathetic pathways to the temperature regulation center in the hypothalamus, causing the patient's temperature to drift toward the temperature of the immediate environment (poikilothermia). The patient is unable to conserve or lower body heat or shiver or perspire below the level of lesion.

NURSING DIAGNOSIS: BOWEL INCONTINENCE

Related To
- Impaired autonomic nervous system function
- Loss of muscular control
- Immobility
- Unopposed vagal stimulation

Defining Characteristics
Decreased/absent bowel sounds
Absence of sensation/control of bowel movements
Abdominal distention

Patient Outcomes
Normal bowel elimination will be maintained/restored.

Nursing Interventions	Rationales
Assess abdomen: bowel sounds, distention, frequency, and character of stool.	
Check rectum daily for impaction. Utilize anesthetic ointment.	Impaction and/or rectal stimulation can trigger autonomic dysreflexia.
Place patient on high-fiber diet with adequate fluid intake (1800–2400 mL/day).	
Insert nasogastric tube if bowel sounds are absent.	The patient is at risk for vomiting and aspiration. An NG tube will help prevent this.

Nursing Interventions	Rationales
Administer stool softeners as ordered.	
Monitor for signs of GI bleeding: guaiac nasogastric drainage; guaiac stools. Administer antacids, histamine H_2 receptor antagonists, and/or sucralfate as prescribed.	Unopposed vagal stimulation increases hydrochloric acid production and puts the patient at risk for ulcer development and GI bleeding.

NURSING DIAGNOSIS: URINARY RETENTION

Related To
- Impaired neural innervation
- Urinary retention

Defining Characteristics
Bladder distention   No urine output
Signs of urinary tract infection

Patient Outcomes
Adequate urinary elimination will be maintained.

Nursing Interventions	Rationales
Assess for bladder distention.	
During acute stage insert indwelling catheter.	This enables more accurate evaluation of fluid balance and renal function.
Place patient on schedule for intermittent catheterization.	This stimulates bladder emptying and prevents infection.
Note color, cloudiness, odor, and sediment in urine.	Cloudiness, foul odor or sediment may indicate the presence of infection.
Provide catheter care once a shift.	Both upper and lower motor neuron lesions produce a flaccid bladder initially. After spinal shock passes, upper motor neuron lesions cause a spastic bladder, while lower motor neuron lesions produce a flaccid bladder.

NURSING DIAGNOSIS: INEFFECTIVE INDIVIDUAL COPING

Related To
- Loss of independence
- Physical disability

Defining Characteristics
Anxiety
Inability to meet basic needs
Inappropriate use of defense mechanisms
Verbalization of inability to cope

Patient Outcomes
The patient will: display coping behaviors that are health promoting. Verbalize feelings indicating the ability to cope.

Nursing Interventions	Rationales
Assess previous coping mechanisms.	These data will help the nurse anticipate patient responses, identify patient strengths and weaknesses, and determine how new coping mechanisms might be developed.
Assess current coping mechanisms. Listen to patient's comments and response to situation. Discuss meaning of loss with patient. Assess current emotional status.	
Assess support systems and family dynamics.	The spinal injury patient will require long-term emotional and physical support and the family plays a key role in this.
Encourage significant others to visit.	This helps provide the patient with support and assists in developing a relationship of trust with significant others.
Provide encouragement for any progress.	
Include patient in decision-making process as much as possible: care routines, relaxing activities, and choice of diet.	This provides the patient with some sense of control.

Nursing Interventions	Rationales
Encourage patient participation in self-care as able. Provide support for expression of grief and loss. Provide consistent, truthful information to patient.	
Encourage patient to express needs.	Patients with severe disabilities will be dependent on others for most of their care and must be able to express their needs.
Encourage participation of significant others in care of the patient.	This will begin to prepare both the patient and family for future role changes.

DISCHARGE PLANNING/CONTINUITY OF CARE

- Assess need for/type of long-term care and follow-up
- If the discharge destination is home, assess existing supports and the need for assistance.
- Determine coping deficits/support needs and institute assistance measures.
- Determine knowledge deficits/teaching needs and document and institute a teaching plan.
- Refer patient to social services as appropriate.
- Communicate coping deficits/support needs and knowledge deficits/ learning needs to unit accepting the patient on transfer.
  NOTE: After the acute stage, patients with spinal injuries will require long-term care/rehabilitation and the use of multiple community supports and resources.

REFERENCES

Coen, S. D. (1992). Spinal cord injury: Preventing secondary injury. *AACN Clinical Issues in Critical Care Nursing, 3*(1), 44–54.

Dillingham, T. R. (1988). Prevention of complications during acute management of the spinal cord-injury patient: First step in the rehabilitation process. *Critical Care Nursing Quarterly, 11*(2), 71–77.

Glick, O. J. (1992). Interventions related to activity and movement. *Nursing Clinics of North America, 27*(2), 541–568.

Hilton, G. & Frei, J. (1991). High dose methylprednisolone in the treatment of spinal cord injuries. *Heart & Lung, 20*(6), 675–680.

Hughes, M. C. (1990). Critical care nursing for the patient with a spinal cord injury. *Critical Care Nursing Clinics of North America, 2*(1), 33–40.

Kiraly, A. M., Carnagie, J., Frazier, C., & Hartner, K. M. (1989). Spinal cord injury. In M. S. Sommers (Ed.), *Difficult diagnoses in critical care nursing,* (pp. 253–276). Rockville, MD: Aspen.

Kocan, M. J. (1990). Pulmonary considerations in the critical care phase. *Critical Care Nursing Clinics of North America, 2*(3), 369–374

Mitchell, M. (1989). *Neuroscience Nursing: A nursing diagnosis approach.* Baltimore, MD: Williams & Wilkins.

Nemeth, L. (1988). Intensive care of the spinal cord-injured patient: Focus on early rehabilitation. *Critical Care Nursing Quarterly, 11*(2), 79–84.

Schwenker, D. (1990). Cardiovascular considerations in the critical care phase. *Critical Care Nursing Clinics of North America, 2*(3), 363–368.

Sullivan, J. (1989). Incomplete spinal cord injuries: Nursing diagnoses. *Dimensions of Critical Care Nursing, 8*(6), 338–346.

Walleck, C. A. (1989). Spinal cord injury. In K. T. VonRueden & C. A. Walleck (Eds.), *Advanced critical care nursing.* (pp. 181–204). Rockville, MD: Aspen.

Walleck, C. A. (1990). Neurologic considerations in the critical care phase. *Critical Care Nursing Clinics of North America, 2*(3), 357–362.

▼

CEREBRAL ANEURYSM

Cerebral aneurysms, caused by weakness in the arterial muscle wall, usually arise at an arterial bifurcation in the circle of Willis. The most commonly occurring cerebral aneuyrsms are saccular or berry aneurysms. Berry aneurysms are thought to be due to a congenital defect in development of the arterial muscle wall. Saccular aneurysms result from congenital hypoplasia of the medial layer of the arterial wall muscle in conjunction with atherosclerosis and hypertension.

When rupture occurs, hemorrhage occurs in the subarachnoid space. Hemorrhage varies in severity, and clinical manifestations may range from milder signs such as nuchal rigidity, photophobia, or ptosis to more severe signs of increased intracranial pressure or even brain death. The major causes of morbidity and mortality are rebleeding and cerebral arterial vasospasm. The greatest danger of rebleeding occurs in the first 24–48 hr and then again 7–14 days after the initial bleed. Cerebral vasospasm may occur 3–4 days, after bleeding, peaks at 4–12 days and resolves over 3 weeks.

ETIOLOGIES

- Contributing factors in development
  - trauma
  - atherosclerosis
  - possibly cocaine use
  - inflammation or infection
  - congenital formation
- Contributing factors to rupture
  - hypertension
  - strenuous physical activity
  - seasonal variation

CLINICAL MANIFESTATIONS

- Warning signs

-headaches   -fatigue   -vomiting
-generalized, transient weakness   -ptosis
-diplopia
- Early indicators
  - headache
  - fever
  - lethargy
  - nuchal rigidity
  - photophobia
  - nausea and vomiting
- Varying manifestations of increased intracranial pressure depending on severity of bleed. (see Increased Intracranial Pressure)

CLINICAL/DIAGNOSTIC FINDINGS

- CT scan: presence of subarachnoid blood within 48 hr
- MRI: same as CT scan
- Cerebral arteriogram: location of bleed; diagnosis of cerebral vasospasm
- Transcranial Doppler ultrasonography: presence of cerebral vasospasm
- No lumbar puncture (potential brain herniation and aneurysmal bleeding)

NURSING DIAGNOSIS: ALTERED TISSUE PERFUSION—CEREBRAL

Related To
- Disruption of blood flow due to rupture of artery
- Increased intracranial pressure (ICP)

Defining Characteristics

Headache
Lethargy
Vomiting
Signs of increased ICP
Photophobia
Ptosis
Diplopia

Patient Outcome
The patient's cerebral tissue perfusion will be maintained/restored.

Cerebral Aneurysm

Nursing Interventions	Rationales
Assess/record clinical signs of increased ICP at least every hour and notify physician immediately with any changes: 1. level of consciousness, orientation, and memory 2. pupil size, position, and response to light 3. verbalization and response to command 4. movement, strength, and sensation in all extremities 5. pathological reflexes 6. vital signs: blood pressure, heart rate, respiratory rate, temperature 7. ICP, cerebral perfusion pressure (CPP), and MAP continuously 8. respiratory pattern 9. ABGs and/or pulse oximetry 10. utilize Glasgow Coma Scale (GCS) to standardize assessment	Increased ICP can occur as the result of hydrocephalus, cerebral vasospasm, cerebral ischemia, or bleeding. The physician must be notified immediately of any changes to prevent herniation and/or irreversible ischemic damage.
Maintain complete bedrest, performing all ADLs for patient. Place in private room, with door closed, blinds drawn, and lights out.	
Discourage coughing, sneezing, and straining at stool. Administer stool softeners and oral laxatives as prescribed and record results.	Straining at stool, coughing, or sneezing increases intrathoracic pressure decreasing cerebral venous return and increasing intracranial pressure.
Administer sedatives as prescribed to decrease restlessness, anxiety, and irritability. Do not use rectal temperatures, medications, enemas, or tubes. Reduce external stimuli: no TV, radio, or reading. Limit visitors to immediate family/significant others.	Activity or any sensory stimuli can increase blood pressure, increasing intracranial pressure and putting the patient at risk for rebleeding.

Nursing Interventions	Rationales
Administer medications as prescribed to control blood pressure and prevent extreme fluctuations. Monitor patient response and notify physician immediately if ineffective.	Adequate blood pressure must be maintained to provide adequate cerebral blood flow. This may mean a higher or lower pressure than the patient's baseline. The optimal blood pressure is determined by the patient's level of consciousness.
Administer analgesics as prescribed to control pain, anxiety, and restlessness.	Pain, anxiety, and/or restlessness will increase blood pressure and release of catecholamines, which can cause rebleeding.
Administer antifibrinolytics as prescribed and monitor for complications (signs of bleeding).	Aminocaproic acid (Amicar) is used to prevent lysis of the clot (occurs 7–14 days postrupture). Its use is controversial.
Prepare patient for surgery, reinforcing physician's explanations and providing support.	Surgery may occur early (within 3 days) or late. In either case, the patient must be prepared/supported emotionally to alleviate anxiety.
Institute hypervolemic hemodilution therapy as prescribed. Administer fluids (colloids or dextrans) to maintain optimal cardiac output and cause hypervolemia (CVP 10–12 mmHg; PCWP 18–20 mmHg; CI 3–5.5 L/min). Administer inotropes/vasoconstrictors as ordered to induce hypertension (within 20 mmHg of patient's normal blood pressure).	Cerebral vasospasm occurs with cerebral aneurysm as the result of release of mediators (serotonin, prostaglandins) that cause vasoconstriction. This vasospasm can lead to decreased cerebral blood flow and ischemia causing decreased neurological functioning and secondary brain injury. Cerebral blood flow is influenced by arterial pressure, cardiac output, intravascular volume, and blood viscosity. In hypervolemic hemodilution cerebral blood flow is optimized and cerebral vasospasm is minimized by manipulating these variables, inducing hypervolemia, hypertension, and lowered blood viscosity. A blood pressure higher than 20 mmHg above the patient's norm will increase ischemia and incidence of bleeding.

Nursing Interventions	**Rationales**
During hypervolemic hemodilution monitor hemodynamic parameters (see previous intervention), hematocrit (Hct), and serum glucose.	The hematocrit is used as a measure of blood viscosity. The range of 30–35% provides the optimum Hct for oxygen transport when blood oxygen content is decreased due to decreased blood viscosity. Hyperglycemia will cause increased blood viscosity due to its hyperosmolar effects.
During hypervolemic hemodilution, monitor closely for signs of rebleeding and neurological response to therapy, i.e., improvement in neurological signs.	Any evidence of neurological deterioration requires immediate discontinuation of hypervolemic hemodilution.
Administer calcium blocking agents as ordered and monitor patient response.	Calcium channel blockers reduce the severity of cerebral vasospasm by inhibiting vascular smooth-muscle contraction.
Prepare patient for cerebral angioplasty: what patient can expect. Reinforce physician explanation of indications, potential risks, and potential outcomes.	Cerebral angioplasty may be indicated in patients with delayed cerebral ischemia who do not respond to hypervolemic hemodilution or calcium blockers.
Monitor serum sodium level. Administer concentrated saline infusions as prescribed and monitor response. Administer fludrocortisone as prescribed and monitor response.	Salt-wasting hyponatremia is believed to occur due to hypothalamic stimulation of the sympathetic nervous system causing release of atrial natriuretic factor and release of natriuretic peptides from the third ventricle. Concentrated saline infusions are used to maintain a serum sodium around 135 mmol/L. Fludrocortisone is used to inhibit sodium excretion.
Monitor the EKG for prolonged Q-T intervals, peaked T waves, peaked P waves, shortened P-R intervals, and large U waves. Treat dysrhythmias per protocols and monitor patient response.	The EKG changes may occur as the result of vagal stimulation due to intracranial hypertension and increased catecholamine release from hypothalamic irritation due to subarachnoid blood.

Nursing Interventions	Rationales
Institute measures to prevent/decrease increased intracranial pressure (see Increased Intracranial Pressure).	

NURSING DIAGNOSIS: HIGH RISK FOR FLUID VOLUME EXCESS

Risk Factors
- Hypervolemic hemodilution

Patient Outcomes
The patient will remain free of complications of fluid volume excess, as evidenced by the absence of
- pulmonary congestion
- pulmonary/peripheral edema
- congestive heart failure
- fluid and electrolyte disturbances

Nursing Interventions	Rationales
Assess for patients at risk for fluid volume problems resulting from hypervolemic hemodilution, that is, the elderly and those with previous cardiac history. Monitor fluid balance: daily weight, intake, and output.	
Monitor cardiovascular status: vital signs, hemodynamics CVP/PCWP, CO/CI), and peripheral pulses/perfusion. Monitor for signs of pulmonary edema: PCWP > 20 mmHg, fine crackles, CO < 4 L/min, shortness of breath/dyspnea, decreased PaO_2, pulse oximetry < 90%, and pink frothy sputum. Monitor for signs of congestive heart failure: decreased CO/CI, urine output < 30 mL/hr, peripheral edema, jugular venous distention, and hepatojugular reflex. Monitor for signs of myocardial ischemia: EKG changes, dysrhythmias, and chest pain.	Hypervolemic hemodilution requires the infusion of large volumes of fluid to maintain cerebral blood flow which can result in compromise of the cardiovascular system.
Monitor laboratory values for hyponatremia, hypochloremia, hypoosmolality, and decreased hematocrit (see previous care plan)	

NURSING DIAGNOSIS: IMPAIRED PHYSICAL MOBILITY

Related To
- Institution of aneurysmal precautions
- Alteration in motor function

Defining Characteristics
Complete bedrest
Complete dependence for ADLs
Decreased muscle strength/paresis/posturing
Inability to move purposefully

Patient Outcomes

The patient will
- maintain full joint range of motion.
- be free of skin breakdown and/or contractures.

Nursing Interventions	Rationales
Assess for physical mobility deficit: leg/arm movement and strength and ability for purposeful movement. Increase/maintain limb mobility. Perform passive range of motion exercises. Support extremities with pillows to prevent or reduce swelling.	
Utilize boots or high-top shoes in patient with altered lower extremity mobility.	Boots or high-top shoes will maintain proper alignment of foot to ankle and prevent foot drop.
Change position at least every 2 hr. Utilize specialized beds that provide pressure relief. Inspect skin every 2 hr for signs of reddening or breakdown. Keep off reddened areas as much as possible.	

▼

DISCHARGE PLANNING/CONTINUITY OF CARE

- Assess need for/type of long-term care and follow-up.
- If the discharge destination is home, assess existing supports and the need for assistance.
- Determine coping deficits/support needs and institute assistance measures.
- Determine knowledge deficits/teaching needs and document and institute a teaching plan.
- Refer patient to social services as appropriate
- Communicate coping deficits/support needs and knowledge deficits/teaching needs to unit accepting the patient on transfer.

REFERENCES

Cook, H. A. (1991). Aneurysmal subarachnoid hemorrhage: Neurosurgical frontiers and nursing challenges. *Clinical Issues in Critical Care Nursing, 2*(4), 665–674.

Flynn, E. P. (1989). Cerebral vasospasm following intracranial aneurysm rupture: A protocol for detection. *Journal of Neuroscience Nursing, 21*(6), 348–352.

Grimes, C. M. (1991). Cerebral balloon angioplasty for treatment of vasospasm after subarachnoid hemorrhage. *Heart & Lung, 20*(5), 431–435.

Hummel, S. K. (1989). Cerebral vasospasm: Current concepts of pathogenesis and treatment. *Journal of Neuroscience Nursing, 21*(4), 216–224.

MacDonald, E. (1989). Aneurysmal subarachnoid hemorrhage. *Journal of Neuroscience Nursing, 21*(5), 313–321.

Manifold, S. L. (1990). Aneurysmal SAH: Cerebral vasospasm and early repair. *Critical Care Nurse, 10*(8), 62–69.

Rea, J. B. & Dunbar, S. B. (1992). Neurogenic electrocardiographic abnormalities in subarachnoid hemorrhage. *Focus on Critical Care, 19*(1), 50–54.

Stewart-Amidei, C. (1989). Hypervolemic hemodilution: A new approach to subarachnoid hemorrhage. *Heart & Lung, 18*(6), 590–598.

Willis, D. & Harbit, M. D. (1989). A fatal attraction: Cocaine related subarachnoid hemorrhage. *Journal of Neuroscience Nursing, 21*(3), 171–174.

▼

GUILLAIN-BARRÉ SYNDROME

Guillain-Barré syndrome is an acute inflammatory demyelinating disease of the peripheral nervous system of unknown cause. It occurs in all ages and both sexes. It is thought to be produced by immunologically mediated demyelination of the peripheral nervous system with Schwann cells and myelin the targets. The response is mediated by both humoral and cellular components, but the exact antigens are unclear. The response involves infiltration of mononuclear cells around the capillaries of the peripheral neurons, edema of the endoneural compartment, and demyelination of ventral spinal roots. The result is slowing or loss of the ability to conduct nerve impulses.

Typically, Guillain-Barré is primarily a motor disorder with weakness developing over hours to days, ascending from the legs to the arms and producing flaccid paralysis. The paralysis may halt at any level. In severe cases weakness may involve respiratory and bulbar muscles requiring ventilatory support. Its clinical course is varied with some patients recovering completely (60%) and others remaining severely disabled.

ETIOLOGIES

- Flulike or diarrheal illness 2–4 weeks before
- Infectious agents
  - cytomegalovirus
  - *Chlamydia psittaci*
  - *Salmonella typhi*
  - Epstein Barr and herpes simplex virus
  - *Mycoplasma pneumoniae*
  - *Campylobacter jejuni*
  - parainfluenza
- Other antecedent events
  - immunization
  - renal transplant
  - general surgery
- Suppressed immune system
  - Hodgkin's disease
  - human immunodeficiency virus
  - lyme disease
  - lupus erythematosus

CLINICAL MANIFESTATIONS

- Neuromuscular: Demyelinization of the peripheral nervous system produces
  - tingling of feet and/or hands
  - decreased/lost deep-tendon reflexes
  - mild to moderate bilateral facial weakness
  - mild weakness of tongue muscles
  - loss of gag reflex
  - decreased ventilation: hypercapnea, hypoventilation, poor cough, hypoxemia
  - hypersensitivity of skin   – muscular pain
  - progressive ascending flaccid paralysis
- Autonomic nervous system disturbance produces
  - increased sympathetic nervous system: diaphoresis, general vasoconstriction, sinus tachycardia
  - decreased sympathetic nervous system: postural hypotension, sensitivity to sedatives and dehydration
  - increased parasympathetics: facial flushing, bradycardia
  - transient/persistent hypertension
  - transient bladder paralysis
  - cardiac dysrhythmias: persistent tachycardia, bradycardia, ventricular tachycardia, atrial flutter, atrial fibrillation, asystole
  - increased or decreased sweating
  - paralytic ileus

CLINICAL/DIAGNOSTIC FINDINGS

- Cerebrospinal fluid (CSF): increased protein, increased WBC count, normal glucose, normal pressure
- Electrodiagnostic studies: marked slowing of nerve conduction velocity
- Evoked motor response decreased
- Electromyography: decreased number of units firing
- Mild increase in erythrocyte sedimentation rate
- Hyponatremia (<135 mEq/L)
- Antibodies to cytomegalovirus or Epstein-Barr virus (25%)
- Evidence of recent viral infection
- EKG: ST-T wave changes

NOTE: There is no specific diagnostic test. Diagnosis is a matter of ruling out other etiologies.

NURSING DIAGNOSIS: INEFFECTIVE BREATHING PATTERN

Related To weakened respiratory muscles

Defining Characteristics

$PaCO_2$ > 45 torr
Hypoventilation
Dyspnea
Tidal volume < 5 mL/kg
Adventitious breath sounds

Decreasing PaO_2
Ineffective cough
Tachypnea
Vital capacity < 10 mL/kg

Patient Outcomes

An adequate breathing pattern will be maintained/restored, as evidenced by
- ABGs within normal ranges
- respirations 12–20 per minute
- tidal volume 5–7 mL/kg
- vital capacity > 10 mL/kg
- lungs clear
- effective cough

Nursing Interventions	Rationales
Assess/record rate, depth, and rhythm of respiration; airway and breathing effort; use of accessory muscles; strength of cough; and ability to mobilize secretions.	Although the patient's respiratory muscles may not initially be affected, this is a progressive disease and requires frequent monitoring for signs of pulmonary involvement. The baseline assessment provides data against which to compare future assessments.
Auscultate breath sounds for decreased/absent breath sounds and adventitious sounds.	
Assess ABGs and pulse oximetry as prescribed and prn respiratory distress.	
Assess/monitor pulmonary function parameters: tidal volume and vital capacity.	
Assess for subjective complaints of shortness of breath (SOB) and dyspnea on exertion (DOE).	

Nursing Interventions	Rationales
Support airway as appropriate: airway, supplementary oxygen, suctioning, and intubation equipment/ventilator.	
Position patient for ease of respiratory effort, that is, head of bed elevated	
Provide quiet, restful environment.	
Allow frequent rest periods during activity. Minimize activity to decrease oxygen need.	
Send sputum for culture and sensitivity and administer antibiotics as prescribed.	
Assist patient with coughing and deep breathing.	Weakened respiratory muscles produce hypoventilation resulting in pooling of secretions, atelectasis, and possible pneumonia.
Provide adequate humidification with oxygen.	Drying of the airways can cause drying of mucous membranes, making secretions more difficult to mobilize.
Assist removal of secretions via nasotracheal or orotracheal suctioning as needed.	Due to weakened respiratory muscles, the patient may not be able to cough up secretions.
Reposition patient every 2 hr.	Frequent repositioning helps prevent pooling of secretions and atelectasis.
Monitor fluid balance closely.	
Use sterile suctioning technique.	These patients are at risk for pulmonary infections due to stress and hypoventilation.
Monitor swallowing closely. Insert NG tube if patient is unable to swallow and/or gag reflex is absent.	Gullain-Barré syndrome may cause weakened pharyngeal muscles and/or loss of gag reflex, placing the patient at risk for aspiration.

NURSING DIAGNOSIS: IMPAIRED PHYSICAL MOBILITY

Related To progressive muscle paralysis

Defining Characteristics
Limited range of motion
Limited muscle strength
Impaired coordination
Inability to move without assistance

Patient Outcomes
Physical mobility will be restored to patient baseline.

Nursing Interventions	Rationales
Assess for physical mobility deficit: leg/arm movement and strength, paresthesias of hands and feet, and ability to perform ADLs.	
Perform range-of-motion exercises.	These measures help to maintain limb mobility.
Support extremities with pillows to prevent or reduce swelling.	
When/if able, encourage patient to perform exercise regimens as prescribed.	
As early as possible get patient out of bed.	
Avoid pillows under knees.	Pillows under the knees can interfere with circulation, increasing the risk for deep-vein thrombosis.
Align legs properly when supine (toes and knees pointed toward ceiling). Utilize boots or high-top shoes.	Proper alignment of legs and feet helps to prevent foot drop.
Avoid prolonged periods of hip flexion.	Hip flexion can interfere with lower extremity venous return, increasing the risk for development of deep-vein thrombosis.

Nursing Interventions	Rationales
Apply elastic hose and/or intermittent pneumatic compression devices to lower extremities.	
Institute preventive measures to maintain skin integrity: turn and reposition; assess pressure points for redness, blanching or breakdown with each position change; keep skin clean, avoiding hot water and overdrying; and provide frequent mouth care.	
Institute/prepare patient for plasmapheresis and monitor for side effects: hypotension, tachycardia, hypovolemia, hypocalcemia, and hypomagnesemia. Withhold drugs during the procedure.	Plasmapheresis is believed to remove antimyelin antibodies, slowing and/or halting progression of the disease. Hypotension and tachycardia can occur as the result of fluid shifts without protein replacement or decreased blood volume. Plasmapheresis will remove drugs from the blood so drugs should be held until after the procedure. Hypocalcemia can occur due to binding of ionized calcium by citrate or albumin. Hypomagnesemia can follow after repeated sessions of plasmapheresis.

NURSING DIAGNOSIS: DECREASED CARDIAC OUTPUT

Related To autonomic nervous system dysfunction causing vasoconstriction/vasodilation and cardiac dysrhythmias

Defining Characteristics
Dysrhythmias
CO < 4 L/min
CVP < 2 mmHg

Hypotension
CI < 2.5 L/min/m^2
PCWP < 8 mmHg

Patient Outcomes
Cardiac output will be maintained/restored, as evidenced by
- CO 4–8 L/min
- CI 2.5–4 L/min/m^2
- heart rate 60–100 bpm

- MAP 60 mmHg or greater
- CVP 2–10 mmHg; PCWP 8–12 mmHg

Nursing Interventions	Rationales
Assess cardiovascular status: heart rate, respiratory rate, blood pressure with postural changes; mean arterial pressure, CO/CI, and CVP/PCWP.	Autonomic disturbances in Guillain-Barré can stimulate the sympathetic nervous system (tachycardia, increased blood pressure), depress the sympathetic nervous system (postural hypotension), or stimulate the parasympathetic nervous system (bradycardia).
Assess for peripheral indicators of altered cardiac output: restlessness, confusion, dizziness, urine output < 30 mL/hr, and weak peripheral pulses.	
Assess for peripheral indicators of autonomic nervous system disturbance: 1. increased sympathetic: diaphoresis; cool, clammy skin 2. decreased sympathetic: increased response to sedatives, dehydration 3. increased parasympathetic: facial flushing	
Monitor EKG for cardiac dysrhythmias.	Rhythm disturbances associated with Guillain-Barré include tachycardia, bradycardia, ventricular tachycardia, atrial flutter, atrial fibrillation, and asystole.
Monitor/record fluid balance: intake and output and daily weight. Monitor for signs of dehydration: postural hypotension, dry mucous membranes, and reflex tachycardia.	Changes in vascular tone, decreased fluid intake, and fluid shifts can compromise volume status.
Administer fluids as prescribed to treat postural hypotension and dehydration.	Decreased sympathetic nervous system stimulation can cause postural hypotension and dehydration.

NURSING DIAGNOSIS: ALTERED SENSORY PERCEPTION

Related To
- Sensorimotor dysfunction due to cranial nerve involvement
- Hyperesthesias
- Paresthesias
- Deep muscle aches

Defining Characteristics
Tingling of feet and/or hands
Hypersensitivity of skin
Loss of gag reflex
Mild to moderate bilateral facial weakness
Progressive ascending paralysis
Muscular pain

Patient Outcomes
Patient sensory perception returns to normal, as evidenced by
- normal facial sensation and movement
- normal chewing and swallowing ability
- normal corneal and gag reflex
- normal head and shoulder movement
- absence of paresthesias, hyperesthesias, and muscle aches

Nursing Interventions	Rationales
Assess/record cranial nerve (CN) function: 1. pupillary light reflex, presence of diplopia, presence of ptosis and extraocular eye movements (CN III, IV, V) 2. corneal reflex, facial sensation and movement, ability to chew (CN V, VII) 3. gag reflex, swallowing, and tongue movement (CN IX, X, XII) 4. ability to turn head and/or shrug shoulders (CN IX)	Demyelinization of the peripheral nervous system can also affect cranial nerve function. A baseline assessment is required to accurately evaluate progression/improvement of the disease.

Nursing Interventions	Rationales
Assess for pain, administer pain medication as prescribed, and monitor effects.	As paresthesia progresses, muscle pain and tenderness occur, especially in the shoulders, back, pelvis, buttocks, and thighs.
Monitor/record changes in neurological status and notify physician of any changes: ability to speak, response to commands/painful stimuli, and sensation (hot/cold, dull/sharp).	
Provide safe environment: siderails up, bed in low position, protect from thermal injury, and place objects where patient can see them.	Changes in sensory perception that can occur with Guillain-Barré make the patient more dependent on nursing care and at higher risk for injury.
Assist patient with ADLs as needed. Provide oral suctioning with oral hygiene.	
Assist patient in positioning for comfort and proper alignment. Explain reasons for discomfort.	
Institute measures to promote relaxation: radio, TV, visitors, relaxation tapes, and massage.	
Provide meaningful sensory stimuli: clock, radio, TV, and conversation.	
Explain procedures and care.	
Do not feed patient if gag reflex or swallowing is affected.	This prevents possible aspiration.
Provide artificial tears for eyes and/or patch eyes as needed.	This prevents overdrying of the eyes and corneal abrasions.
Encourage significant others to talk to and touch patient.	This may reduce the patient's anxiety and provides significant others with involvement in the patient's care.

NURSING DIAGNOSIS: ALTERED BOWEL/URINARY ELIMINATION

Related To
- Abdominal muscle weakness
- Loss of sensation and reflexes
- Altered gastric motility

Defining Characteristics
Decreased bowel sounds
Bowel incontinence
Urinary incontinence
Nausea/vomiting

Patient Outcomes
Normal bowel and urinary elimination will be maintained/restored.

Nursing Interventions	Rationales
Assess normal bowel/urinary elimination patterns.	This provides a baseline and enables individualization of care.
Assess GI function: presence/decrease/absence of bowel sounds; character, amount, and frequency of bowel movements; abdominal tenderness, distention, or softness; and nausea, and vomiting.	Progressive paralysis may affect GI muscles and bowel, producing ileus, impaction, or bowel obstruction.
Assess for contributing factors to impaired bowel/urinary elimination: medications, age, and fluid status.	
Assess and monitor hydration status. If able to swallow, fluids should be pushed to 2,000 mL per 24 hr. If unable to swallow, maintain adequate fluids via NG tube or intravenously.	Inadequate hydration can produce hard, impassable stools, resulting in impaction and/or inadequate urine output to maintain renal function.
Insert/maintain NG tube as needed.	Because of decreased bowel function and impaired gag reflex, these patients are at risk for aspiration.
Administer laxatives and stool softeners as ordered and monitor/record results.	These measures assist in regulating bowel function and preventing impaction.

Nursing Interventions	Rationales
Maintain high-fiber/high-bulk foods and/or tube feeding.	This helps maintain fecal consistency.
Insert/maintain Foley catheter or provide intermittent catheterization as needed.	

NURSING DIAGNOSIS: HIGH RISK FOR IMPAIRED SKIN INTEGRITY

Risk Factors
- Immobility
- Changes in sensory perception
- Paresis

Patient Outcomes
Skin integrity will be maintained.

Nursing Interventions	Rationales
Inspect skin for signs of reddening/breakdown.	
Provide pressure relief measures: special mattress/bed.	
Reposition patient every 2 hr.	
Keep skin clean, warm, and dry.	
Provide frequent mouth care.	See Appendix C.

DISCHARGE PLANNING/CONTINUITY OF CARE

- Assess need for/type of long-term care and follow-up.
- If the discharge destination is home, assess existing supports and the need for assistance.
- Determine coping deficits/support needs and institute assistance measures.
- Determine knowledge deficits/teaching needs and document and institute a teaching plan.
- Refer patient to social services as appropriate.

- Communicate coping deficits/support needs and knowledge deficits/teaching needs to unit accepting the patient on transfer.

REFERENCES

Anderson, S. B. (1992). Guillain-Barré syndrome: Giving the patient control. *Journal of Neuroscience Nursing, 24*(3), 158–162.

Chad, D. (1991). The Guillain-Barré syndrome. In J. M. Rippe, R. S. Irwin, J. S. Alpert, & M. P. Fink (Eds.), (pp. 1591–1596). *Intensive care medicine*. Boston, MA: Little, Brown.

Eichner, S. & Curtis, R. L. (1990). Alterations in motor function. In C. M. Porth (Ed.), *Pathophysiology: Concepts of altered health states* (3rd ed., pp. 910). Philadelphia, PA: Lippincott.

Mascarella, J. J. & Hudson, D. C. (1991). Dysimmune neurologic disorders. *AACN Clinical Issues in Critical Care Nursing, 2*(4), 677–678.

Mitchell, M. (1989). Guillain-Barré syndrome and myasthenia gravis. In M. Mitchell (Ed.), *Neuroscience nursing: A nursing diagnosis approach*. Baltimore, MD: Williams & Wilkins.

Pfister, S. M. & Bullas, J. B. (1990). Acute Guillain-Barré syndrome. *Criticial Care Nurse, 10*(10), 68–73.

HEAD TRAUMA

Head trauma can produce a spectrum of different types of injuries with varying levels of permanence and incapacity. The mechanisms that produce neurological changes in the head injury victim include (1) actual structural damage to neurons causing focal neurological signs, (2) damage to blood vessels resulting in hemorrhage and/or vasospasm, (3) destruction of brain tissue causing necrosis, and (4) reactive edema.

Head trauma can result in injuries to coverings of the brain, intrinsic brain injury, and/or traumatic intracranial hematomas. Injuries to the coverings of the brain range from scalp injuries, linear skull fractures, depressed skull fractures, compound skull fractures, and basal skull fractures. Intrinsic brain injury may include cerebral concussions, cerebral contusions, or brain stem contusions. Intracranial hematomas include epidural, subdural, and intracerebral hematomas. The degree of neurological deficit and/or damage depends on the severity of the trauma.

ETIOLOGIES

- Motor vehicle accidents
- Gunshot wounds
- Falls
- Acceleration/deceleration injuries
- Blows to the head
- Stab wounds

CLINICAL MANIFESTATIONS

- Basal skull fracture
  - bleeding from ears/blood behind eardrum
  - rhinorrhea or otorrhea
  - Battle's sign (mastoid ecchymosis)
  - periorbital ecchymosis

- Cerebral concussion
  - unconsciousness less than 10–15 min
  - retrograde or antegrade amnesia
  - confusion, restlessness, irritability
  - headache
  - nausea, vomiting
- Cerebral contusion
  - varies depending on severity and location
  - loss of consciousness/decreased level of consciousness
  - memory loss
  - motor/sensory dysfunction
  - cranial nerve dysfunction
  - seizures
- Brain stem contusion
  - comatose and tend to remain so
  - hyperactivity of autonomic nervous system
  - hyperthermia
  - diaphoresis
  - motor deficits
  - abnormal pupil size, reaction
  - tachycardia
  - varying respiratory pattern
  - abnormal reflexes
- Epidural hematoma
  - short period of unconsciousness, followed by lucid interval and then rapid deterioration
  - signs and symptoms of increased ICP
- Subdural hematoma
  - may not develop symptoms for days to months
  - signs and symptoms of increased ICP
- Intracerebral hematoma
  - signs and symptoms vary with area of brain involved, size of hematoma, and rate of bleeding
  - signs and symptoms of increased ICP

CLINICAL/DIAGNOSTIC FINDINGS

- EEG: brain wave abnormalities
- Skull x-ray: fractures, hemispheric shifts
- CT scan: edema, hemorrhage, hemispheric shifts
- Cerebral angiography: vasospasm, aneurysm

NURSING DIAGNOSIS: ALTERED TISSUE PERFUSION— CEREBRAL

Related To
- Hematoma/hemorrhage in brain
- Cerebral edema
- Cerebral vasospasm

Defining Characteristics

CPP < 60 mmHg ICP > 15 mmHg
Plateau waves on ICP monitor
Signs and symptoms of increased ICP

Patient Outcomes

Cerebral tissue perfusion will be maintained/restored, as evidenced by
- CPP > 60 mmHg
- ICP < 15 mmHg
- absence of plateau waves
- neurological signs returning to patient baseline

Nursing Interventions	Rationales
Assess/record for clinical signs of increased ICP at least every hour and notify physician immediately of any changes (see Increased Intracranial Pressure).	
Assess for signs of herniation (see Increased Intracranial Pressure).	
Test drainage from nose or ears for presence of cerebrospinal fluid (CSF).	Bloody drainage encircled by a yellowish ring on linen or dressing is highly suggestive of CSF drainage. When fluid is tested with Dextrostix, CSF will test positive for glucose.
If there is CSF drainage from nose or ears, place sterile mustache dressing (nose) or loose 4 x 4 covering (ears) allowing free drainage.	
Instruct patient to avoid coughing, sneezing, nose blowing, or Valsalva-type maneuvers, that is, bearing down and turning in bed without assistance. Avoid nasal suctioning.	These activities can cause further damage of the dura.
Administer antibiotics as prescribed and monitor for side effects.	Patients with skull injuries, especially if associated with lacerations, are prone to the development of infections and meningitis.

Nursing Interventions	Rationales
Maintain ICP monitoring devices (see Increased Intracranial Pressure).	
Institute interventions to prevent/decrease increased ICP (see Increased Intracranial Pressure).	
Institute measures to prevent cerebral vasospasm (see Cerebral Aneurysm).	

NURSING DIAGNOSIS: IMPAIRED PHYSICAL MOBILITY

Related To
- Requirement for complete bedrest
- Alterations in motor function
- Alteration in mental function

Defining Characteristics
Limited range of movement
Decreased spontaneous/purposeful movement
Decreased muscle strength/paresis/posturing
Confusion, restlessness, lethargy, stupor, coma

Patient Outcomes
The patient will
- maintain full joint range of motion.
- be free from skin breakdown and/or contractures.

Nursing Interventions	Rationales
See Increased Intracranial Pressure	•

NURSING DIAGNOSIS: HIGH RISK FOR INJURY

Risk Factors
- Seizures
- Decreased level of consciousness
- Stress ulcer
- Immobility

Patient Outcome
The patient will remain free of injury.

Nursing Interventions	Rationales
See Appendix C	

DISCHARGE PLANNING/CONTINUITY OF CARE

- Assess need for/type of long-term care and follow-up.
- If the discharge destination is home, assess existing supports and the need for assistance.
- Determine coping deficits/support needs and institute assistance measures.
- Determine knowledge deficits/teaching needs, document and institute a teaching plan.
- Refer patient to social services as appropriate.
- Communicate coping deficits/support needs and knowledge deficits/learning needs to unit accepting the patient on transfer.

REFERENCES

Aumick, J. E. (1991). Head trauma: Guidelines for care. *RN. 54*(4), 26–31.

Coburn, K. (1992). Traumatic brain injury: The silent epidemic. *Clinical Issues in Critical Care Nursing, 3*(1), 9–18.

Dettbarn, C. L., & Davidson, L. J. (1989). Pulmonary complications in the patient with acute head injury: Neurogenic pulmonary edema. *Heart & Lung, 18*(6), 583–589.

Mitchell, M. (1989). *Neuroscience nursing: A nursing diagnosis approach.* Baltimore, MD: Williams & Wilkins.

Rudy, E. B., Turner, B. S., Baum, M., Stone, K. S., & Brucia, J. (1991). Endotracheal suctioning in adults with head injury. *Heart & Lung, 20*(6), 667–674.

Sisson, R. (1990). Effects of auditory stimuli on comatose patients with head injury. *Heart & Lung, 19*(4), 373–378.

Susi, E. A., & Walls, S. K. (1990). Traumatic cerebral vasospasms and secondary head injury. *Critical Care Nursing Clinics of North America, 2*(1), 15–20.

Walleck, C. A. (1989). Controversies in the management of the head-injured patient. *Critical Care Nursing Clinics of North America, 1*(1), 67–74.

Walleck, C. A. (1992). Preventing secondary brain injury. *AACN Clinical Issues in Critical Care Nursing, 3*(1), 19–28.

INCREASED INTRACRANIAL PRESSURE

Intracranial pressure (ICP) is determined by the pressure exerted by the intracranial volumes of brain mass, blood, and cerebrospinal fluid (CSF). An increase in ICP can occur with any pathology that causes an increase in any one of these volumes. Normal ICP (0–15 mmHg) is maintained via autoregulatory mechanisms that maintain a constant cerebral blood flow and compensatory mechanisms that are initiated if ICP increases.

When ICP begins to rise, limited compensation can occur via displacement of CSF, increased absorption of CSF, and compression of the venous system. As the intracranial volume continues to increase, these compensatory mechanisms fail, resulting in significant increases in ICP. The more rapid the increase in volume (i.e., an acute bleed), the sooner decompensation will occur.

Autoregulatory mechanisms maintain cerebral blood flow via vasoconstriction or vasodilation over a MAP range of 50–150 mmHg. Cerebral perfusion pressure (CPP), utilized to measure cerebral blood flow (CPP = MAP − ICP), must be maintained at greater than 60 mmHg to prevent brain tissue ischemia and cell damage. When ICP is increased, any factor that increases cerebral blood flow (acidosis, hypoxia, increased metabolic rate) will only further increase ICP and decrease CPP. Uncorrected increases in ICP can cause brain tissue ischemia and/or herniation of a portion of the brain through openings within the intracranial cavity, resulting in irreversible brain damage and brain death.

ETIOLOGIES

- Hydrocephalus
  - obstruction of CSF pathways
  - deficient CSF absorption
  - oversecretion of CSF
- Craniocerebral trauma

- Infectious processes
  - meningitis
  - ventriculitis
  - Reye's syndrome
  - encephalitis
  - intracranial abscess
- Neoplasms
- Metabolic disorders
  - water intoxication
  - dehydration and thrombosis of venous sinuses
  - exogenous poisons: alcohol, lead
  - metabolic encephalopathy: acidosis, hypoxia, hypercapnea
  - systemic encephalopathy: uremia, hepatic, pancreatic, endocrine disorders
  - hyperthermia
- Vascular disorders
  - emboli
  - cerebral infarction
  - cerebral vasculitis
  - DIC
- Venous outflow obstruction
  - compression of jugular veins
  - increased intrathoracic and/or intra-abdominal pressure
- Idiopathic

CLINICAL MANIFESTATIONS

- Cerebrovascular: Pressure on the vasomotor center produces
  - increased systolic BP
  - widened pulse pressure
  - decreased heart rate
- Neurovascular: Increased intracranial pressure produces
  - decreased level of consciousness
  - headache
  - change in vision
  - change in reflexes
  - change in pupil size/reaction
  - change in motor response
  - seizures
- Pulmonary: Pressure on the respiratory center produces
  - Cheyne-Stokes respirations
  - neurogenic hyperventilation
  - apneustic respiration
  - Biot's respiration
- Gastrointestinal: Pressure on the emetic center produces
  - vomiting
  - stress ulcer

CLINICAL/DIAGNOSTIC FINDINGS

- CT scan: edema, tumor, infarction, contusion, cyst, hemorrhage, hydrocephalus, shifts
- Cerebral angiography: aneurysms, arteriovenous malformation (AVM), vascular tumors, vasospasm
- Skull x-ray: fractures, shift of pineal gland, changes in sella turcica, changes in cranial convolution
- EEG: brain wave activity

- Evoked responses/potentials: BAER: (brain-stem auditory evoked response) assessment of brain stem integrity, VER: (visual evoked response) lesion on visual pathways
- Spinal tap: usually not done if hemorrhage suspected

NURSING DIAGNOSIS: ALTERED TISSUE PERFUSION—CEREBRAL

Related To
- Decreased CPP
- Increased volume of brain mass and/or blood
- Increased CSF volume
- Cerebral edema
- Cerebral vasospasm

Defining Characteristics
CPP < 60 mmHg ICP > 15 mmHg
Plateau waves on ICP monitor
Clinical signs of increased intracranial pressure

Patient Outcomes
Cerebral tissue perfusion will be maintained/restored, as evidenced by
- CPP > 60 mmHg
- ICP < 15 mmHg
- absence of plateau waves
- return of neurological signs to patient baseline

Nursing Interventions	Rationales
Assess for/record clinical signs of increased ICP at least every hour and notify physician immediately of any changes.	
Assess level of consciousness, orientation, and memory.	Consciousness is mediated by the reticular activating system, which sends sensory stimuli from the environment to the cortex, maintaining wakefulness. Increased ICP causes decreased stimulation of the cortex, decreasing wakefulness. Level of consciousness is the most sensitive indicator of ICP and is the first to change as ICP rises.

Nursing Interventions	Rationales
Assess pupil size, position, shape, symmetry, and reactivity.	Pupillary changes indicate pressure on the third cranial nerve. This occurs when the temporal lobe's medial side is pushed over the edge of the tentorium. Pupillary changes indicate impending herniation and require immediate intervention.
Assess verbalization (fluency, aphasia, word difficulty) and response to command.	
Assess movement, strength, and sensation in all extremities.	Pressure on the cortex or upper pyramidal pathways will decrease movement and strength on the opposite side. Pressure on the cortex or upper sensory pathways will decrease pain, temperature, and pressure perception on the opposite side.
Assess for pathological reflexes (see Table 21.1)	
Assess vital signs: blood pressure, heart rate, respiratory rate, and temperature.	The vasomotor center in the lower pons and upper medulla of the brain stem controls blood pressure and heart rate. Initially, pressure on the vasomotor center will cause a rise in systolic blood pressure, a widening pulse pressure, and a decrease in heart rate. As ICP continues to rise, blood pressure will fall and heart rate will increase. Because of the vasomotor center's location, changes in vital signs generally occur late and indicate herniation.

Nursing Interventions	Rationales
Monitor ICP, MAP, and CPP continuously.	Intracranial pressure monitoring allows early detection and intervention to prevent sustained increases in ICP. Prolonged increases of ICP > 15 mmHg can result in herniation and brain death. An adequate MAP and normal ICP are necessary to maintain a CPP > 60 mmHg. Cerebral blood flow begins to fail at 40 mmHg.
Monitor respiratory pattern (see Table 21.2).	The respiratory centers are located in the pons and the medulla in the brain stem. Depending on the level of pressure on this center, a variety of respiratory patterns may be seen.
Monitor ABGs/pulse oximetry as ordered or prn respiratory changes or distress.	Changes in the respiratory pattern may cause changes in the acid-base balance. Hypoventilation produces hypercapnea, acidosis, and cerebral vasodilatation and can further increase ICP. Hyperventilation produces alkalosis and cerebral vasoconstriction, reducing ICP.
Utilize the GCS to standardize assessment (see Table 21.3).	
Assess for signs of cingulate herniation and notify physician immediately if present, that is, changes in mental status and level of consciousness.	Cingulate herniation occurs when pressure in the supratentorial space forces the cingulate gyrus under the falx cerebri, causing compression of the internal cerebral vein.
Assess for signs of uncal herniation and notify physician immediately if present. Early signs are unilateral pupil dilatation and contralateral hemiplegia. Late signs are decerebrate posturing, absence of oculocephalic and oculovestibular reflexes, and midposition fixed pupils.	Uncal herniation occurs when pressure exerted by a lateral lesion of the middle fossa forces the uncus (inner basal medial edge of temporal lobe) over the tentorial notch, displacing the midbrain and exerting pressure on the third cranial nerve.

Nursing Interventions	Rationales
Assess for signs of central herniation and notify physician immediately if present. Early signs are decreased level of consciousness, altered respiratory pattern with yawns, pauses and deep sighs, small reactive pupils, and increased motor spasticity with bilateral Babinski. Late signs are doll's eyes, Cheyne-Stokes respiration, coma, and decorticate posturing.	Central herniation occurs when the diencephalon, thalamus, hypothalamus, subthalamus, and/or epithalamus are pushed downward through the tentorial notch.
Maintain ICP monitoring devices (see Table 21.4). Place transducer at level of foramen of Monro (intraventricular catheter), that is, anterior upper ear/outer canthus of eye. Relevel with each position change. Calibrate and zero transducer/monitor at least once every 8 hr or with position change. Assess catheter patency: quality of waveform and accuracy of pressures. Monitor connections for leaks and tubing for air and/or kinks.	Improper positioning and calibration make the pressure readings inaccurate. Leaks can cause excessive drainage of CSF (ventricular catheter) or herniation (screw). Air in the tubing can cause an air embolus and/or inaccurate pressure readings.
Monitor and record amount of CSF drainage and record patient/pressure response. Avoid excessive drainage of CSF from ventricular catheter.	Drainage of CSF may be utilized to decrease ICP. Excessive drainage can cause the ventricles to collapse.
Monitor pressure-monitoring device for signs of infection: cloudy CSF fluid and inflammation at insertion site.	
Monitor ICP waveform (see Table 21.5) and record pressures.	
Calculate and record CPP (MAP-ICP) and notify physician of decrease.	Cerebral perfusion pressure indicates blood flow to the brain. Significant decreases can cause irreversible ischemic damage.
Correlate ICP values with neurological status.	

Nursing Interventions	Rationales
Notify physician immediately with any increase in ICP/change in neurological status not responsive to ordered measures, for example, hyperventilation, drainage of CSF, and mannitol.	
Notify physician immediately with occlusion of catheter/screw, system integrity problem, displacement/detachment of system, signs and symptoms of infection, fluid blood tinged, or excessive drainage.	
Maintain sterile system: 1. Change tubing/system every 48–72 hr. 2. Change dressing every 24–72 hr. 3. Monitor site for signs of infection.	
Monitor serum sodium level.	Sodium may be lost with CSF drainage.
Flush subarachnoid screw with 0.1-mL sterile saline every 6–8 hr or as ordered. Avoid if ICP is elevated or there is decreased compliance.	This maintains patency of system.
Monitor/record activities that cause change in ICP.	
Elevate head of bed 30° at all times.	Placing the head flat increases blood flow to the brain and can increase ICP.
Avoid neck flexion/rotation and hip/knee flexion.	Neck flexion or rotation can cause venous outflow obstruction, increasing ICP. Hip/knee flexion can cause increased abdominal pressure and increased ICP.

Nursing Interventions	Rationales
Monitor oxygenation via continuous pulse oximetry.	Oxygenation must be maintained between 80 and 100 torr because hypoxia causes significant cerebral vasodilation and increases in cerebral blood flow, increasing ICP.
Hyperventilate and oxygenate (FiO_2 100%) pre- and postsuctioning. Limit suctioning passes to less than 15 s.	Even transient periods of hypoxia produced by suctioning can cause cerebral vasodilation and worsen increased ICP.
Monitor blood pressure continuously and maintain in low normal range utilizing pharmacological drips if necessary.	Hypotension will decrease CPP, endangering brain tissue, and should be maintained with dopamine. Hypertension will increase ICP and should be prevented with sedation or medications such as nitroprusside.
Prevent/correct hyperthermia	An increase of 1 °C increases the metabolic demands of the brain by 10% and causes vasodilation, increasing ICP.
Administer hyperosmolar agents as prescribed and monitor effects.	One of the consequences of intracranial pathology and injury may be cerebral edema which increases ICP. Hyperosmolar agents such as mannitol increase serum osmolality and pull water from the brain into the bloodstream. Mannitol is also thought to decrease production of CSF.
Administer diuretics as prescribed and assess effects.	Diuretics facilitate loss of water, decrease brain volume, and decrease CSF production, which can minimize increases in ICP due to edema.
Monitor fluid balance closely and maintain fluid restriction.	Patients are kept on the dry side to minimize cerebral edema and decrease ICP. However, too little fluid can decrease CPP, resulting in cerebral ischemia.

Nursing Interventions	Rationales
Maintain hypocapnea and/or hyperventilate with increases in ICP.	Cerebral blood flow changes about 2% for every 1 mmHg change in $PaCO_2$. Hyperventilation causing decreased $PaCO_2$ should decrease ICP in 30 s with effects lasting for 15–20 min. In mechanically ventilated patients, $PaCO_2$ is generally maintained around 25–30 mmHg.
Administer glucocorticoids as prescribed and monitor for side effects such as GI bleeding, infection, and hyperglycemia.	Glucocorticoids (usually dexamethasone) are thought to decrease brain edema, decrease CSF production, and increase release of oxygen.
Administer drugs as prescribed to paralyze and/or sedate patients and monitor response	Restlessness, agitation, or severe posturing can increase intrathoracic pressure (decrease cerebral venous return) and blood pressure (increase CPP), causing increases in ICP. If the patient is paralyzed, sedation is important to minimize anxiety.
Institute barbiturate therapy to induce coma and monitor blood pressure, ICP, ventilation, and cardiac function closely.	Barbiturate therapy (usually pentobarbital) is used for severe refractory or persistent increased ICP. It decreases ICP by decreasing the brain's metabolic demands and by decreasing blood pressure. It can cause decreased blood pressure, CO, contractility, ventilation, and dysrhythmias.
Instruct patient to avoid Valsalva maneuver, straining, coughing, and sneezing. Administer stool softeners.	The Valsalva maneuver and straining both decrease venous outflow from the brain and can increase ICP. Coughing and sneezing indirectly increase ICP, as does hip/knee flexion when turning in bed without assistance.

Nursing Interventions

Avoid excessive stimulation or emotional arousal. Avoid talking about patient at bedside. Space out nursing care.

Rationales

Excessive stimulation (painful stimuli, loud noises, patient cares done all at the same time) can causes increases in ICP. Conversation at the bedside, even in the comatose patient, has been shown to cause increases in ICP.

Table 21.1 • Pathologic Reflexes

Reflex	Level of Abnormality	Abnormal Response
Abnormal flexion Decorticate posturing	Destructive lesion of corticospinal tracts near cerebral hemispheres	Arms flexed on chest, legs extended and internally rotated; plantar flexion
Abnormal extension Decerebrate posturing	Lesion in diencephalon midbrain or pons	Arms adducted and stiffly extended; legs extended; plantar flexion
Plantar reflex Babinski reflex	Upper motor neuron lesion	Dorsiflexion of great toe and fanning of other toes
Oculocephalic/doll's eyes	Lesion of midbrain or pons Very deep coma	One or both eyes remain fixed with head movement, i.e., loss of doll's eyes
Pupillary reflex, CN 3	Lesion of midbrain	Abnormal size, unequal, no response to light
Blink reflex, CN 5 and 7	Lesion of pons	Absent
Gag reflex CN 9 and 10	Lesion of medulla	Absent
Oculovestibular	Brain stem lesion	No response to caloric stimulation

Note: CN = cranial nerve.

Table 21.2 • Respiratory Patterns Related to Brain Pathology

Type	Level of lesion	Description
Cheyne-Stokes	Bilateral deep cerebral lesions Some cerebellar lesions	Brief periods of apnea with rhythmic hyperventilation and hypoventilation
Central neurogenic hyperventilation	Lesions of midbrain and upper pons	Very rapid, deep respirations; no apnea
Apneustic breathing	Lesions of mid to lower pons	Prolonged 2–3 s inspiratory and/or expiratory pause
Cluster breathing	Lesions of lower pons or upper medulla	Irregular gasping respirations with long apneic periods
Ataxic (Biot's) breathing	Lesions of medulla	Completely irregular respiratory and apneic periods

Table 21.3 • Glascow Coma Scale

Eye opening	
Spontaneously	4
To voice	3
To noxious stimuli	2
No response	1
Motor response	
Obeys commands	6
Localizes pain	5
Flexion withdrawal	4
Abnormal flexion	3
Abnormal extension	2
No response	1
Verbal response	
Oriented	5
Confused	4
Inappropriate words	3
Incomprehensible words	2
No response	1

Scoring: 15 = normal; > 9 = no coma; < 7 = coma; 3 = compatible with brain death.

Table 21.4 • Intracranial Pressure Monitoring Devices

Intraventricular

Location	Anterior horn of one of lateral ventricles
Advantages	Direct measurement, most accurate
	Can drain CSF
	Able to determine compliance
	Access to instill drugs
Disadvantages	Infection risk
	Difficult to insert
	Leakage of CSF
	Can cause bleeding

Subarachnoid screw

Location	Subarachnoid space
Advantages	Direct ICP measurement
	Can evaluate compliance
	Easy to insert
	Lower risk of infection
Disadvantages	Unable to withdraw CSF
	Unreliable if pressure high

Epidural

Location	Epidural space
Advantages	Easy to insert
	Avoid dural penetration
	Lowest risk of infection
Disadvantages	Least accurate
	Cannot drain CSF; cannot measure compliance

Table 21.5 • Intracranial Pressure Waveforms

Plateau (A) waves	Increases in ICP 50–100 mmHg lasting 5–20 min; significant indicators of increased ICP; cause ischemia and brain damage
B waves	Oscillations occur with changes in respiration; range 20–50 mmHg; clinical significance unclear
C waves	No known clinical correlation, possibly associated with changes in blood pressure; pressures up to 20 mmHg

NURSING DIAGNOSIS: IMPAIRED GAS EXCHANGE

Related To
- Altered breathing pattern
- Neurogenic pulmonary edema

Defining Characteristics
Abnormal breathing pattern (see Table 21.2)
Adventitious breath sounds
Decreased lung compliance
Decreased PaO_2 (<80 torr)
SaO_2 < 90%

Patient Outcomes
Adequate gas exchange will be maintained/restored as evidenced by
- normal breathing pattern
- clear lungs
- PaO_2 80–100 torr
- SaO_2 > 90%
- normal lung compliance

Nursing Interventions	Rationales
Assess respiratory function: rate, rhythm, and depth of respiration; breath sounds; and ability to handle oral and pulmonary secretions.	Neurogenic pulmonary edema can develop due to sympathetic discharge from pressure on the hypothalamus. This can result in decreased pulmonary compliance, pulmonary hypertension, pulmonary congestion, and atelectasis, producing an ARDS-like syndrome.
Assess ABGs and pulse oximetry as ordered and prn changes in respiratory function.	
Assess for signs of respiratory distress: use of accessory muscles.	
Support airway as appropriate: oral/nasal airway, supplementary oxygen, suctioning, intubation, and mechanical ventilation.	

Nursing Interventions	Rationales
Position patient for ease of respiratory effort, that is, head of bed elevated.	
Administer sedation as prescribed to maintain effective breathing pattern.	Altered breathing patterns produced by increased ICP may interfere with oxygenation. This is especially true if the patient is being mechanically ventilated and is "bucking" the ventilator.
Reposition patient at least every 2 hr.	
Monitor fluid balance closely.	The use of osmotic diuretics can pull fluid out of the brain into the vascular space and contribute to the development of neurogenic pulmonary edema. At the same time, if kept too dry, the patient will be unable to mobilize secretions.
If PEEP is utilized, monitor for hypotension and increases in ICP and withdraw gradually.	Positive end-expiratory pressure causes increased intrathoracic pressure, reducing systemic venous return (hypotension, decreased CPP) and cerebral venous return (increased ICP). Abrupt withdrawal of PEEP can cause increased ICP due to rebound increases in blood pressure.

NURSING DIAGNOSIS: INEFFECTIVE AIRWAY CLEARANCE

Related To
- Altered level of consciousness
- Depression/absence of normal protective mechanisms
- Paralyzing agents/barbiturate coma
- Sedation

Defining Characteristics
Weak/absent cough reflex
Abnormal breath sounds

Absent gag reflex

Patient Outcomes
Airway clearance will be maintained/restored, as evidenced by
- clear breath sounds
- patent airway

Nursing Interventions	Rationales
Provide adequate humidification with oxygen.	Humidification will prevent drying of airways and assist in mobilizing secretions.
Monitor swallowing and gag reflex closely. Insert NG tube if swallow and/or gag reflex absent.	Swallowing, cough, and gag reflexes may be lost with increased ICP, placing the patient at risk for aspiration.
Utilize sterile suctioning technique.	The use of corticosteroids depresses the immune system making these patients particularly vulnerable to infections.
Hyperoxygenate and hyperventilate before and after suctioning and monitor ICP closely.	Hypercapnea and/or hypoxia can trigger plateau waves and increase ICP.
Suction only when necessary and limit duration to 15 s.	Prolonged and/or frequent suctioning can produce hypoxia and rises in systemic blood pressure, both of which can cause increased ICP.

NURSING DIAGNOSIS: IMPAIRED PHYSICAL MOBILITY

Related To
- Requirement for complete bed rest
- Alterations in motor function
- Need for restraints to protect patient
- Barbiturate coma
- Use of paralyzing agents/sedatives

Defining Characteristics
Limited range of motion
Decreased muscle strength/paresis/posturing
Inability to move purposefully

Patient Outcomes
The patient will
- maintain full joint range of motion
- be free of skin breakdown and/or contractures

Nursing Interventions	Rationales
Assess for physical mobility deficit: leg/arm movement and strength and ability for purposeful movement.	
Increase/maintain limb mobility. Perform active/passive range-of-motion exercises. Support extremities with pillows to prevent or reduce swelling. Encourage the patient to get out of bed two to four times a day when condition is stabilized.	
Utilize boots or high-top shoes to prevent foot drop.	
Change position at least every 2 hr.	
Utilize specialized beds that provide pressure relief.	
Inspect skin every 2 hr for signs of reddening or breakdown. Keep off reddened areas as much as possible.	

NURSING DIAGNOSIS: ALTERED SENSORY PERCEPTION

Related To
- Altered level of consciousness
- Sensory overload
- Hospital environment

Defining Characteristics
Disorientation   Confusion
Restlessness   Irritability
Inability to speak (due to intubation or neurological changes)
Cranial nerve change

Patient Outcomes
Sensory perception will be maintained/restored to optimum level.

Nursing Interventions	Rationales
Assess for preexisting sensory deficits, that is, hearing loss, sight loss, and previous CVA.	This prevents misjudgment of sensory deficits such as judging a patient who needs a hearing aide as unresponsive.
Assess for/record present alterations in sensory perception.	
Increase meaningful stimuli: familiar objects within site, clocks and calendars, favorite music, and TV shows.	
Structure routines as much as possible.	
Orient patient with each contact: 1. Call patient by name. 2. Orient to person, place, time, and situation. 3. Explain all procedures and cares. 4. Maintain eye contact when speaking with patient. 5. Explain all equipment. 6. Speak calmly and quietly. 7. Present information in simple and small amounts.	
Encourage significant others to dialogue with patient even if unresponsive.	Hearing may be one of the last senses lost: so the presence and dialogue of significant others may be comforting and meaningful to the patient.

NURSING DIAGNOSIS: HIGH RISK FOR INJURY

Risk Factors
- Seizures
- Decreased level of consciousness
- Stress ulcer
- Immobility

Patient Outcomes
The patient will remain free of injury.

Nursing Interventions	Rationales
See Appendix C.	

DISCHARGE PLANNING/CONTINUITY OF CARE

Assess need for/type of long-term care and follow-up.
If the discharge destination is home, assess existing supports and the need for assistance.
Determine coping deficits/support needs and institute assistance measures.
Determine knowledge deficits/teaching needs and document and institute a teaching plan.
Refer patient to social services as appropriate.
Communicate coping deficits/support needs and knowledge deficits/learning needs to unit accepting the patient on transfer.

REFERENCES

Drummond, B. L. (1990). Preventing increased intracranial pressure: Nursing care can make the difference. *Focus on Critical Care, 17*(2), 116–122.

Hickman, K. M., Mayer, B. L., & Muwaswes, M. (1990). Intra-cranial pressure monitoring: Review of risk factors associated with infection. *Heart & Lung, 19*(1), 84–91.

Johnson, S. M., Omery, A., & Nikas, D. (1989). Effects of conversation on intracranial pressure in comatose patients. *Heart & Lung, 18*(1), 56–63.

Luchka, S. (1991). Working with ICP monitors. *RN, 54*(4), 34–37.

Marano Morrison, C. A. (1987). Brain herniation syndromes. *Critical Care Nurse, 7*(5), 34–38.

McQuillan, K. A. (1991). Intracranial pressure monitoring: Technical imperatives. *Clinical Issues in Critical Care Nursing, 2*(4), 623–636.

Mitchell, M. (1989). *Neuroscience nursing: A nursing diagnosis approach*, Baltimore, MD: Williams & Wilkins.

Shepard, R. & Hotter, A. N. (1989). Evaluating an ICP epidural catheter. *Critical Care Nurse, 9*(2), 74–80.

Stewart-Amidei, C. (1991). Assessing the comatose patient in the intensive care unit. *Clinical Issues in Critical Care Nursing, 2*(4), 613–622.

Thelan, L. A., Davie, J. K., & Urden, L. D. (1990). *Textbook of critical care nursing: Diagnosis and management*. St. Louis, MO: Mosby.

INTRACRANIAL INFECTIONS

Intracranial infections may be the result of neurological injury, such as head trauma, or may occur without injury. The most common infecting organisms are bacteria, parasites, or viruses. Infection may result in cerebral or spinal edema, neuronal injury, or infarction. Contributing factors may include immunosuppression due to steroids, chemotherapy or radiation therapy, surgical incisions, and nutritional depletion. The result of intracranial infections ranges from full recovery to brain tissue injury and/or death from increased ICP, decreased cerebral blood flow, arteritis, thrombophlebitis, and toxic factors.

Meningitis is an acute inflammation of the pia mater and arachnoid meninges caused by an infection carried via the cerebrospinal fluid (CSF) to the entire brain and spinal cord. The infection is most often introduced from the bloodstream or from contiguous infected areas (sinuses, middle ear, penetrating head injuries). The bacteria and their toxins can lead to vasculitis with necrosis of cortical parenchyma, hydrocephalus, petechial hemorrhages within the brain, cranial nerve neuritis, and ependymitis. Adults who develop meningitis (most frequently pneumococcal), usually have some predisposing/underlying disease such as alcoholism, malignancy, immunodeficiency, diabetes, pneumonia, or renal disease.

Encephalitis is an inflammation of the parenchyma of the brain and meninges in response to infection. It may be caused by a virus, bacteria, rickettsia, fungus, or parasite. Acute viral encephalitis is most commonly caused by arbovirus and herpes simplex infections. Arbovirus causes widespread nerve cell degeneration, edema, and areas of necrosis while herpes causes hemorrhagic necrosis usually in the temporal or frontal lobes. Herpes simplex has a high fatality rate, and diagnosis may be difficult because symptoms are similar to acute functional psychosis, meningitis, subarachnoid hemorrhage, tumor, or abscess.

Brain abscesses most commonly form in the cerebrum and subdural and epidural space via direct extension (osteomyelitis or spread along the wall of a vein) or infective emboli (metastatic abscess). Infection can be introduced via the middle ear, mastoid cells, nasal cavity, nasal sinuses, heart and lung infections, open trauma, or neurosurgery. The infectious agent produces an inflammatory response causing liquefactive necrosis with surrounding cerebral edema. Within 2 weeks the area is usually encapsulated with granulation tissue. The clinical course varies significantly, but the mortality rate is 30–60%.

ETIOLOGIES

- Meningitis
  - 80–90% of cases: *Hemophilus influenzae* (children), *Neisseria meningitidis* (meningococcal), *Streptococcus pneumoniae* (pneumococcal)
  - other bacteria: *Klebsiella, Escherichia coli, Stapyhlococcus aureus, Pseudomonas, Mycobacterium tuberculosis, Listeria monocytogenes*
  - fungi: cryptococcosis, coccidioidomycosis, mucormyocosis, candidiasis, aspergillosis
  - viruses: mumps, enterovirus, herpes simplex, adenovirus, California virus
  - diseases causing immunological suppression: lymphomas, cirrhosis, renal transplant, steroid therapy, AIDS
- Encephalitis
  - arbovirus encephalitis (mosquitoes or ticks)
  - herpes simplex encephalitis
  - postviral: rubella, rubeola, mumps, chickenpox, mononucleosis
  - postvaccination: measles, mumps, rubella
- Brain abscess
  - middle-ear and mastoid infections (40%)
  - sinus infections (10%)
  - metastatic abscesses (50%)

CLINICAL MANIFESTATIONS

- Meningitis: Infection produces
  - fever/chills
  - skin rash
  - tachycardia
  - petechiae
- Meningeal irritation produces
  - headache
  - nuchal rigidity
  - positive Brudzinski's sign
  - positive Kernig's sign
  - exaggerated deep-tendon reflexes
- Increased intracranial pressure produces
  - photophobia
  - altered mental status
  - focal deficits
  - seizures
  - nausea and vomiting

- Encephalitis: Inflammation, infection and increased intracranial pressure produce
  - fever
  - seizures
  - nuchal rigidity
  - dysphasia
  - diplopia
  - ocular paralysis
  - facial muscle weakness
  - headache
  - hemiparesis
  - ataxia
  - blurred vision
  - nystagmus
  - altered mental status
  - difficulty chewing or swallowing
- Brain abscess: Infection, inflammation, and increased intracranial pressure produce
  - headache
  - chills/fever
  - speech disorders
  - irritability
  - stupor
  - localized deficits
  - malaise
  - lethargy
  - seizures
  - confusion
  - motor/sensory impairment
  - signs of increased ICP

CLINICAL/DIAGNOSTIC FINDINGS

- Meningitis
  - lumbar puncture: elevated opening pressure, elevated protein, increased cell count (polymorphonuclear neutrophils [PMNs]), decreased glucose, cloudy
  - CAT scan: hydrocephalus, middle-ear or sinus pus collection, abscess
  - skull films: skull fracture, sinus/mastoid disease
  - positive blood cultures
  - positive CSF cultures
- Encephalitis
  - lumbar puncture: elevated or normal opening pressure, elevated protein and WBC count (monocytes), normal or low glucose, RBCs (herpes)
  - EEG: focal or generalized slowing, seizure activity, paroxysmal burst activity
  - CT scan: low-density lesions in temporal area (herpes)
  - brain biopsy
  - antibody titers

  Brain abscess
  - CAT scan: localized changes in brain density
  - EEG: area of high-voltage, slow wavy activity or phase reversal and electrical silence at abscess location
  - arteriogram: of limited value until abscess encapsulated
  - lumbar puncture: increased opening pressure, elevated WBC count (lymphocytes), elevated protein, normal glucose

NURSING DIAGNOSIS: ALTERED THOUGHT PROCESSES

- Irritation of meninges
- Increased ICP

Defining Characteristics
Confusion
Restlessness
Incoherence
Signs of increased intracranial pressure
Lethargy
Stupor
Disorientation

Patient Outcome
The patient's thought processes will return to patient baseline.

Nursing Interventions	Rationales
Identify patients at risk for meningitis: history of otitis media, mastoiditis, sinusitis, tonsilitis, sepsis, pleuropulmonary infections, head trauma, and craniotomy.	By identifying patients at risk, early diagnosis of intracranial infection may be made.
Identify patients at risk for encephalitis: history of measles, mumps, chickenpox, herpes virus, and mosquito or tick bites.	
Identify patients at risk for brain abscess: history of ear or sinus infection, bacterial endocarditis, and lung infection or acute abdominal infection.	
Assess/monitor neurological status: establish baseline normal; alertness and orientation; clarity of speech; movement of extremities; sensation intactness; appropriateness of behavior; and cranial nerve function. Record and report changes to physician.	

Intracranial Infections

Nursing Interventions	Rationales
Minimize effects of environment on mental status: 1. Reorient patient as needed. 2. Maintain quiet environment, minimizing extraneous stimuli. 3. Provide simple, brief explanations of activities, procedures, or equipment. 4. Provide meaningful, relaxing stimuli to patient. 5. Provide consistent caregivers when possible.	The stresses of the critical care environment (sensory overload, sensory deprivation, and sleep deprivation) can aggravate mental status changes produced physiologically. Taking preventive measures may minimize these environmental effects.
Keep head of bed elevated 30°–45°.	The patient with altered mental status is at risk for vomiting and aspiration. This will also help decrease ICP.
Obtain an order for a NG tube in patients with altered level of consciousness.	The patient with altered level of consciousness is at risk for vomiting and aspiration. Inserting a NG tube and keeping the stomach empty will minimize this risk.
Administer antibiotics as prescribed and monitor effect.	
Control patient temperature with cooling measures.	A fever will increase the metabolic demands of the brain, increase cerebral blood flow, and can lead to increased ICP.

NURSING DIAGNOSIS: ALTERED TISSUE PERFUSION—CEREBRAL

Related To increased ICP

Defining Characteristics
CPP < 60 mmHg
Plateau waves on ICP monitor
Clinical signs of increased ICP

ICP > 15 mmHg

Patient Outcomes

The patient's cerebral tissue perfusion will be maintained/restored, as evidenced by
- CPP > 60 mmHg
- ICP < 15 mmHg
- absence of plateau waves
- neurological signs returning to baseline

Nursing Interventions	Rationales
See Increased Intracranial Pressure	

NURSING DIAGNOSIS: IMPAIRED PHYSICAL MOBILITY

Related To
- Bedrest
- Motor impairment
- Pain with movement
- Altered level of consciousness

Defining Characteristics
Limited range of motion
Impaired coordination
Limited muscle strength
Inability to perform ADLs/move without assistance

Patient Outcomes
Physical mobility will be restored to patient baseline.

Nursing Interventions	Rationales
Assess for physical mobility deficit: leg/arm movement and strength, pain with movement, and ability to perform ADLs.	
Institute measures to maintain limb mobility. Perform range-of-motion exercises. Support extremities with pillows. Encourage patient to perform exercise regimens as prescribed when able. Get patient out of bed as early as possible.	This will maintain muscle strength and tone and prevent or reduce swelling which could interfere with mobility.

Nursing Interventions	Rationales
Avoid pillows under knees. Avoid prolonged periods of hip flexion.	Pillows under knees and/or hip flexion may interfere with lower extremity venous return, increasing the risk for development of deep-vein thrombosis.
Align legs properly when supine (toes and knees pointed toward ceiling). Utilize boots or high-top shoes to maintain foot alignment.	
Apply elastic hose and/or intermittent compression devices to lower extremities.	
Reposition every 1–2 hr. Assess pressure points for redness, blanching or breakdown with each position change.	
Utilize special mattress or bed that will minimize pressure points.	
Keep skin clean, avoiding hot water and overdrying.	
Provide frequent mouth care.	

NURSING DIAGNOSIS: HIGH RISK FOR INJURY

Risk Factors
- Seizures
- Altered level of consciousness

Patient Outcomes
The patient will remain free from injury.

Nursing Interventions	Rationales
Describe and record seizure activity: onset, duration, progression, and type; frequency; presence of aura, incontinence, eye/head deviation, and tongue biting; and postictal state, if any.	

Nursing Interventions	Rationales
Prevent injury during seizure activity: 1. Pad siderails and keep siderails up and bed in low position. 2. Stay with patient during seizure. 3. Remove objects from the environment that may cause patient injury. 4. Do not try to force anything into patient's mouth.	
Maintain/protect airway. If possible, insert oral airway in mouth. Assess need for intubation and have equipment/ventilator on standby. Suction as needed. Keep patient on side if possible.	
Administer medications as prescribed to control seizure activity and monitor effect	

DISCHARGE PLANNING/CONTINUITY OF CARE

- Assess need for/type of long-term care and follow-up.
- If the discharge destination is home, assess existing supports and the need for assistance.
- Determine coping deficits/support needs and institute assistance measures.
- Determine knowledge deficits/teaching needs and document and institute a teaching plan.
- Refer patient to social services as appropriate.
- Communicate coping deficits/support needs and knowledge deficits/teaching needs to unit accepting the patient on transfer.

REFERENCES

Barzaga, R. A., Klen, N. C., & Cunho, B. A. (1992). Herpes simplex meningoencephalitis. *Heart & Lung*, 21(4), 405–406.

Boss, B. J., Heath, J., & Sunderland, P. M. (1990). Alterations in neurologic function. In K. L. McCance & S. E. Huether (Eds.), *Pathophysiology: The biologic basis for disease in adults and children* (pp. 505–508). St. Louis, MO: Mosby.

Mitchell, M. (1989). *Neuroscience nursing: A nursing diagnosis approach*. Baltimore, MD: Williams & Wilkins.

Morgenthaler, D. & Cunha, B. A. (1992). *Listeria monocytogenes* meningoenchephalitis. *Heart & Lung 21*(2), 189–191.

Roos, K. L. & Scheld, W. M. (1988). The management of fulminant meningitis in the intensive care unit. *Critical Care Clinics, 4*(2), 375–392.

MYASTHENIA CRISIS

Myasthenia gravis is an autoimmune disorder causing a reduction in the number of acetylcholine receptors at neuromuscular junctions. The reduced number of receptors is believed to be caused by an antiacetylcholine receptor antibody. The result is decreased muscle depolarization with subsequent muscle weakness.

Crises in myasthenia gravis occur when there is a rapid decrease in neuromuscular function with profound weakness of the respiratory muscles. Such a crisis may be myasthenic or cholinergic. Myasthenic crisis is the result of insufficient acetylcholine. Cholinergic crisis is the result of excess acetylcholine. Both types can produce acute severe muscle weakness and respiratory failure.

ETIOLOGIES

- Infectious or neoplastic process within the thymus
- Myasthenic crisis
  - change/withdrawal of medication
  - emotional/physical stress
  - infection
  - surgery
  - progression of underlying autoimmune disorder
  - drugs: quinidine, aminoglycoside antibiotics, quinine, procainamide, phenothiazines, narcotics, barbiturates, tranquilizers
- Cholinergic crisis: drug overdose

CLINICAL MANIFESTATIONS

- Myasthenic crisis: Insufficient acetylcholine produces
  - increased blood pressure
  - restlessness
  - dyspnea
  - tachycardia
  - apprehension
  - absent cough reflex

- difficulty swallowing
- generalized muscle weakness
- increased bronchial secretions, sweating, or lacrimation
- Cholinergic crisis: Excess acetylcholine produces
  - decreased blood pressure
  - bradycardia
  - restlessness
  - apprehension
  - dyspnea
  - fasciculations
  - difficulty swallowing
  - generalized muscle weakness
  - increased bronchial secretions, sweating, or lacrimation
  - difficulty speaking
  - blurred vision
  - nausea and vomiting
  - abdominal cramps and diarrhea

CLINICAL/DIAGNOSTIC FINDINGS

- Increase in muscle strength with edrophonium chloride (Tensilon) or neostigmine methylsulfate (Prostigmine)
- Electromyography: decrementing muscle response to low-frequency stimulation
- Positive serum antiacetylcholine receptor antibodies

NURSING DIAGNOSIS: INEFFECTIVE BREATHING PATTERN
Related To severe muscle weakness

Defining Characteristics
Hypoventilation
Dyspnea
Tidal volume < 5 mL/kg
PaO_2 < 80
SaO_2 < 90%
Vital capacity < 10 mL/kg

Patient Outcomes
The patient's breathing pattern will be maintained/restored, as evidenced by
- respirations 12–20 per minute
- PaO_2 > 80 torr
- SaO_2 > 90%
- tidal volume 5–7 mL/kg
- vital capacity > 10 mL/kg
- absence of dyspnea

Nursing Interventions	Rationales
Identify underlying condition that may have precipitated crisis.	In order to be able to treat the crisis and prevent future crises, the etiology (cholinergic vs. myasthenic, other triggering factors) must be identified.

Nursing Interventions	Rationales
Assess weakened muscle effect on breathing pattern and record: rate, depth, and rhythm of respiration; airway and breathing effort; and use of accessory muscles. Auscultate breath sounds: adventitious sounds and decreased/absent sounds. Assess ABGs and pulse oximetry as ordered and prn respiratory distress. Assess pulmonary function parameters: tidal volume and vital capacity. Assess for subjective complaints of SOB and DOE. Assess strength of cough/ability to mobilize secretions.	This assessment provides the baseline data against which to gauge deterioration or improvement.
Support airway as appropriate: oral/nasal airway, supplementary oxygen, suctioning, and intubation equipment/ventilator.	
Position patient for ease of respiratory effort, that is, head of bed elevated.	
Provide quiet, restful environment. Allow frequent rest periods during activity. Minimize activity.	Adequate rest and controlled activity decrease oxygen need.
Administer steroids as prescribed and monitor for adverse effects (GI irritation, increased glucose, infection).	Steroids are believed to interrupt the autoimmune response.
Administer anticholinesterase agents as prescribed in myasthenic crisis, hold in cholinergic crisis, and note muscular response.	Anticholinesterase agents such as pyridostigmine increase the response of the muscle to nerve impulses by reducing the action of cholinesterase, allowing acetylcholine to build up at the junction.

Nursing Interventions	Rationales
Administer atropine as prescribed and monitor response.	Anticholinesterase drugs can increase salivation and bronchial secretions. Atropine may be used to control secretions but may mask a cholinergic crisis. Use with caution.
Institute/prepare patient for plasmapharesis and monitor for side effects: hypotension, tachycardia, hypocalcemia, and hypomagnesemia. Withhold drugs during procedure.	Plasmapharesis clears the plasma of antibodies that interfere with acetylcholine receptors. Hypotension and tachycardia can occur as the result of fluid shifts without protein replacement or decreased blood volume. Hypocalcemia can occur due to binding of ionized calcium by citrate or albumin. Hypomagnesemia can follow after repeated sessions of plasmapharesis. Plasmapharesis will remove drugs from the blood.

NURSING DIAGNOSIS: INEFFECTIVE AIRWAY CLEARANCE

Related To
- Muscle weakness
- Inability to manage secretions
- Difficulty swallowing

Defining Characteristics
Absent/decreased cough reflex
Increased secretions
Adventitious lung sounds
Decreased/absent gag reflex

Patient Outcomes
The patient's airway will be maintained, as evidenced by
- clear lung sounds
- intact cough and gag reflexes
- minimal secretions

Nursing Interventions	Rationales
Assess swallowing and gag reflex closely. Insert nasogastric tube if swallow and/or gag reflex absent.	Swallowing and cough and gag reflexes may be lost, placing the patient at risk for aspiration.
Auscultate lung sounds.	
Assess amount/consistency of secretions and ability to mobilize secretions.	Anticholinesterase drugs can increase salivation and bronchial secretions. Muscle weakness may affect the patient's ability to mobilize secretions.
Provide adequate humidification of oxygen.	Humidification will prevent drying of airways and assist in mobilizing secretions.
Assist patient with coughing and deep breathing.	Weakened respiratory muscles produce hypoventilation resulting in pooling of secretions, atelectasis, and possible pneumonia.
Assist removal of secretions via nasotracheal or orotracheal suctioning as needed.	Due to weakened respiratory muscles and increased secretions, the patient may not be able to cough up secretions.
Reposition patient every 2 hr.	
Monitor fluid balance closely.	Adequate fluid balance is an influential factor in the ability to mobilize secretions.
Use sterile suctioning technique.	The use of steroids depresses the immune system, making the patient more prone to infections.

NURSING DIAGNOSIS: IMPAIRED PHYSICAL MOBILITY

Related To
- Severe muscle weakness
- Bedrest

Defining Characteristics
Limited range of motion
Limited muscle strength
Impaired coordination
Inability to move without assistance

Patient Outcomes
The patient's physical mobility will be restored to patient baseline.

Nursing Interventions	Rationales
Assess for physical mobility deficit: leg/arm movement and strength and ability to perform ADLs.	
Perform range-of-motion exercises. When/if able, encourage patient to perform exercise regimens as prescribed. Get patient out of bed as early as possible.	
Support extremities with pillows	This prevents or reduces swelling.
Space/pace activities to prevent overtiring. Encourage most demanding activities in early morning. Allow for periods of rest between activities.	Clinical manifestations grow more prominent throughout the day as the patient fatigues.
Avoid pillows under knees. Avoid prolonged periods of hip flexion.	Pillows under knees and hip flexion can interfere with lower extremity venous return, increasing the risk for the development of deep-vein thrombosis.
Align legs properly when supine (toes and knees pointed toward ceiling). Utilize boots or high-top shoes to maintain foot alignment.	
Apply elastic hose and/or intermittent pneumatic compression devices to lower extremities.	
Turn and reposition every 2 hr. Assess pressure points for redness, blanching or breakdown with each position change.	
Keep skin clean, avoiding hot water and overdrying.	
Provide frequent mouth care.	

▼

NURSING DIAGNOSIS: CARDIAC OUTPUT

Related To
- Insufficient acetylcholine
- Excess acetylcholine

Defining Characteristics
Myasthenic crisis: increased blood pressure, tachycardia
Cholinergic crisis: decreased blood pressure, bradycardia

Patient Outcomes
The patient's cardiac output will be maintained, as evidenced by
- blood pressure return to patient baseline
- heart rate 60–100 bpm

Nursing Interventions	Rationales
Assess/monitor cardiovascular status: vital signs and hemodynamic parameters (CVP/PCWP, CO/CI, MAP)	
Monitor heart rhythm continuously.	
Assess effects of abnormal heart rhythm on hemodynamics, that is, CO, blood pressure, and CVP/PCWP.	
Treat cardiac dysrhythmias according to established protocol.	
Administer treatments/medications to combat crisis (see appropriate interventions under Ineffective Breathing Pattern).	
If necessary, administer medications to maintain blood pressure within normal range as ordered and monitor effects.	

DISCHARGE PLANNING/CONTINUITY OF CARE

- Assess need for/type of long-term care and follow-up.
- If the discharge destination is home, assess existing supports and the need for assistance.

- Determine coping deficits/support needs and institute assistance measures.
- Determine knowledge deficits/teaching needs and document and institute a teaching plan.
- Refer patient to social services as appropriate.
- Communicate coping deficits/support needs and knowledge deficits/learning needs to unit accepting the patient on transfer.

REFERENCES

Bell, J. (1989). Understanding and managing myasthenia gravis. *Focus on Critical Care*, *16*(1), 57–65.

Chipps, E. (1991). Myasthenia gravis: The patient in crisis. *Critical Care Nurse*, *11*(7), 18–26.

Hickey, J. V. (1991). Myasthenia crisis—your assessment counts. *RN*, *54*(5), 54–58.

Hood, L. J. (1990). Myasthenia gravis: Regimens and regimen-associated problems in adults. *Journal of Neuroscience Nursing*, *22*, 358–363.

Litchfield, M. & Norolan E. (1989). Changes in selected pulmonary functions in patients diagnosed with myasthenia gravis. *Journal of Neuroscience Nursing*, *21*, 375–381.

Mascarella, J. J. & Hudson, D. C. (1991). Dysimmune neurologic disorders. *AACN Clinical Issues in Critical Care Nursing*, *2*(4), 675–677.

▼

STATUS EPILEPTICUS

Status epilepticus exists when seizures last for more than 30 min or sequential seizures occur without return to baseline between attacks. These seizures can take multiple forms (see below). Status epilepticus is dangerous because sustained seizure activity can cause hypoxemia or anoxia, hypoglycemia, cardiac dysrhythmias, acidosis, and respiratory failure. If not corrected within 1–2 hr, these sequelae can result in permanent neurological damage or death.

Convulsive status epilepticus consists of tonic-clonic partial seizures that generalize or primary generalized seizures (less common). These seizures are usually of a few minutes duration followed by a prolonged period of unconsciousness leading to the next seizure. With recurrent seizures the tonic activity (generalized contractions of muscles) is lengthened and clonic activity (violent, rhythmic jerking muscle contractions) is shortened.

Partial status epilepticus is the second most common type of seizure and is characterized by focal clonic or tonic-clonic activity localized to the face or an extremity but may spread. Consciousness is usually intact. Epilepsia partialis continua is a form of partial motor status with continuous localized seizures that do not generalize and consciousness is maintained.

Myoclonic status epilepticus consists of repetitive, asynchronous myoclonus (spasm of a muscle or group of muscles) with variable clouding of consciousness. They may evolve into generalized tonic-clonic seizures. In the adult these types of seizures are usually secondary to acute or subacute encephalopathies with toxic, metabolic, viral, or degenerative origins.

Nonconvulsive status epilepticus consists of absence seizures and complex partial status seizures. They may resemble psychiatric fugue states. Absence seizures consist of variable levels of alertness with subtle myoclonic movements of the face (fluttering of eyelids) and occasional automatisms of the face (lip smacking, chewing, swallowing) and hands. Complex partial status consists of a series of complex partial seizures with staring, unresponsiveness, and motor automatisms separated by a twilight state OR a more prolonged state of partial responsiveness and semipurposeful automatisms.

ETIOLOGIES

- Central nervous system infection
  - meningitis
  - encephalitis
- Toxic drugs
  - theophylline
  - xylocaine
  - penicillin
  - withdrawal states (alcohol, barbiturates)
- Structural brain lesion
  - trauma
  - tumor
  - CVA
- Metabolic
  - hypocalcemia
  - hyponatremia
  - hypomagnesemia
  - anoxia
  - uremia
  - hyperosmolar state
  - hyper- or hypoglycemia
- Degenerative diseases
  - Alzheimer's
  - multiple sclerosis
  - Huntington's chorea
  - Pick's
- Precipitating factors
  - change in anticonvulsant blood levels: change in drug therapy, change in drug absorption, noncompliance, errors in medication
  - underlying infection
  - alcohol excess or withdrawal

CLINICAL MANIFESTATIONS

Convulsive status epilepticus
- Tachycardia
- Hypertension
- Positive Babinski
- Hyperthermia
- Memory impairment
- Hypoxia
- Loss of corneal and pupil reflexes

Systemic complications (after 30 min)
- Cardiovascular
  - early (due to increased sympathetic activity): tachycardia, hypertension
  - late: bradycardia, cardiac arrest, hypotension, shock (lactic acidosis) dysrhythmias (autonomic overactivity, acidosis, hyperkalemia)
- Pulmonary
  - early: tachypnea, apnea with CO_2 retention
  - late (related to mechanical impairment from tonic muscle contraction, disturbed respiratory center function, and massive autonomic discharge producing bronchial constriction and secretions): apnea, aspiration, Cheyne-Stokes respirations, neurogenic pulmonary edema (increase in pulmonary circulation with transcapillary fluid flux)

- Renal
  - late (related to combination of rhabdomyolysis with myoglobinuria and hypotension with poor renal perfusion): uremia, myoglobinuria, ATN
- Autonomic nervous system
  - early: mydiasis, excessive sweating, salivary and tracheobronchial hypersecretion, bronchial constriction
  - late: hyperpyrexia, hyperthermia (excessive muscle activity and hypothalamic dysfunction)

CLINICAL/DIAGNOSTIC FINDINGS

- EEG depends on type of seizure
- Lactic acidosis (>2.2 mEq/L)
- Hyperkalemia (>5 mEq/L)
- Glucose > 115 mg/dL (early catecholamine and glucagon release); glucose < 60 mg/dL (late increased plasma insulin consumption and excess muscle activity)
- Prolactin > 23 ng/mL (women); > 20 ng/mL (men)

NURSING DIAGNOSIS: ALTERED TISSUE PERFUSION—CEREBRAL AND CARDIOPULMONARY

Related To
- Continuous seizure activity
- Increased oxygen demand
- Decreased blood flow

Defining Characteristics
Continuous/repetitive seizure activity
Tachycardia   Hypertension/hypotension
Dysrhythmias   Tachycardia/bradycardia
Hyperthermia

Patient Outcomes
Cerebral and cardiopulmonary perfusion will be maintained/restored as evidenced by
- heart rate 60–100 bpm
- blood pressure return to patient baseline
- normothermia
- absence of seizure activity
- absence of dysrhythmias

Nursing Interventions	Rationales
Assess for possible etiologies: 1. omission of anticonvulsant medication 2. precipitating factors, that is, fever, emotional or physical stress, hypoxia 3. previous conditions: head injury, drug/alcohol abuse, CNS infections, toxic drugs, metabolic problems, preexisting neurological conditions 4. electrolyte abnormalities: hypocalcemia, hyponatremia, hypomagnesemia, hypoglycemia, hyperosmolar state	Determining the underlying cause enables correct long-term treatment.
Assess neurological status: Establish baseline normal, alertness and orientation, clarity of speech, movement of extremities, sensation intactness, and appropriateness of behavior. Record and report changes to physician.	Assessing neurological status allows for early detection of deterioration.
Describe and record seizure activity: onset, duration, progression, and type; frequency; presence of aura, incontinence, and eye/head deviation; tongue biting; and postictal state, if any.	This helps establish baseline data against which to compare subsequent/ongoing seizure activity.
Monitor/record cardiovascular status before, during and after seizure activity: vital signs (including temperature) and dysrhythmias.	Seizure activity can cause tachycardia, hyper- or hypotension, hyperthermia, and dysrhythmias. The drugs utilized to treat seizures can also cause hypotension and dysrhythmias.
Administer 50% dextrose and thiamine 100 mg IV as prescribed and monitor patient response.	These drugs are used to prevent hypoglycemia and support the high metabolic demands created by continuous seizure activity.

Nursing Interventions	Rationales
Administer lorazepam (Ativan) as prescribed (0.1 mg/kg IV bolus; < 2 mg/min if seizing) and monitor for respiratory depression	Lorazepam is a benzodiazepine sedative that interrupts seizure activity by inhibiting neurotransmitters. It has a longer duration than diazepam but will not prevent more seizures.
Administer diazepam (Valium) as prescribed (0.25–0.4 mg/kg; 5–10 mg IV); up to 30 mg in 1 hr; may repeat in 2–3 hr). Monitor for hypotension and respiratory depression.	Diazepam is a benzodiazepine sedative that interrupts seizure activity by inhibiting presynaptic activity. It will not prevent future seizures.
Administer phenytoin (Dilantin) as prescribed (usual dose: 15–20 mg/kg IV at <50 mg/min; additional doses 5 mg/kg up to 30 mg/kg). Monitor for hypotension, EKG changes and respiratory depression. Use normal saline only for flush.	Phenytoin limits seizure activity by altering ion transport and decreasing synaptic transmission. It can prolong the Q-T interval and produce dysrhythmias in patients with underlying cardiac disease.
Administer phenobarbital as prescribed (usual loading dose: 20 mg/kg IV at <100 mg/min). Monitor for respiratory depression, increased secretions, and prolonged coma.	Phenobarbital limits seizure activity by inhibiting transmission in the nervous system and raising the seizure threshold.
Administer pentobarbital (Nembutal) as prescribed (usual dose: 5 mg/kg IV load; 0.5–2 mg/kg/hr maintenance). Induces coma; patient must be intubated. Infiltration may cause local tissue injury.	If unable to control seizures with the above medications, it will be necessary to induce a coma to halt seizure activity.

NURSING DIAGNOSIS: IMPAIRED GAS EXCHANGE

Related To
- Hypoventilation/apnea
- Decreased respiratory rate
- Increased oxygen need
- Aspiration
- Antiseizure medications

Defining Characteristics
Bradypnea
$PaCO_2 > 45$ torr
$SaO_2 < 90\%$
$PaO_2 < 80$ torr
$pH < 7.35$

Patient Outcomes
Gas exchange will be maintained/restored as evidenced by
- ABG pH 7.35–7.45, $PaCO_2$ 35–45 torr, $PaO_2 > 80$ torr
- normal respiratory pattern
- SaO_2/pulse oximetry > 90%

Nursing Interventions	Rationales
Assess/record respiratory status: rate, depth, and rhythm of respirations; use of accessory muscles; breath sounds; ability to handle secretions; and amount/quality of secretions.	Prolonged seizure activity can cause respiratory depression or respiratory arrest.
Monitor ABGs and/or pulse oximetry as indicated.	
Monitor effects of antiseizure medications on respirations.	Most of the drugs used to control seizure activity also cause respiratory depression.
Maintain/protect airway. If possible, insert oral airway in mouth. Assess need for intubation; have equipment/ventilator on standby. Suction as needed. Turn patient on side as soon as possible.	Continuous seizure activity can cause closure of the patient's airway and respiratory arrest. The patient will be unable to swallow secretions during seizure activity, and suctioning and/or turning the patient may prevent aspiration.
Administer oxygen as prescribed and monitor patient response.	Continuous seizure activity increases the demand for oxygen.

NURSING DIAGNOSIS: ALTERED TISSUE PERFUSION—RENAL

Related To
- Rhabdomyolysis with myoglobinuria
- Hypotension with decreased renal perfusion

Defining Characteristics
Uremia
Urine output < 30 mL/hr
Myoglobinuria

Patient Outcomes

Renal tissue perfusion will be maintained/restored, as evidenced by
- BUN 5–20 mg/dL; creatinine 0.6–1.2 mg/dL
- urine output > 30 mL/hr
- absence of myoglobinuria

Nursing Interventions	Rationales
Monitor fluid balance and notify physician of abnormalities: intake and output, daily weight, and serum electrolytes.	
Monitor renal function and notify physician of abnormalities: BUN, creatinine, hourly urine output, and color of urine.	Vigorous muscle contraction can cause muscle cell breakdown, releasing large amounts of myoglobin into the blood. Myoglobin can occlude the kidneys and precipitate renal failure. Red- or cola-colored urine may indicate the presence of myoglobin.
Administer fluids and diuretics as prescribed and monitor response.	Fluids and diuretics help flush the renal system and thus flush out the myoglobin.

NURSING DIAGNOSIS: HIGH RISK FOR INJURY

Risk Factors
- Seizure activity
- Altered level of consciousness

Patient Outcomes
The patient will remain free of injury.

Nursing Interventions	Rationales
Pad siderails.	
Stay with patient during seizure. Remove objects from environment that may cause patient injury; loosen clothing.	
Do not try to force anything into patient's mouth.	

Nursing Interventions	Rationales
Keep siderails up and bed in low position.	
Turn patient to side if possible.	If the patient vomits during the seizure, this helps prevent aspiration.
Reorient patient when seizure is over.	
Assess patient for injury when seizure is over, that is, bruises, and biting of tongue.	
Avoid excessive stimulation after seizure.	Bright lights and abrupt movement or sudden noises could reactivate seizure activity.
Maintain patient on bedrest.	

DISCHARGE PLANNING/CONTINUITY OF CARE

- Assess need for/type of long-term care and follow-up.
- If the discharge destination is home, assess existing supports and the need for assistance.
- Determine coping deficits/support needs and institute assistance measures.
- Determine knowledge deficits/teaching needs and document and institute a teaching plan.
- Refer patient to social services as appropriate.
- Communicate coping deficits/support needs and knowledge deficits/learning needs to unit accepting the patient on transfer.

REFERENCES

Miller, J. A. & Hallenbeck, J. M. (1989). Pharmacologic approach to acute seizures. In B. Chernow (Ed.), *Essentials of critical care pharmacology* (pp. 222–235). Baltimore, MD: Williams & Wilkins.

Mitchell, M. (1989). Seizures. *Neuroscience nursing: A Nursing diagnosis approach.* Baltimore, MD: Williams & Wilkins.

Phillips, C. & Blumenfeld, A. M. (1991). Status epilepticus. In J. M. Rippe, R. S. Irwin, J. S. Alpert, & M. P. Fink (Eds.), *Intensive care medicine* (2nd ed., pp. 1565–1570). Boston, MA: Little Brown.

Vallerand, A. H. & Deglin, J. H. (1991). *Nurse's guide for IV medications.* Philadelphia, PA: Davis.

Pulmonary Care

▼

ACUTE RESPIRATORY DISTRESS SYNDROME

Acute respiratory distress syndrome (ARDS), also known as high-permeability pulmonary edema, is a form of noncardiogenic pulmonary edema. When the alveolar-capillary membrane is damaged, large molecules escape from the vascular space into the interstitial space, increasing oncotic pressure and pulling fluid with them. The fluid that accumulates in the alveolar and interstitial space and small airways impairs ventilation and oxygenation of capillary blood. Severe hypoxemia is a hallmark of this physiological condition.

The management of ARDS is supportive, with the goal of allowing the injured lungs time to recover while maintaining oxygenation to organ systems. Therapies are aimed at treating the underlying cause of ARDS as well as preventing multisystem complications.

ETIOLOGIES

- Sepsis syndrome
- Cardiopulmonary bypass
- Surgery
- Burns
- Hypertransfusions
- Fractures
- Disseminated intravascular coagulation
- Pneumonia
- Pulmonary aspiration
- Fat embolism

CLINICAL MANIFESTATIONS

- Pulmonary: Impaired ventilation and oxygenation can produce
  - dyspnea
  - pink, frothy sputum
  - cough
  - decreased lung compliance

- shortness of breath
- use of accessory muscles
- fine crackles
- decreased/absent breath sounds
- tachypnea
- thin, frothy sputum
- wheezes
- Cardiovascular: Noncardiogenic pulmonary edema and hypoxemia can produce
  - tachycardia
  - hypotension or hypertension
  - dysrhythmias
  - diaphoresis
- Neurological: Decreased oxygenation can produce
  - confusion
  - changes in orientation
  - fatigue
  - restlessness
  - agitation

CLINICAL/DIAGNOSTIC FINDINGS

- Chest x-ray
  - ground-glass appearance or white-out without signs of cardiac failure
  - diffuse alveolar/interstitial infiltrates
- Arterial blood gases
  - respiratory alkalosis ($PaCO_2$ < 35 torr; pH > 7.45)
  - refractory hypoxemia (PaO_2 < 55 torr)
  - increased intrapulmonary shunt [arterial to alveolar oxygen (a/A) ratio <0.75]
- Hemodynamics
  - CO < 4 L/min
  - CVP > 10 mmHg
  - PCWP normal (8–12 mmHg) or low
  - pulmonary hypertension (increased pulmonary artery pressure, i.e., >25–30/8–12 mmHg)

NURSING DIAGNOSIS: IMPAIRED GAS EXCHANGE

Related To
- Alveolar-capillary injury
- Alveolar edema
- Ventilation/perfusion mismatch

Defining Characteristics
SaO_2 < 90%
Cyanosis
Confusion
Irritability

PaO_2 < 60 torr
Tachycardia
Restlessness
Dizziness

Patient Outcomes

Gas exchange will be restored, as evidenced by
- ABGs within normal range
- $SaO_2 > 90\%$
- $PaO_2 > 60$ torr
- $CO > 4$ L/min
- absence of cyanosis
- absence of confusion, restlessness, irritability, dizziness
- heart rate 60–100 bpm

Nursing Interventions	Rationales
Assess for changes in level of consciousness and anxiety (restlessness, O_2 hunger).	Anxiety or changes in level of consciousness may indicate oxygen desaturation.
Monitor hemoglobin, PaO_2 and SaO_2.	Hemoglobin is the major oxygen-carrying compound. The PaO_2 reflects how much oxygen is in the blood. The saturation of hemoglobin is reflected by SaO_2. Oxygen transport is compromised with oxygen saturation less than 90%.
Monitor arterial pH and blood lactate levels.	These levels reflect overall acid-base balance.
Administer oxygen as prescribed and make changes as needed according to blood gas analysis or pulse oximeter changes.	Supplementary oxygen may be required to provide for adequate gas exchange.
Determine cardiac output.	Cardiac output is the primary determinant of oxygen delivery to the tissues.
Maintain patient on continuous positive pressure ventilation (positive pressure tidal ventilation with positive end-expiratory pressure).	By increasing the degree of alveolar recruitment and distention, continuous positive pressure ventilation lessens intrapulmonary shunt and improves arterial oxygenation.

Nursing Interventions	Rationales
Consider pressure control inverse ratio ventilation.	Increased inspiratory time and decreased expiratory time increases functional residual capacity and lowers peak airway pressures. Pressure control inverse ratio ventilation is thought to reduce the likelihood of iatrogenic lung damage from positive pressure ventilation (high peak inspiratory pressure).
Maintain patency of endotracheal tube by suctioning.	Endotracheal suctioning removes secretions and debris from the tracheobronchial tree and promotes airway patency facilitating ventilation.
Turn patient every 2 hr.	Position changes reduce pooling of secretions in the dependent areas of the lung.
Consider use of prone or semi-prone position.	The prone position has been found to improve oxygenation.
Consider paralytics. Administer sedatives as prescribed and monitor patient response.	Paralytic agents decrease oxygen requirements of muscles.
Administer therapies to reduce intravascular volume.	These therapies help to reduce lung edema and improve gas exchange.
Consider administration of exogenous surfactant as prescribed and monitor patient response.	Loss of surfactant activity is thought to be a component of ARDS.
Consider administration of anti-inflammatory agents as prescribed and monitor patient response.	A generalized inflammatory response is thought to underlie ARDS associated with septic shock.

NURSING DIAGNOSIS: INEFFECTIVE BREATHING PATTERN

Related To increased work of breathing due to increased resistance and decreased compliance

Defining Characteristics
Increased $PaCO_2$ with decreasing pH
Decreasing PaO_2
Increased respiratory rate
Use of accessory muscles of ventilation
Paradoxic breathing pattern/asymmetrical chest expansion
Diminished breath sounds
Atelectatic crackles

Patient Outcomes
An effective breathing pattern will be restored, as evidenced by
- absence of cyanosis
- respiratory rate 12–20 at rest
- absence of crackles or wheezes
- ability to breathe independent of ventilator
- equal, full breath sounds
- minimal or absent atelectatic crackles
- vital capacity > 10 mL/kg or 20–25% of predicted normal
- inspiratory force -20 to -25 cm H_2O
- resting spontaneous minute ventilation < 10 L/min

Nursing Interventions	Rationales
Monitor $PaCO_2$ via ABGs or capnography.	Interstitial fibrosis and capillary obliteration with ARDS causes increased dead space and CO_2 retention.
Administer ventilation to patient via intubation with positive pressure ventilation.	Assisted ventilation will improve the ventilatory pattern, returning pH and $PaCO_2$ to within normal limits.
Consider providing inverse ratio ventilation.	Increased inspiratory time and decreased expiratory time increase functional residual capacity and lower peak airway pressures.
Position patient with head of bed elevated.	This facilitates diaphragmatic descent for the best use of ventilatory muscles.
Administer theophylline as prescribed and monitor drug levels.	Theophylline has been reported to improve contractility of the diaphragm and other respiratory muscles, although this is not well defined.

NURSING DIAGNOSIS: INEFFECTIVE AIRWAY CLEARANCE

Related To
- Airway closure
- Excess or retained secretions
- Alveolar congestion

Defining Characteristics
Adventitious breath sounds
Lung fields congested on chest x-ray
Diminished breath sounds
Decreasing PaO_2
Ineffective cough
$PaCO_2 > 45$ torr

Patient Outcomes
Effective airway clearance is restored, as evidenced by
- ability to cough up secretions
- ability to breathe off ventilator
- ABGs within normal range or returned to baseline
- thin mucus produced by cough or suctioning
- absence of clinical manifestations of infection
- clear lung fields on chest x-ray

Nursing Interventions	Rationales
Auscultate lung fields for presence of adventitious sounds.	Adventitious breath sounds indicate the need for suctioning.
Monitor ABGs as prescribed and prn respiratory distress.	The ABGs provide an accurate method to assess for adequate ventilation and oxygenation.
Monitor serial chest x-rays.	
Apply humidified oxygen.	Humidified oxygen prevents drying of secretions.
Suction with presence of adventitious lung sounds.	Suctioning can remove secretions from the trachea and main bronchi.
Reposition patient frequently.	Repositioning helps match ventilation with perfusion.
Administer medications as prescribed and monitor patient response: beta adrenergics, methylxanthines, anticholinergics, mucolytics, antibiotics, and expectorants.	These medications may be used to improve mucociliary clearance.

Nursing Interventions	Rationales
Implement measures to prevent respiratory infections (strict aseptic technique).	Depressed mucociliary clearance provides an environment conducive to the development of infection.

NURSING DIAGNOSIS: DECREASED CARDIAC OUTPUT

Related To
- Hypoxemia
- Increased PEEP (increased intrathoracic pressure)
- Positive pressure ventilation
- Heart failure

Defining Characteristics
Hypotension
Bradycardia
CO < 4 L/min
Cardiovascular collapse
Warm flushed skin
Dysrhythmias
CI < 2.5 L/min/m^2

Patient Outcomes
Cardiac output is restored, as evidenced by
- CO 4–8 L/min; CI 2.5–4 L/min/m^2
- blood pressure within 10 mmHg of patient baseline
- heart rate 60–100 bpm
- PCWP 8–12 mmHg
- absence of cardiovascular collapse

Nursing Interventions	Rationales
Assess and document cardiovascular status: vital signs, hemodynamics, and peripheral pulses. Assess for signs of cardiovascular collapse: bradycardia, hypotension, increased CVP/PCWP, decreased CO/CI, decreased MAP, and weak peripheral pulses.	Positive pressure ventilation and PEEP cause decreased venous return to the heart and decreased cardiac output.
Administer vasoactive drugs to support cardiac output as needed.	Positive inotropic agents may be needed to support cardiac output.

Nursing Interventions	Rationales
Reduce myocardial oxygen consumption by providing calm environment and administering sedatives/paralytics and comfort measures.	
Administer fluids as necessary.	Fluid administration is used to augment preload.
Identify causes of dysrhythmias and treat according to protocol. Assess effect on cardiac output.	Dysrhythmias may further decrease cardiac output.
Administer vasodilators to reduce pulmonary vascular resistance.	Increased right ventricular afterload is common due to pulmonary vasoconstriction, endothelial edema, and intravascular microembolism or fibrosis. Prostaglandin E_1 acts as a pure pulmonary vasodilator and has been shown to lower pulmonary vascular resistance and increase cardiac output. Nitroprusside has been shown to impair hypoxic pulmonary vasoconstriction and may worsen arterial oxygenation.

DISCHARGE PLANNING/CONTINUITY OF CARE

- Assess need for/type of long-term care and follow-up.
- If the discharge destination is home, assess existing supports and the need for assistance.
- Determine coping deficits/support needs and institute assistance measures.
- Determine knowledge deficits/teaching needs and document and institute teaching plan.
- Refer patient to social services as appropriate.
- Communicate coping deficits/support needs and knowledge deficits/teaching needs to unit accepting patient on transfer.

REFERENCES

Ahrens, T. (1989). Blood gas assessment of intrapulmonary shunting and deadspace. *Critical Care Nursing Clinics of North America*, 1(4), 641–648.

East, T. D., Bohm, S. H., Wallace, J., Clemmer, T. P., Weaver, L. K., Orme, J. F., & Morris, A. H. (1992). A successful computerized protocol for clinical management of pressure control inverse ratio ventilation in ARDS patients. *Chest, 101*(3), 697–710.

Hudson, L. D. (1990). The prediction and prevention of ARDS. *Respiratory Care, 35*(2), 161–171.

Humphrey, H., Hall, J., Sznajder, I., Silverstein, M., & Wood, L. (1990). Improved survival in ARDS patients associated with a reduction in pulmonary capillary wedge pressure. *Chest, 97*(5), 1176–1179.

Idell, S. (1989). The deadly danger of ARDS. *Emergency Medicine, 21*(7), 67–72.

Lanken, P. N. (1990). New therapeutic approaches for ARDS. *Hospital Practice, 1*, 42–45.

Maunder, R. J. & Hudson, L. D. (1990). Pharmacologic strategies for treating the adult respiratory distress syndrome. *Respiratory Care, 35*(3), 241–245.

Mims, B. C. (1989). Fat embolism: A variant of ARDS. *Orthopaedic Nurse, 8*(3), 22–27.

Roberts, S. L. (1990). High permeability pulmonary edema: Nursing assessment, diagnosis and intervention. *Heart & Lung, 19*(3), 287–299.

Schmitz, T. M. (1991). The semi-prone position in ARDS: Five case studies. *Critical Care Nurse, 11*(5), 22–33.

Vaughan, P. & Brooks, C. (1990). Adult respiratory distress syndrome. *Critical Care Clinics of North America, 2*(2), 235–253.

White, B. S., & Roberts, S. L. (1991). Nursing management of high permeability pulmonary edema. *Intensive Care Nursing, 7*, 11–22.

▼

ACUTE RESPIRATORY FAILURE

The respiratory system consists of two parts: the lung as a gas-exchanging organ and the ventilatory pump that ventilates the lung. Failure of the lung leads mainly to failure of gas delivery and cellular function, which results in hypoxemia (respiratory failure). Failure of the ventilatory pump leads mainly to alveolar hypoventilation. Failure of the pump can occur from central nervous system disorders which drive the pump of the lung to the muscles which are responsible for inspiration. Early signs of acute respiratory failure are the result of inadequate gas exchange and include primarily symptoms of respiratory distress. Acute respiratory acidosis (carbon dioxide retention) is a late manifestation of respiratory failure and is usually preceded by dyspnea, tachypnea, and uncoordinated chest wall movements.

ETIOLOGIES

- Respiratory dysfunction and failure of gas exchange in the lung secondary to
  - ventilation/perfusion mismatch
  - intrapulmonary shunts
  - failure of diffusion across alveolar capillary membrane
  - decreased oxygen transport (decreased cardiac output, decreased hemoglobin, decreased partial pressure of dissolved oxygen in the arteries)
- Ventilatory dysfunction secondary to
  - chronic obstructive pulmonary disease (COPD)
  - restrictive lung disease
  - neuromuscular disease: stroke, extrapyramidal disorders, spinal cord injuries (above C4), lower motor neuron disease (paralytic poliomyelitis, amyotrophic lateral sclerosis)
  - neurological dysfunction
  - acute respiratory distress syndrome (ARDS)
  - asthma
  - thorax deformities

- bronchiectasis
- viral or bacterial pneumonia
- inhalation injuries
- cor pulmonale with pulmonary edema
- central respiratory drive depression (drug induced)
- abnormal chest wall function
- thoracic surgery

CLINICAL MANIFESTATIONS

- Pulmonary: Impaired ventilation and gas exchange can produce
  - dyspnea
  - tachypnea
  - tachycardia
  - use of accessory muscles
  - paradoxic breathing pattern
  - intercostal retractions
  - neck vein distention
- Central nervous system: Impaired ventilation and gas exchange can produce
  - altered level of consciousness
  - seizures
  - papilledema
  - sleep disturbances
- Cardiovascular: Impaired gas exchange can produce
  - dysrhythmias
  - tachycardia
  - hypertension (systolic)
  - palpitations
  - chest pain
- Skin: Impaired ventilation and gas exchange can produce
  - pallor
  - cyanosis
  - clammy skin
  - cool skin
  - flushed skin

CLINICAL/DIAGNOSTIC FINDINGS

- $SaO_2 < 90\%$
- $PaO_2 < 60$ torr
- Acidosis (pH < 7.35)
- Vital capacity < 10 mL/kg
- Hemoglobin < 13 g/dL
- CO < 4 L/min

NURSING DIAGNOSIS: INEFFECTIVE BREATHING PATTERN

Related To
- Inspiratory muscle fatigue
- Respiratory muscle deconditioning from mechanical ventilation
- Chronic airflow limitations

- Chest wall restrictions
- Abdominal pain

Defining Characteristics
Increased $PaCO_2$ with decreasing pH
Decreasing PaO_2
Respiratory rate > 30
Subjective complaints of dyspnea
Subjective complaints of fatigue
Use of accessory muscles of ventilation
Paradoxic breathing pattern/asymmetrical chest expansion
Diminished breath sounds
Atelectatic crackles

Patient Outcomes
The breathing pattern is restored/returned to baseline, as evidenced by
- respiratory rate 12–20 at rest
- $PaCO_2$ return to baseline
- pH 7.35–7.45
- equal, full breath sounds
- symmetric chest expansion
- minimal or absent atelectatic crackles
- vital capacity > 10 mL/kg or 20–25% of predicted normal
- inspiratory force -20 to -25 cm H_2O
- resting spontaneous minute ventilation < 10 L/min

Nursing Interventions	Rationales
Assess patient fear/anxiety and assist with coping strategies	Fear and anxiety are a common response to breathing difficulties. However, if not dealt with adequately, they can also worsen the patient's respiratory status.
Monitor ventilation and oxygenation by use of arterial blood gas analysis or capnography and/or pulse oximetry.	Monitoring $PaCO_2$ is the primary assessment used to evaluate ventilation. The assessment parameters PaO_2 and SaO_2 are used to evaluate oxygenation. Capnography can track trending in CO_2 levels. It needs to be correlated with arterial pH, $PaCO_2$, and clinical assessment findings.

Nursing Interventions	Rationales
Monitor criteria for weaning from mechanical ventilation: vital capacity, inspiratory force, forced expiratory volume in 1 s, and respiratory rate.	
Administer ventilation to patient via 1. intubation with mechanical ventilation 2. pressure support ventilation 3. continuous positive airway pressure (CPAP) mask 4. nasal mask	Assisted ventilation will improve the ventilatory pattern, returning the pH and $PaCO_2$ to within normal limits. Underlying disorders which have impaired the breathing pattern can then be treated.
Position patient with head of bed elevated.	This facilitates diaphragmatic descent for the best use of ventilatory muscles.
Administer theophylline as prescribed and monitor drug levels and patient response.	Theophylline has been reported to improve contractility of the diaphragm and other respiratory muscles, although this is not well defined.
Endotracheal suction patient as needed.	Endotracheal suctioning removes secretions and debris from the tracheobronchial tree and promotes airway patency, facilitating ventilation.
Select sedatives if needed with minimal muscle relaxant effects.	Most sedatives cause some degree of respiratory depression and must be used judiciously and with caution.
Treat pain according to its cause.	Pain causes splinting of the muscles of ventilation, adversely affecting the breathing pattern.
Provide adequate nutritional support (see Appendix A).	Effective ventilation requires adequate calories.
Teach pursed-lip breathing.	This maneuver keeps airways open longer during exhalation and evacuates trapped air.
Teach diaphragmatic breathing (use abdominal muscles for breathing).	The diaphragm uses less energy than accessory muscles.

NURSING DIAGNOSIS: IMPAIRED GAS EXCHANGE

Related To
- Ventilation/perfusion mismatch
- Intrapulmonary shunting (right-left shunting)
- Failure of diffusion across alveolar-capillary membrane

Defining Characteristics
Restlessness
Irritability
Hypoxia (PaO_2 < 60 torr; SaO_2 < 90%)
Confusion
Cyanosis

Patient Outcomes
Gas exchange and oxygen balance are restored, as evidenced by
- PaO_2 > 80 torr or return to baseline
- SaO_2 > 90%
- absence of cyanosis
- absence of restlessness, confusion, irritability, dizziness
- heart rate 60–100 bpm
- airways clear of mucous

Nursing Interventions	Rationales
Assess respiratory rate and depth and use of accessory muscles. Assess/monitor for symptoms of dyspnea, fatigue, drowsiness, headache, and apathy. Assess/monitor for sudden changes or absence of breath sounds, fine or coarse crackles, wheezing, stridor, and pleural rubs.	Baseline and ongoing assessment permits early determination of problems with airway clearance/oxygenation and provides data for evaluation of therapies.
Assess for changes in level of consciousness and anxiety.	Altered/decreased level of consciousness and anxiety (restlessness, air hunger) may indicate oxygen desaturation.
Assess nailbeds, lips, and buccal mucosa for cyanosis.	
Monitor for sudden changes in temperature and increased heart rate.	An increased temperature and heart rate may indicate pulmonary infection.

Nursing Interventions	Rationales
Monitor hemoglobin, PaO_2 and SaO_2.	Hemoglobin is the major oxygen-carrying compound. The PaO_2 reflects how much oxygen is in the blood. The saturation of hemoglobin is reflected by SaO_2. Oxygen transport is compromised with oxygen saturation less than 90%.
Monitor arterial pH and blood lactate levels.	These levels reflect overall acid-base balance.
Administer oxygen as prescribed and make changes as needed according to blood gas analysis or pulse oximeter changes.	Oxygen may be needed to improve gas exchange.
Determine cardiac output.	Cardiac output is the most important component determining oxygen delivery.
Consider application of CPAP or mechanical ventilation with PEEP.	Continuous positive airway pressure and PEEP cause alveolar hyperinflation, increasing surface area available for gas exchange.
Tracheal suction prn.	Endotracheal suctioning removes secretions and debris from the tracheobronchial tree and promotes airway patency, facilitating ventilation.
Encourage patient to turn, cough, and deep breathe.	Position changes, coughing, and breathing deeply maximize alveolar ventilation.
Limit patient activities. Provide an environment conducive to rest. Provide uninterrupted rest periods.	Inadequate rest and excess activity increase oxygen consumption.

Clinical Clip

Acid-Base Balance in Acute Respiratory Failure

Early in acute respiratory failure, the patient will present with respiratory alkalosis (carbonic acid deficit) in response to decreasing arterial oxygen content. As respiratory failure continues, respiratory acidosis will predominate as ventilatory muscles fail and carbonic acid is retained.

▼

NURSING DIAGNOSIS: INEFFECTIVE AIRWAY CLEARANCE

Related To
- Excess, thick secretions
- Cognitive impairment
- Immobility/bedrest
- Chest wall restrictions
- Bronchospasm/bronchial edema
- Decreased energy/fatigue
- Neuromuscular dysfunction
- Artificial airway
- Pulmonary fibrosis
- Pain

Defining Characteristics
Verbal statements by patient of inability to clear airway
Adventitious breath sounds
Dyspnea
Weak/ineffectual cough
Lung fields congested on chest x-ray

Patient Outcomes
The patient will maintain a patent airway through a controlled cough technique, as evidenced by
- patient not having respiratory distress
- clear breath sounds or return to baseline
- pH 7.35–7.45; $PaCO_2$ 35–45 torr; PaO_2 > 80 torr; SaO_2 > 90% or ABG's return to baseline
- thin mucus produced by coughing or suctioning
- absence of clinical manifestations of infection
- clear lung fields on chest x-ray

Nursing Interventions	Rationales
Assess lung fields for presence of adventitious sounds or wheezing. Administer bronchodilator as prescribed and monitor patient response.	Adventitious sounds are thought to be caused by abnormal motion of the walls of the airways or substances within the airways during breathing and indicate the need for coughing or suctioning. Wheezing indicates bronchospasm and may require bronchodilators for correction.
Monitor ABGs	Arterial blood gases allow evaluation for adequate ventilation ($PaCO_2$) and oxygenation (PaO_2).
Monitor serial chest x-rays.	

Nursing Interventions	Rationales
Monitor for signs of infection: progressive dyspnea; increasing cough; fever; and changes in amount, color, viscosity, and odor of pulmonary secretions. Obtain sputum culture and sensitivity with above signs.	
Consider endotracheal/nasotracheal intubation of patient.	Intubation may be needed to protect the airway from occlusion by accumulation of secretions, aspiration, or airway edema.
Apply humidified oxygen. Maintain hydration (in the absence of renal or cardiac disease) to 30 mL/hr plus insensible loss.	Humidification prevents drying of secretions and increases the water content of mucus and reduces its viscosity. This allows easier clearance from the respiratory tract. Artificial airways bypass the body's normal humidification system.
Perform chest physiotherapy and postural drainage as prescribed and evaluate patient response.	Chest physiotherapy helps loosen dry secretions and mucus plugs. Postural drainage brings these secretions into the larger airways where they can be coughed up.
Suction patients with ineffective cough or with presence of adventitious lung sounds.	Suctioning can remove secretions from the trachea and main bronchi.
Reposition patient frequently.	Repositioning helps match ventilation with perfusion.
Alleviate any pain or discomfort with medication and/or splinting.	Relief of pain will provide for maximal thoracic expansion.
Provide for rest between airway clearance maneuvers.	Intermittent respiratory muscle exercises and rest periods can improve muscle function.
Administer medications as prescribed to improve mucociliary clearance and monitor patient response: beta adrenergics, methylxanthines, anticholinergics, mucolytics, antibiotics, and expectorants.	

Nursing Interventions	Rationales
Implement measures to prevent respiratory infection. Use strict aseptic techniques in suctioning and other activities as appropriate.	Depressed mucociliary clearance provides an environment conducive to the development of infection.
Encourage deep-breathing exercises (maximal inhalation for 3–10 s) every hour with incentive spirometer or other mechanical aid. Teach COPD patients pursed-lip breathing.	Deep breathing assists in reinflating collapsed alveoli. Reinflated alveoli stay inflated for 1 hr. Pursed-lip breathing will decrease CO_2 retention and air trapping and will enhance secretion clearance.
Encourage patient to cough. Teach series coughing (three short coughs).	When the normal mucociliary clearance mechanism is impaired or overloaded, coughing is the primary mechanism of sputum removal. Coughing generates high intrathoracic pressure and compresses small airways. Secretions are moved to larger airways where they can be removed. Three short coughs use less energy and produce less wheezing and airway collapse.

NURSING DIAGNOSIS: ANXIETY

Related To
- Dyspnea
- Fear of dying

Defining Characteristics
Verbalization of anxiety
Restlessness
Decreased attention span
Tachycardia

Patient Outcomes
The patient's behavior demonstrates a decreased level of anxiety, as evidenced by
- patient verbalization of decreased anxiety
- heart rate 60–100 bpm
- absence of restlessness

Nursing Interventions	Rationales
Assess level and cause of anxiety.	This provides baseline data that enable the development of effective interventions.
Monitor oxygenation status (PaO_2 via ABGs, SaO_2 via pulse oximetry). Provide oxygen therapy as needed.	Hypoxia is a physiological trigger which promotes restlessness and anxiety.
Employ therapeutic use of self to reassure patient of proximity of nursing staff.	Provision of emotional support during periods of dyspnea can decrease associated anxiety.
Encourage verbalization of anxiety associated with dyspnea. Provide a caring, concerned attitude in interacting with patient.	
Encourage participation in care as tolerated.	This helps alleviate feelings of powerlessness that may be contributing to anxiety.
Administer sedatives judiciously.	Most sedatives produce some degree of respiratory depression and must be given with caution in patients having respiratory difficulty.
Explain ongoing assessments, procedures, and treatments.	
Teach and encourage pursed-lip breathing.	This is an active coping strategy for dyspnea.

NURSING DIAGNOSIS: ALTERED NUTRITION—LESS THAN BODY REQUIREMENTS

Related To
- Decreased appetite from dyspnea and weakness
- Prolonged debilitating lung disease

Defining Characteristics
Weight loss
Albumin < 3.5 g/dL
Lack of interest in food
Negative nitrogen balance

Patient Outcomes

Nutritional status is restored, as evidenced by
- weight within 20% of ideal or return to baseline
- albumin 3.5–5 g/dL
- positive nitrogen balance

Nursing Interventions	Rationales
See Appendix A	

Clinical Clip

Nutrition in Patients with Pulmonary Disease

1. It is important to limit the amount of calories supplied by glucose. Glucose produces CO_2 as it is metabolized and therefore may cause problems in patients who normally retain CO_2 or in patients weaning from mechanical ventilation. Increased lipogenesis can also augment CO_2 production.
2. Malnutrition causes impaired repletion of epithelial tissue which can lead to laryngeal ulcerations and pulmonary infection, lengthening the intubation period. Starvation also reduces the response to hypoxia and hypercapnia.
3. With a hypermetabolic stress state, patients are often insulin resistant and protein is broken down for gluconeogenesis, increasing oxygen consumption and causing negative nitrogen balance. As malnutrition continues, serum albumin levels are reduced, which augments pulmonary edema because of reduced interstitial pressure.
4. There are commercially prepared enteral nutritional supplements which contain a greater percentage of essential amino acids in relation to glucose to provide calories. This will decrease CO_2 metabolism. Total parenteral nutrition may also be prepared with less glucose.

DISCHARGE PLANNING/CONTINUITY OF CARE

- Assess need for/type of long-term care and follow-up.
- If the discharge destination is home, assess existing supports and the need for assistance.
- Determine coping deficits/support needs and institute assistance measures.
- Determine knowledge deficits/teaching needs and document and institute a teaching plan.
- Refer patient to social services as appropriate.
- Communicate coping deficits/support needs and knowledge deficits/teaching needs to unit accepting patient on transfer.

REFERENCES

Pennock, B. F., Kaplan, P. D., Carlin, B. W., Sabangan, J. S., & Magovern, J. A. (1991). Pressure support ventilation with a simplified ventilatory support system administered with a nasal mask in patients with respiratory failure. *Chest*, *100*(5), 1371–1376.

Portier, F., Defouilloy, C., & Muir, J. F. (1991). Determinants of immediate survival among chronic respiratory insufficiency patients admitted to an intensive care unit for acute respiratory failure. *Chest*, *99*(3), 204–210.

Rothkoph, M. M., Stanislaus, G., Haverstick, L. (1989). Nutritional support in respiratory failure. *Nutrition in Clinical Practice*, *4*, 166–172.

Stone, K. S. & Turner, B. (1989). Endotracheal suctioning. *Annual Review of Nursing Research*, *7*, 27–49.

Szaflarski, N. L. & Cohen, N. H. (1991). Use of capnography in critically ill adults. *Heart and Lung*, *20*(4), 363–374.

Ward, M. & Macklem, P. T. (1990). The act of breathing and how it fails. *Chest*, *97*(3), 36S-39S.

▼

CHEST TRAUMA

Chest trauma is associated with a high mortality rate because resulting injuries may cause fatal intrathoracic or extrathoracic hemorrhage, tamponade, and cardiac failure. Such injuries may include traumatic aortic rupture or tear, avulsions or tears of other great vessels of the chest (innominate artery, subclavian artery, carotid artery), rib and clavicular fractures, flail chest, hemopneumothorax, pulmonary contusion, pulmonary lacerations, and airway rupture. Varying degrees of shock are present with chest trauma. Proper evaluation and immediate supportive interventions are critical to caring for these patients immediately after injury. The principal pathological problem caused by chest injury is compromise of respiratory function because adequate ventilation and oxygenation depend on an intact chest wall.

ETIOLOGIES

- Blunt trauma
  - motor vehicle accidents
  - falls
  - pedestrian accidents
- Penetrating trauma
  - gun shot wounds
  - stab wounds
- Blast trauma

CLINICAL MANIFESTATIONS

- Pulmonary: Impaired ventilation and gas exchange can produce
  - hypoxemia (PaO_2 < 60 torr)
  - stridor
  - uneven chest movement
  - decreased/absent breath sounds
  - fine crackles
  - cyanosis
  - bloody secretions
  - subcutaneous emphysema

- craniofacial edema
- bubbling from the wound
- tachypnea and shallow breathing (or apnea)
- facial petechiae
- Cardiovascular: Decreased tissue perfusion and hemorrhage can produce
  - hypotension
  - pale mucous membranes
  - pulsus paradoxus
  - neck vein distention
  - cardiac arrest
  - tachycardia
  - cold, clammy skin
  - muffled/distant heart sounds
  - narrowed pulse pressure

CLINICAL/DIAGNOSTIC FINDINGS

- $PaO_2 < 60$ torr
- $PaCO_2 > 45$ torr
- $SaO_2 < 90\%$
- Acidosis (pH < 7.35)
- CO < 4 L/min
- Radiographic confirmation of injury
- Radiographic densities

NURSING DIAGNOSIS: IMPAIRED GAS EXCHANGE

Related To
- Damage to alveolar and capillary structures
- Tissue edema
- Ventilation/perfusion mismatch
- Intrapulmonary shunting
- Airway obstruction from blood clots

Defining Characteristics
Hypoxemia ($PaO_2 < 60$ torr; $SaO_2 < 90\%$)
Restlessness
Radiographic density
Cyanosis
Fine crackles

Patient Outcomes
Gas exchange and oxygen balance are restored, as evidenced by
- $PaO_2 > 80$ torr or return to baseline
- $SaO_2 > 90\%$
- absence of cyanosis
- absence of restlessness, confusion, irritability, dizziness
- heart rate 60–100 bpm
- airway clear of mucus

Nursing Interventions	Rationales
Assess respiratory rate, depth, and use of accessory muscles. Assess/monitor for sudden change/absence of breath sounds, fine or coarse crackles, wheezing, stridor, and pleural rub.	
Assess chest for cutaneous wounds, symmetry of movement, and contusion or hematoma. Palpate for subcutaneous air or point tenderness. Examine the position of the trachea.	
Assess for changes in level of consciousness and anxiety.	Altered/decreased levels of consciousness and/or anxiety may indicate oxygen desaturation.
Monitor arterial pH and blood lactate levels.	These parameters relect overall acid-base balance and the adequacy of oxygen delivery to tissues.
Monitor hemoglobin, PaO_2 and SaO_2.	Hemoglobin is the major oxygen-carrying compound. The PaO_2 reflects how much oxygen is in the blood. The saturation of hemoglobin is reflected by SaO_2. Oxygen transport is compromised with oxygen saturation less than 90%.
Monitor cardiac output.	Cardiac output is the most important determinant of oxygen delivery.
Administer oxygen as prescribed and make changes as needed according to blood gas analysis or oximeter changes.	Oxygen may be required for adequate gas exchange.
Occlude any defect in the chest wall with a gauze dressing. Tape dressing on three sides only.	To prevent a tension pneumothorax, it is necessary to seal any communication between the atmosphere and the intrapleural space.

Nursing Interventions	Rationales
Administer fluids carefully.	Too rapid/too much fluid administration can increase pulmonary artery pressure, causing deterioration of pulmonary function.
Manage the chest tube system of patients with tube thoracotomy.	Pneumothorax/hemothorax is a common presenting clinical problem with chest trauma and tube thoracotomy is used to decompress the pleural space and/or drain blood.
Administer diuretics as prescribed and monitor effects.	Interstitial edema associated with vascular damage in chest trauma is common.
Consider use of PEEP in patients with lung contusion.	Positive end-expiratory pressure causes alveolar hyperinflation, increasing the surface area available for gas exchange.
Tracheal suction as needed.	Endotracheal suctioning removes secretions and debris from the tracheobronchial tree and promotes airway patency, facilitating ventilation and oxygenation.
Provide an environment conducive to rest.	Decreasing patient activities reduces oxygen consumption and therefore oxygen requirements.

NURSING DIAGNOSIS: INEFFECTIVE BREATHING PATTERN

Related To
- Unstable chest wall
- Airway obstruction
- Thoracic pain

Defining Characteristics
Increased $PaCO_2$ (>45 torr) with decreasing pH (<7.35)
Subjective complaints of dyspnea
Use of accessory muscles of ventilation
Decreasing PaO_2 Tachypnea
Paradoxic breathing pattern   Diminished breath sounds
Atelectatic crackles

Patient Outcomes
The breathing pattern will be restored, as evidenced by
- respiratory rate 12–20 at rest
- $PaCO_2$ return to baseline
- pH 7.35–7.45
- equal, full breath sounds
- symmetric chest expansion
- minimal or absent atelectatic crackles

Nursing Interventions	Rationales
Monitor ventilation and oxygenation by use of arterial blood gas analysis.	The $PaCO_2$ is the assessment parameter used to evaluate ventilation. Assessment parameters PaO_2 and SaO_2 are used to evaluate oxygenation.
Establish a secure airway.	
Administer ventilation to patient via intubation with mechanical ventilation.	Mechanical ventilation will improve the ventilatory pattern, returning pH and $PaCO_2$ to within normal limits. Underlying disorders which have impaired the breathing pattern can then be treated.
Position patient with head of bed elevated if other injuries permit.	Head elevation facilitates diaphragmatic descent for the best use of ventilatory muscles.
Consider use of neuromuscular blocking agents.	These drugs are used long term to paralyze patients for optimal ventilatory support and to reduce patient energy demands.

NURSING DIAGNOSIS: INEFFECTIVE AIRWAY CLEARANCE

Related To
- Chest wall restrictions
- Bronchospasm/bronchial edema
- Decreased energy/fatigue
- Excess thick secretions
- Pain
- Immobility/bedrest
- Artificial airway

Defining Characteristics
Adventitious breath sounds　　　Dyspnea
Lung field consolidation on chest x-ray

Patient Outcomes

Airway clearance will be restored, as evidenced by
- clear breath sounds or return to baseline
- AGBs: pH 7.35–7.45, $PaCO_2$ 35–45 torr, PaO_2 > 80 torr, SaO_2 > 90% or return to baseline
- suctioning that produces thin mucous/effective cough
- clear lung fields on chest x-ray

Nursing Interventions	Rationales
Consider endotracheal/nasotracheal intubation of airway.	Intubation may be necessary to protect the airway from occlusion by accumulation of secretions, aspiration, or airway edema.
Provide chest physiotherapy and postural drainage over uninvolved lung segments.	These measures are taken to ensure normal lung function of these segments or lobes. Chest physiotherapy loosens dry secretions and mucous plugs. Postural drainage brings them into the larger airways where they can be coughed up.
Gently provide chest physiotherapy to involved lung segments.	
Consider positioning patient on the involved lung side, alternating with the back if actively bleeding, otherwise turn side to side.	This position allows for postural drainage of active bleeding and avoids blood spilling into the unaffected lung segments or lobes.
Administer bronchodilators as prescribed and monitor patient response.	Bronchodilators may be used to assist in removal of secretions or blood.
Administer medications as prescribed to improve mucociliary clearance and monitor patient response: beta adrenergics, methylxanthines, anticholinergics, mucolytics, and antibiotics.	
Administer measures to prevent respiratory infections. Use a strict aseptic technique in suctioning and other activities as appropriate.	Depressed mucociliary clearance provides an environment conducive to the development of infection.

Nursing Interventions	Rationales
Correlate physical assessment findings with serial chest x-ray.	Physical assessment and chest x-ray findings allow for monitoring of changes in airway clearance and evaluation of the effectiveness of interventions.

NURSING DIAGNOSIS: ACUTE PAIN

Related To
- Chest wall fractures
- Penetrating injuries
- Lung contusion
- Skeletal muscle injury

Defining Characteristics
Patient subjective reports of acute pain
Patient nonverbal cues of acute pain: restlessness, "beaten look," alteration in muscle tone, hypertension, pupillary dilation, increased/decreased respiratory rate, lack luster eyes, grimacing, diaphoresis, tachycardia

Patient Outcomes
Acute pain is relieved or reduced to a tolerable level, as evidenced by
- patient's subjective report that acute pain is relieved or tolerable (0–3 on pain-rating scale of 0–10)
- absence of nonverbal signs of acute pain

Nursing Interventions	Rationales
Assess pain using verbal as well as nonverbal cues. Utilize a pain-rating scale for verbal ranking of pain.	Multiple injuries or intubation may prevent the patient from being able to provide verbal cues of acute pain.
Assess for anxiety. Administer sedatives with analgesics if needed and monitor patient response.	Anxiety may heighten pain perception.
Administer analgesics (intravenous, epidural, or intercostal) as prescribed and monitor patient response.	Pharmacological intervention is usually required to treat acute pain.
Schedule pain medications on a routine schedule initially (as opposed to prn).	Scheduled doses or continuous infusion of an analgesic prevents severe pain episodes.

Nursing Interventions	Rationales
Reposition patient frequently.	The pain response may be heightened by immobility.
Splint chest wall fractures while moving patient.	This minimizes pain caused by manipulation of the chest wall.
Provide for general comfort measures: mouth care, positioning, and hygiene.	

NURSING DIAGNOSIS: HIGH RISK FOR FLUID VOLUME DEFICIT

Risk Factors
- Hemothorax
- Damage to great vessels in chest (aorta, innominate artery, subclavian artery, carotid artery)
- Pulmonary laceration

Patient Outcomes
Fluid volume will be maintained, as evidenced by
- blood pressure within 10 mmHg of patient baseline
- heart rate 60–100 bpm
- CVP 2–10 mmHg; PCWP 8–12 mmHg
- warm, dry skin
- peripheral pulses that remain at patient baseline
- urine output > 30 mL/hr

Nursing Interventions	Rationales
Monitor cardiovascular status: blood pressure and heart rate, including orthostatic changes; hemodynamic measurements; and peripheral pulses.	Increased heart rate; decreased blood pressure and/or orthostatic changes; low CVP, PCWP, CO, CI, and MAP; and weak peripheral pulses indicate hypovolemia. Normalization of these measurements will reflect adequate fluid replacement. Fluid overload is prevented through continuous assessments during fluid administration.

Nursing Interventions	Rationales
Monitor/record fluid balance: daily weight and intake and output.	Daily weights and intake and output provide a means to trend and evaluate fluid balance.
Monitor renal function: BUN, creatinine, and hourly urine output.	BUN and creatinine reflect renal function and their increase indicates prolonged decreased renal perfusion. Decreased urine output (<30 mL/hr) is an early sign of decreased perfusion and inadequate fluid replacement. Blood urea nitrogen may also rise with hemorrhage and dehydration.
Monitor coagulation studies and complete blood count.	These studies are used to monitor patient response to treatment and prevent complications related to coagulation defects.
Initiate fluid resuscitation via large-bore intravenous line. Administer intravenous colloids, crystalloids, or blood products as prescribed until signs and symptoms of hypovolemia stabilize. Monitor for signs of fluid overload such as increased CVP/PCWP, adventitious breath sounds, jugular venous distention, and respiratory distress.	Initially colloids or cystalloids are used for fluid resuscitation. Blood losses of greater than 1500 mL require blood replacement in addition to fluids.

NURSING DIAGNOSIS: HIGH RISK FOR DECREASED CARDIAC OUTPUT

Risk Factors
- Blood loss
- Decreased venous return (decreased preload)
- Decreased contractility
- Increased afterload

Patient Outcome
Cardiac output will be maintained, as evidenced by
- CO 4–8 L/min
- CI 2.5–4 L/min/m^2
- MAP > 60 mmHg

- blood pressure within 10 mmHg patient baseline
- heart rate 60–100 bpm
- peripheral pulses at patient baseline

Nursing Interventions	**Rationales**
Assess/document cardiovascular status: vital signs, hemodynamic measurements, and cardiac rhythm.	
Monitor for signs of cardiovascular collapse: bradycardia or tachycardia, hypotension, decreased CO/CI, decreased MAP, weak peripheral pulses, and cold, clammy skin.	
Monitor for changes in mental status.	Decreases in cardiac output may produce changes in mental status due to decreased cerebral perfusion.
Monitor urine output hourly.	Decreased urine output is an early sign of decreased cardiac output with decreased perfusion to the kidney.
Monitor peripheral circulation: Inspect skin, noting color and temperature and check quality of peripheral pulses and capillary refill time (CRT).	Cold, clammy, pale skin, weak peripheral pulses, or increased CRT indicate decreased cardiac output with decreased peripheral perfusion.
Elevate lower extremities 20°–30° degrees from the horizontal position.	Elevation of the lower extremities will increase venous return.
Administer inotropic agents as prescribed and monitor patient response.	Inotropic drugs such as dobutamine, dopamine, or inocor may be used to increase cardiac output by increasing cardiac contractility.
Administer fluids as prescribed (see Fluid Volume Deficit).	

DISCHARGE PLANNING/CONTINUITY OF CARE

- Assess need for/type of long-term care and follow-up.
- If the discharge destination is home, assess existing supports and the need for assistance.

- Determine coping deficits/support needs and institute assistance measures.
- Determine knowledge deficits/teaching needs and document and institute a teaching plan.
- Refer patient to social services as appropriate.
- Communicate coping deficits/support needs and knowledge deficits/teaching needs to unit accepting patient on transfer.

REFERENCES

Anderson, F. D. (1987). Chest trauma in the military scenario. *Emergency Care Quarterly, 2*(4), 37–46.

Cogbill, R. H. & Landercasper, J. (1991). Injury to the chest wall. In E. Moore (Ed.), *Trauma* (2nd ed.). Norwalk, CT: Appleton.

Cowley, R. A., Conn, A., & Dunham, C. M. (1987). *Trauma care: surgical management.* Maryland Institute for Emergency Medical Services Systems, Baltimore, MD.

Jarpe, M. B. (1992). Nursing care of patients receiving long-term infusion of neuromuscular blocking agents. *Critical Care Nurse, 12*(7), 58–63.

O'Malley, K. F. & Spence, R. K. (1990). Emergency department initial evaluation and resuscitation in chest trauma. *Topics in Emergency Medicine, 12*(1), 7–15.

Unkle, D. (1988). Traumatic injury to the thorax. *Today's OR Nurse, 10*(11), 12–33.

▼

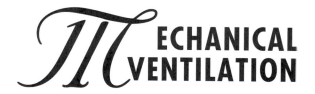

MECHANICAL VENTILATION

Mechanical ventilation is a process by which positive pressure is used to move gases into and out of the pulmonary system. The ventilator is a device that inflates the lungs by positive pressure. Humidified oxygen is also delivered.

Controlled ventilation delivers a preset tidal volume at a preset rate. The machine is set so the patient is unable to generate a breath from the machine. With assist-control ventilation, the patient can initiate each breath by creating negative intrathoracic pressure, and the ventilator delivers a positive pressure breath at a preset tidal volume. With intermittent mandatory ventilation, the patient is allowed to spontaneously breathe humidified, oxygenated air from the system at his or her own rate and tidal volume. In addition, intermittent positive pressure breaths are delivered from the ventilator at preset intervals and with a preset volume to ensure adequate alveolar ventilation. Positive end-expiratory pressure (PEEP) can also be delivered to increase functional residual capacity and improve gas exchange. Pressure support ventilation allows the clinician to select a preset level of positive airway pressure to assist the patient's own spontaneous inspiratory effort. The patient determines the length of inspiration, inspiratory flow, and respiratory rate. Tidal volume is dependent on the level of pressure support as well as airway and chest compliance.

ETIOLOGIES

Preexisting conditions that alter lung mechanics, including
- Acute respiratory failure (gas delivery/cellular failure)
- Acute ventilatory failure (respiratory muscle failure/CNS disorders)
- Impending ventilatory failure
- Inadequate oxygenation
- Airway obstruction
- Severe trauma
- Neurological disease
- Active pulmonary problems (infection, atelectasis)

- General anesthesia
- Obesity
- Chest wall deformities
- Renal failure

CLINICAL MANIFESTATIONS

- Pulmonary: Impaired ventilation and gas exchange produce
  - dyspnea
  - use of accessory muscles
  - paradoxic breathing pattern
  - tachypnea
  - tachycardia
  - neck vein distention
- Neurological: Impaired ventilation and gas exchange produce
  - altered level of consciousness
  - sleep disturbances
  - papilledema
  - seizures
- Cardiovascular: Impaired gas exchange produces
  - dysrhythmias
  - systolic hypertension
  - chest pain
  - tachycardia
  - palpitations
- Skin: Impaired ventilation and gas exchange produce
  - pallor
  - clammy skin
  - flushing
  - cyanosis
  - cool skin

CLINICAL/DIAGNOSTIC FINDINGS

- SaO_2 < 90%
- PaO_2 < 60 torr
- Acidosis (pH < 7.35)
- $PaCO_2$ > 45 torr
- Vital capacity < 10 mL/kg
- CO < 4 L/min

NURSING DIAGNOSIS: INEFFECTIVE BREATHING PATTERN

Related To
- Respiratory muscle fatigue
- Airway obstruction caused by a kinked ventilator tube, mucous plug, biting of endotracheal tube
- Chronic airflow limitations
- Chest wall restrictions
- Accidental extubation
- Ventilator malfunction
- Barotrauma

Defining Characteristics
Respiratory rate > 30
Minute volume > 12 L/min

Abdominal paradox
Respiratory alternans

Increasing $PaCO_2$ with decreasing pH
Decreasing PaO_2
Subjective complaints of dyspnea
Use of accessory muscles of ventilation
 – Asymmetrical chest expansion
Atelectatic crackles
Subjective complaints of fatigue
 – Diminished breath sounds

Patient Outcomes

Breathing pattern is restored/returned to baseline, as evidenced by
- respiratory rate 12–20 at rest
- $PaCO_2$ return to baseline
- pH 7.35–7.45
- equal, full breath sounds
- symmetric chest expansion
- minimal or absent atelectatic crackles
- vital capacity > 10 mL/kg or 20–25% predicted normal
- inspiratory force −20 to −25 cmH_2O
- resting spontanous minute ventilation < 10 L/min

Nursing Interventions	Rationales
Assess pulmonary system: respiratory effort, spontaneous effort, breath sounds, and equality of respiratory excursion.	
Assess endotracheal tube cuff pressure every 8 hr. Use minimal leak method for cuff inflation (slight air leak heard with a sigh).	The cuff must be checked regularly to ensure patency of the airway and adequate ventilation. The minimal leak method prevents alteration in tracheal integrity (stenosis) related to increased cuff pressure.
Monitor respiratory rate every hour and prn.	Increased respiratory rate is the first clinical indication of respiratory muscle fatigue.
Monitor tidal volume the patient actually receives.	Factors such as total compliance of the breathing circuit, circuit leakage, resistance in the patient's airways and in the circuit, and dead space in the system affect the mechanics of the patient's ventilation and thus tidal volume delivery.

Nursing Interventions	Rationales
Monitor for airway obstruction related to kinked tube or patient biting of the endotracheal tube. Prevent airway obstruction by maintaining oral airway to prevent biting on tube, securing endotracheal tube, and positioning tubing to prevent water buildup.	Maintaining/ensuring patency of the endotracheal tube is essential for airway and breathing maintenance.
Monitor ventilation by use of arterial blood gas analysis or capnography.	The $PaCO_2$ is the primary value reflecting the adequacy of ventilation.
Monitor for signs of tension pneumothorax, including increased airway pressures, unequal breath sounds, decreased breath sounds, subcutaneous emphysema, asymmetrical chest expansion, tracheal deviation, decreased cardiac output, distended neck veins, and decreased compliance with hand ventilation.	Barotrauma from positive pressure mechanical ventilation and high levels of PEEP may cause a tension pneumothorax. If pneumothorax occurs, disconnect from ventilator, manually ventilate, reassure patient, set up chest tube system, and obtain chest x-ray.
Assist in establishing airway with endotracheal tube and cuff inflation.	A cuffed tube is required with positive pressure ventilation.
Check physician orders for ventilator settings every shift (mode of ventilation, tidal volume, respiratory rate, FiO_2, PEEP, pressure support).	
Check position of endotracheal tube at lip or nares every shift and document. Secure tube and observe at points of potential disconnection. Allow slack on tubing to accommodate patient movement. Keep spare endotracheal tube at bedside.	There is always the danger of endotracheal tube displacement, accidental extubation, or disconnection. Correct positioning is necessary to ensure a patent airway and equal expansion of both lungs.
Endotracheal suction patient according to physical assessment.	Endotracheal suctioning removes secretions and debris from the tracheobronchial tree and promotes airway patency, facilitating ventilation.

Nursing Interventions	Rationales
Position patient with head of bed elevated.	Head elevation facilitates diaphragmatic descent for the best use of ventilatory muscles.
Sedate patient as needed.	Sedation may be needed to help the patient relax and breathe in cycle with the ventilator or to prevent auto-peep.
Provide adequate nutritional support (see Appendix A).	Effective ventilation requires calories. More calories supplied by fat rather than glucose are needed to minimize CO_2 production.

NURSING DIAGNOSIS: IMPAIRED GAS EXCHANGE

Related To
- Ventilation/perfusion mismatch
- Intrapulmonary shunting
- Failure of diffusion across alveolarcapillary membrane
- Atelectasis
- Oxygen toxicity from high inspired oxygen concentration

Defining Characteristics
Restlessness
Irritability
Hypoxia (PaO_2 < 60 torr; SaO_2 < 90%)
Confusion
Cyanosis

Patient Outcomes
Gas exchange and oxygen balance are restored, as evidenced by
- PaO_2 > 80 torr or return to baseline
- SaO_2 > 90%
- absence of cyanosis
- absence of restlessness, confusion, irritability, dizziness
- heart rate 60–100 bpm
- airways clear of mucous

Nursing Interventions	Rationales
Assess/monitor respiratory rate and depth and use of accessory muscles; symptoms of dyspnea, fatigue, drowsiness, headache, and apathy; breath sounds; and sudden changes/absence of breath sounds, fine or coarse crackles, wheezing, stridor, or pleural rub.	Regular ongoing assessment is necessary to determine early problems with oxygenation and establishes a baseline for evaluation of therapy.
Assess for changes in level of consiousness and anxiety (restlenssness, air hunger).	Anxiety or decreased level of consiousness may indicate oxygen desaturation.
Assess nailbeds.	The color of nailbeds indicate peripheral tissue perfusion.
Monitor hemoglobin, PaO_2 and SaO_2.	Hemoglobin is the major oxygen-carrying compound. The PaO_2 reflects how much oxygen is in the blood. The saturation of hemoglobin is reflected by SaO_2. Oxygen transport is compromised with oxygen saturation less than 90%.
Monitor arterial pH and blood lactate levels.	These measures reflect overall acid-base balance.
Administer oxygen as prescribed and make changes as needed according to blood gas analysis or pulse oximeter changes.	Oxygen may be necessary to provide adequate oxygen for gas exchange.
Determine cardiac output.	Cardiac output is the primary determinant of oxygen delivery to the cells.
Identify patients with increased minute volume.	Patients with increased minute volume (i.e., COPD, asthma patients) are at risk for the development of auto-peep. Auto-peep is unintentional positive end-expiratory pressure in patients on mechanical ventilation when time provided for exhalation is inadequate. Complications may include hemodynamic compromise, increased work of breathing, miscalculation of compliance, and barotrauma.

Nursing Interventions	Rationales
Hyperoxygenate with 100% oxygen before suctioning using manual ventilation or by increasing FiO$_2$ for 2 min. Limit suctioning to 10 s.	These measures prevent hypoxemia related to suctioning.
Consider application of continuous positive airway pressure (CPAP) or mechanical ventilation with positive end-expiratory pressure (PEEP).	Continuous positive airway pressure and PEEP cause alveolar hyperinflation, increasing the surface area available for gas exchange.
Encourage patient to turn, cough, and deep breathe.	Position changes, coughing, and breathing deeply maximize alveolar ventilation.
Tracheal suction as needed.	Endotracheal suctioning removes secretions and debris from the tracheobronchial tree and promotes airway patency facilitating ventilation.
Limit patient activities. Provide an environment conducive to rest.	Adequate rest decreases oxygen consumption.

NURSING DIAGNOSIS: INEFFECTIVE AIRWAY CLEARANCE

Related To
- Thick secretions
- Cognitive impairment
- Immobility/bedrest
- Pulmonary fibrosis
- Improper positioning of endotracheal tube
- Bronchospasm
- Decreased energy/fatigue
- Neuromuscular dysfunction
- Chest wall restrictions
- Pain

Defining Characteristics
Verbal statements by patient of inability to clear airway
Adventitious breath sounds
Weak/ineffectual cough
Dyspnea
Lung fields congested on chest xray

Patient Outcomes
Effective airway clearance is restored, as evidenced by
- patent airway
- effective mobilization of secretions

- proper positioning of endotracheal tube
- absence of/resolution of bronchospasm
- clear breath sounds or return to baseline
- ABGs: pH 7.35–7.45, $PaCO_2$ 35–45 torr, PaO_2 > 60 torr, SaO_2 > 90% or return to baseline
- cough or suctioning that produces thin mucus
- clear lung fields on x-ray

Nursing Interventions	Rationales
Auscultate lungs for presence of adventitious sounds.	Auscultation ascertains bilateral lung expansion and presence of adventitious sounds which indicate secretions in the airway and the need for suctioning.
Monitor peak inspiratory pressures.	Increased peak inspiratory pressure may reflect airway obstruction from secretions or mucous plugs or patient biting on the endotracheal tube.
Monitor for bronchospasm: increased peak inspiratory pressure, wheezing, and decreased PaO_2.	
Apply humidified secretions. Maintain hydration.	Adequate humidification/hydration prevents drying of secretions, increases the water content of the mucous, and reduces its viscosity, thereby allowing easier clearance from the respiratory tract.
Perform chest physiotherapy and postural drainage as tolerated.	Chest physiotherapy loosens dry secretions and mucous plugs. Postural drainage brings them into the larger airways where they can be suctioned.
Administer medications to improve mucociliary clearance: beta adrenergics, methylxanthines, anticholinergics, mucolytics, antibiotics, and expectorants.	Depressed mucociliary clearance provides an environment conducive to the development of infection.
Reposition patient frequently.	Repositioning facilitates matching ventilation with perfusion.
Place oral airway or bite block as needed.	The patient with an orotracheal tube must be prevented from biting or gumming the tube.

Nursing Interventions	Rationales
Initiate interventions for bronchospasm as needed: manual bag ventilation, reassurance, sedatives, aminophylline, and/or bronchodilators.	

NURSING DIAGNOSIS: DYSFUNCTIONAL VENTILATORY WEANING RESPONSE

Related To
- Ineffective airway clearance
- Uncontrolled episodic energy demands
- Inappropriate pacing of diminished ventilatory support
- Sleep pattern disturbance
- Uncontrolled pain/discomfort
- Knowledge deficit
- Fear
- Hopelessness
- Insufficient trust in caregiver
- Infection
- Inadequate nutrition
- Heart failure
- Decreased motivation
- Anxiety
- Anemia
- Body position

Defining Characteristics
Subjective complaints of increased oxygen need, breathing discomfort, apprehension or pain/discomfort
Restlessness
Decreased level of consciousness
Increased respiratory muscle use
Paradoxical abdominal breathing
Discoordinated breathing with the ventilator
Increasing $PaCO_2$
Decreasing SaO_2
Increased systolic blood pressure
Increased heart rate
Diaphoresis
Agitation
Increased respiratory rate
Shallow chest excursion
Adventitious breath sounds
Decreasing PaO_2
Decreasing pH
Dysrhythmias
Pale/cyanosis
Eye widening
Patient queries about possible machine malfunction
Patient hypervigilence to activities
Increased patient concentration on breathing

Patient Outcomes
Ventilatory weaning is accomplished, as evidenced by
- pH 7.35–7.45
- $PaCO_2$ 35–45 torr or return to baseline
- PaO_2 > 60 torr

- $SaO_2 > 90\%$
- weaned off mechanical ventilation

Nursing Interventions	Rationales
Assess ventilatory parameters for physiological readiness to wean: tidal volume, minute volume, negative inspiratory pressure, respiratory rate, and vital capacity (when obtainable).	Tests that evaluate pulmonary functioning are necessary for assessing weaning potential. Successful weaning requires that the patient possess adequate respiratory muscle function to maintain tidal volume, to cough effectively, and to breathe deeply.
Assess nonventilatory parameters for physiological readiness to wean: absence of muscle fatigue, hemodynamic stability, nutrition, and absence of fever/infection.	The patient's overall condition is important in considering weaning ability.
Assess oxygenation.	Hemoglobin, cardiac outut and PaO_2 must be optimized before weaning is begun.
Assess psychological readiness to wean.	Weaning is a stressful event that is accompanied by release of catecholamines.
Assess psychological status. Institute nursing measures to facilitate coping during weaning: allow patient control, provide a communication method, decrease environmental stress, provide mental stimulation/distraction, teach relaxation, provide rewards for short-term goals, and encourage self-care.	
Monitor vital signs and cardiac rhythm.	Intolerance to weaning may cause hypertension, hypotension, tachycardia, and dysrhythmias.

Nursing Interventions	Rationales
Monitor response to weaning schedule. Alternate weaning with rest.	This promotes muscle conditioning and endurance.
Prepare patient psychologically to be weaned. Address patient stressors. Reduce number of activities during or before weaning. Deal with emotions exhibited by patient.	The patient who is psychologically prepared to wean will have a sense of control over his or her environment.
Suction airway as needed based on pulmonary assessment.	Retained secretions increase the work of breathing.
Institute weaning protocol according to physician's order.	Intermittent mandatory ventilation, pressure support, T-piece, and CPAP weaning may be used in weaning patients from ventilatory support.
Document weaning schedule and patient response through respiratory assessment (respiratory rate, pattern, breath sounds, and ABGs).	A progressive weaning schedule allows for breathing retraining in debilitated patients.
Administer bronchodilators as prescribed.	Bronchospasm increases the work of breathing.
Provide chest physiotherapy: coughing exercises followed by deep inhalation, postural drainage, and suctioning.	Chest physiotherapy, coughing exercises, and suctioning prevent accumulation of secretions, atelectasis, and/or mucous plugging.
Systematically hydrate patient depending on fluid balance.	Adequate hydration helps prevent accumulation of secretions or mucous plugging.
Assist patient to position for weaning which maximizes diaphragm excursion, that is, dangling, leaning forward, and getting out of bed and into a chair.	Functional residual capacity decreases in supine position and can impair gas exchange.

Nursing Interventions	Rationales
Support cardiac output. Provide volume replacement. Monitor hemoglobin.	Drugs and fluid to increase contractility, increase or decrease preload, and decrease afterload optimize cardiovascular stability. Tissue oxygenation is dependent on adequate oxygen transport (cardiac output), metabolic rate, and oxygen-carrying capacity (hemoglobin). Pump failure can be exacerbated by weaning trials.
Identify potential ventilator-related infection sites.	Infection increases metabolic demand, which contributes to failure to wean.
Provide nutrition. Moderate carbohydrate loading.	Weaning requires energy. Excess carbohydrate administration can lead to increased CO_2 production and therefore retention.
Administer fluids/fiber to prevent constipation. Monitor for ileus or abdominal distention.	Abdominal distention secondary to gas, ileus, or constipation prevents adequate diaphragm function.
Provide for uninterrupted sleep.	Adequate sleep and rest is essential to successful weaning.
Provide judicious analgesia.	Pain can contribute to anxiety, inhibit chest movement, and restrict coughing.
Assist with range-of-motion exercises.	Exercise increases muscle function.

NURSING DIAGNOSIS: FLUID VOLUME EXCESS

Related To
- Fluid overload from retention of inspired water
- Decreased insensible loss
- Increased secretion of ADH while on ventilator

Defining Characteristics

Weight gain
CVP > 10 mmHg
Adventitious breath sounds
Haziness on chest x-ray

Jugular venous distention
PCWP > 12 mmHg
Hypoxemia
Ankle edema

Patient Outcomes
Fluid balance is restored, as evidenced by
- optimal fluid balance
- stable weight
- clear breath sounds
- CVP 2–10 mmHg; PCWP 8–12 mmHg
- absence of edema
- normal neck veins
- clear chest x-ray
- PaO$_2$ > 60 torr

Nursing Interventions	Rationales
Monitor fluid balance: daily weights, ankle edema, and intake and output.	Ongoing monitoring and assessment allow for early detection of positive fluid balance.
Monitor for pulmonary edema: fine crackles, wheezing, changes in airway pressure, deceasing PaO$_2$, increased PCWP, pink frothy sputum, and haziness on chest x-ray.	
Administer fluids as prescribed to keep hemodynamic and fluid balance parameters within normal limits.	
Administer therapies as prescribed to reduce fluid overload: diuretics, fluid restriction, and vasodilators.	

NURSING DIAGNOSIS: DECREASED CARDIAC OUTPUT

Related To
- Increased intrathoracic pressures associated with positive pressure mechanical ventilation
- Intentional use of PEEP
- Auto-peep

Defining Characteristics
Hypotension
Bradycardia or tachycardia
Dysrhythmias
CI < 2.5 L/min/m^2

Warm flushed skin
CO < 4 L/min
Cardiovascular collapse

Patient Outcomes

Cardiac output will be maintained/restored, as evidenced by
- blood pressure within normal limits for patient
- heart rate 60–100 bpm
- urine output > 30 mL/hr
- CVP 2–10 mmHg; PCWP 8–12 mmHg
- CO 4–8 L/min; CI 2.5–4 L/min/m²
- absence of dysrhythmias
- absence of cardiovascular collapse

Nursing Interventions	Rationales
Assess and document cardiovascular status: vital signs, hemodynamic parameters, peripheral pulses, and cardiac rhythm.	Mechanical ventilation with positive pressure increases thoracic pressure, decreasing venous return and cardiac output.
Assess for signs of cardiovascular collapse: bradycardia or tachycardia, hypotension, increased CVP/PCWP, decreased CO/CI, decreased MAP, and weak peripheral pulses.	
Monitor patient response to PEEP.	Positive end-expiratory pressure further decreases cardiac output by increasing intrathoracic pressure.
Administer fluids as prescribed.	Fluid administration is necessary to prevent hypovolemia.
Administer inotropic agents as prescribed and monitor patient response.	Inotropic agents increase cardiac output by increasing contractility.
Administer sedatives as prescribed/needed and monitor patient response.	Sedation may be necessary to prevent the patient from fighting mechanical ventilation.
Elevate lower extremities 20°–30° from the horizontal position.	Elevation of the lower extremities will increase venous return and thus cardiac output.

NURSING DIAGNOSIS: HIGH RISK FOR INFECTION

Risk Factors
- Fever
- Purulent pulmonary secretions
- Increased secretions
- Increased WBC count
- Adventitious breath sounds

Patient Outcomes
Patient will be free of infection.

Nursing Interventions	Rationales
Monitor for signs of infection: fever, elevated WBC count, and change in secretion color, amount, consistency, and odor.	
Prevent infection potential by 1. observing sterile technique when suctioning. 2. practicing meticulous handwashing. 3. draining tubing condensation away from patient. 4. changing manual breathing bag every 72 hr. 5. performing frequent oral hygiene. 6. ensuring ventilator tubing changes according to protocol.	
Change patient position every 2 hr.	Changes in patient position will help to mobilize secretions.
If infection is suspected, send sputum, blood, and urine for culture and sensitivity. Administer antibiotics as prescribed.	

NURSING DIAGNOSIS: ANXIETY

Related To
- Mechanical ventilation
- Sensory overload/deprivation
- Diagnosis
- Inability to talk
- Sleep deprivation
- Disorientation

Defining Characteristics
Verbalizations/communications of anxiety
Decreased attention span   Tachycardia
- Restlessness

Patient Outcomes
Patient's behavior demonstrates a decreased level of anxiety, as evidenced by
- patient communication of decreased anxiety
- maintenance of communication within limitation using alternate methods of communication

Nursing Interventions	Rationales
Assess noise levels. Minimize noise as possible.	
Monitor oxygenation status. Provide oxygen therapy as needed.	Hypoxia is a physiological trigger which promotes restlessness and anxiety.
Plan nursing care to provide periods of uninterrupted sleep.	Fatigue can contribute to anxiety.
Reduce sensory overload.	
Orient to time, place, and person.	
Explain all procedures. Provide reassurance to patient.	
Sedate as needed and monitor patient response.	Sedation may be necessary to help the patient relax and breathe in cycle with the ventilator. Administer sedatives judiciously due to possible respiratory depression.
Develop a system of communication: touch, communication board, and phrasing yes/no questions. Include the family.	The inability to speak/communicate is a great source of anxiety.

NURSING DIAGNOSIS: ALTERED NUTRITION—LESS THAN BODY REQUIREMENTS

Related To
- Decreased nutrient intake
- Altered gastrointestinal motility

Defining Characteristics
Weight loss
Albumin < 3.5 g/dL
Lack of interest in food
Negative nitrogen balance

Patient Outcomes

Nutritional balance will be restored, as evidenced by
- weight within 20% of ideal or return to baseline
- albumin 3.5–5 g/dL
- positive nitrogen balance

Nursing Interventions	Rationales
See Appendix A.	

Clinical Clip

In patients with pulmonary disease, especially those who retain CO_2 it is important to limit the amount of calories supplied by glucose. Glucose as it is metabolized produces CO_2 and therefore may cause problems in patients who normally retain CO_2 or in patients weaning from mechanical ventilation.

DISCHARGE PLANNING/CONTINUITY OF CARE

- Assess need for/type of long-term care and follow-up.
- If the discharge destination is home, assess existing supports and the need for assistance.
- Determine coping deficits/support needs and institute assistance measures.
- Determine knowledge deficits/teaching needs and document and institute a teaching plan.
- Refer patient to social services as appropriate.
- Communicate coping deficits/support needs and knowledge deficits/teaching needs to unit accepting patient on transfer.

REFERENCES

Ashton, J. & Black, L. (1991). Quality monitor implementation for standards of care of the mechanically ventilated patient. *AACN Clinical Issues in Critical Care Nursing, 2*(1), 77–81.

Bolgiano, C. S. & Saah, M. L. (1990). Measurement of bedside ventilatory parameters. *Critical Care Nurse, 10*(1), 60–66.

Briones, T. L. (1992). Pressure support ventilation, New ventilatory technique. *Critical Care Nurse, 12*(4), 51–59.

Burns, S., Fahey, S. A., Barton, D. M. (1991). Weaning from mechanical ventilation: A method for assessment and planning. *AACN Clinical Issues in Critical Care Nursing, 2*(3), 372–387.

Henneman, E. A. (1991). The art and science of weaning from mechanical ventilation. *Focus on Critical Care, 18*(6), 490–500.

Ingersoll, G. L. (1989). Respiratory muscle fatigue research: Implications for clinical practice. *Applied Nursing Research*, 2(1), 6–15.

Kastens, V. M. (1991). Nursing management of autopeep. *Focus on Critical Care*, 18(5), 419–421.

Kohlman, V. C. (1991). Dyspnea in the weaning patient: Assessment and intervention. *AACN Clinical Issues in Critical Care Nursing*, 2(3), 462–473.

Logan, J. & Jenny, J. (1990). Deriving a new nursing diagnosis through qualitative research: Dysfunctional weaning response. *Nursing Diagnosis*, 1(1), 37–43.

Norton, L. C. & Neureuter, A. (1989). Weaning long-term ventilatory-dependent patient: Common problems and management. *Critical Care Nurse*, 9(1), 42–52.

Shekleton, M. E. (1991). Respiratory muscle conditioning and the work of breathing: A critical balance in the weaning patient. *AACN Clinical Issues in Critical Care Nursing*, 2(3), 405–414.

St. John, R. E. & Eisenberg, P. (1991). Nutrition and the use of metabolic assessment in the ventilator dependent patient. *AACN Clinical Issues in Critical Care Nursing*, 2(3), 453–461.

Witta, K. (1990). New techniques for weaning difficult patients from mechanical ventilation. *AACN Clinical Issues in Critical Care Nursing*, 1(2), 260–266.

▼

PULMONARY EMBOLISM

Development of deep-vein thrombosis can result in a clot breaking loose from the vein and traveling up through the vena cava to the right side of the heart and into the pulmonary artery. The embolus disrupts blood flow to the alveoli in the area of the embolus. The obstruction may be partial or complete. It can affect the right or left pulmonary artery or both or a branch of either vessel. Pulmonary embolus is not a distinct disease entity, but rather a complication of medical and surgical disorders.

Once the embolus is settled in the pulmonary vasculature, compounds released from the clot, including serotonin, histamine, prostaglandin, and thromboxane, cause bronchial constriction, vasoconstriction, and increasing capillary permeability. When the capillary around an alveolus is blocked or narrowed, oxygen continues to enter the alveolus, but since there is decreased blood flow, hyoxemia results. Hypoxemia results in the loss of surfactant, causing alveoli to collapse. A right-to-left shunt occurs and oxygen is not available for diffusion into the capillary. Massive pulmonary embolism may result in cor pulmonale and cardiogenic shock.

In chronic cases, surgery is considered in patients with recurrent emboli that persist despite heparin therapy or for whom anticoagulation is contraindicated. Blood flow is interrupted through the inferior vena cava to prevent emboli from reaching the pulmonary circulation. Complete ligation of the inferior vena cava can result in many complications, including edema of the legs. A vena caval plication, in which a filter is inserted into the vein, allows normal blood flow while preventing large emboli from getting through.

ETIOLOGIES

- Venous stasis secondary to
  - prolonged bedrest
  - obesity
  - pregnancy
  - postpartum state
  - orthopedic casts

- Vein wall damage secondary to
  - surgery
  - leg and pelvic fractures
  - diabetes
  - burns
  - intravenous drug abuse
- Hypercoagulability secondary to
  - dehydration
  - cancer
  - polycythemia
  - sepsis
  - estrogen replacement therapy/oral contraceptives
  - deficiencies in antithrombin III, protein C, protein S (heredity)

CLINICAL MANIFESTATIONS

- Pulmonary: Decreased perfusion in relation to ventilation produced
  - increased respiratory rate
  - rales per auscultation
  - dyspnea
  - chest or upper back pain
  - cough
  - hemoptysis
  - hypoxemia
- Neurological: Impaired gas exchange and activation of the sympathetic nervous system produce
  - elevated temperature
  - new-onset syncope
  - fever
  - anxiety/restlessness
  - sweats
- Cardiovascular: Impaired gas exchange and tissue perfusion produce
  - tachycardia
  - cor pulmonale
  - clinical signs of deep-vein thrombosis (swelling, calf pain)
  - excessive/unusual facial skin color changes (pallor, flushing, perioral cyanosis)
  - phlebitis
  - cardiogenic shock

  Acute right ventricular failure produces
  - hepatomegaly
  - distended neck veins
  - CVP > 10 mmHg
  - loud pulmonic valve closure (P_2)
- Vascular: Fat emboli produce
  - neck, chest, axillae, and conjunctival petechiae

CLINICAL/DIAGNOSTIC FINDINGS

- High probability ventilation-perfusion lung scan
- Positive pulmonary angiogram
- Abnormal findings on lower extremity venography, duplex ultrasonography, or Doppler flow mapping
- Respiratory alkalosis (pH > 7.45, $PaCO_2$ < 35 torr)

- EKG: right ventricular strain and ischemia
- Chest x-ray
  - nonspecific infiltrates initially
  - atelectasis with decreased ventilation
  - pleural effusion
  - prominent pulmonary arteries

NURSING DIAGNOSIS: IMPAIRED GAS EXCHANGE

Related To
- Reduced cardiac output with widening alveolar arterial oxygen tension difference
- Overperfusion of the nonembolized lung zones not sufficiently ventilated to maintain adequate oxygenation of blood

Defining Characteristics

$PaO_2 < 60$ torr
$SaO_2 < 90\%$
Confusion
Dizziness
Cyanosis
Restlessness
Irritability
Tachycardia

Patient Outcomes

Gas exchange and oxygen balance is restored, as evidenced by
- $PaO_2 > 80$ torr or return to baseline
- $SaO_2 > 90\%$
- absence of cyanosis
- absence of restlessness, confusion, irritability, dizziness
- heart rate 60–100 bpm
- airways clear of secretions

Nursing Interventions	Rationales
Assess breath sounds. Monitor for sudden changes/absence of breath sounds, fine or coarse crackles, wheezing, stridor, or pleural rubs.	
Assess for changes in level of consciousness and anxiety.	Anxiety and decreased level of consciousness may indicate oxygen desaturation.

Nursing Interventions	Rationales
Monitor hemoglobin, PaO_2 and SaO_2.	Hemoglobin is the major oxygen-carrying compound. The PaO_2 reflects how much oxygen is in the blood. The saturation of hemoglobin is reflected by SaO_2. Oxygen transport is compromised with oxygen saturation less than 90%.
Monitor respiratory rate and depth and use of accessory muscles. Monitor for symptoms of dyspnea, fatigue, drowsiness, headache, and apathy.	
Monitor for sudden changes in temperature and heart rate.	Increased temperature may indicate infection or retained secretions which may represent problems with airway clearance or atelectasis. Tachycardia may occur with problems of airway clearance or oxygenation.
Monitor physiological dead space.	The difference between end-tidal and arterial $PaCO_2$ (gradient) is increased with pulmonary embolus.
Administer oxygen therapy as prescribed and make changes as needed according to blood gas analysis or pulse oximeter changes.	Enough oxygen must be administered to provide oxygen for potential gas exchange.
Determine cardiac output.	Cardiac output is the most important determinant of oxygen delivery.
Consider assisted ventilation if PaO_2 does not respond.	Mechanical ventilation with positive end-expiratory pressure can improve gas exchange.
Encourage patient to turn, cough, and deep breathe.	Position changes, coughing, and breathing deeply maximize alveolar ventilation.
Tracheal suction prn.	Suctioning removes secretions and debris from the tracheobronchial tree and promotes airway patency, facilitating ventilation.

Nursing Interventions	Rationales
Limit patient activities. Provide an environment conducive to rest and provide uninterrupted rest periods.	Rest and limited activities will decrease oxygen consumption.
Instruct patient regarding diagnostic procedures.	

NURSING DIAGNOSIS: ALTERED TISSUE PERFUSION—PULMONARY

Related To embolus in pulmonary artery

Defining Characteristics
Excessive/unusual facial skin color changes (pallor, flushing, perioral cyanosis)
Increased respiratory rate   Dyspnea
Chest pain   Cough
Hemoptysis   Tachycardia
Hypoxemia
Right ventricular strain pattern on EKG
Accentuated pulmonic component of second heart sound (P_2)

Patient Outcomes
Perfusion is restored to the lung, as evidenced by
- respiratory rate 12–20
- resolution of dyspnea
- absence of chest pain
- absence of cough
- clear sputum
- heart rate 60–100 bpm
- PaO_2 > 80 torr
- absence of right ventricular strain or ischemic pattern on EKG
- normal heart sounds (S_2)
- normalization of end-tidal CO_2 and $PaCO_2$

Nursing Interventions	Rationales
Monitor for bleeding. Check for occult blood in stool or urine.	Bleeding may be a complication of anticoagulant and fibrinolytic therapy.

Nursing Interventions | Rationales

Nursing Interventions	Rationales
Monitor EKG.	With severe pulmonary artery obstruction, the EKG will show transient changes consistent with right ventricular strain and ischemia, including tall, peaked P waves, ST-segment elevation, and T-wave inversion.
Monitor heart sounds.	An accentuated pulmonic component of the second heart sound (P_2) indicates pulmonary hypertension associated with massive embolism.
Monitor PTT (heparin therapy) and PT (warfarin therapy).	Adequate anticoagulation is measured by PTT or PT 2–2½ times control.
Administer anticoagulant therapy as prescribed (heparin, warfarin sodium) to maintain PTT or PT to twice normal levels.	Anticoagulation is used to prevent formation of additional clots and propagation of existing clots. It also permits the body's own fibrinolytic system mechanisms to lyse clots already formed. Heparin therapy is the drug of choice initially because it inhibits coagulation immediately, preventing more thrombi from forming while inhibiting platelet aggregation. Warfarin is started for long-term therapy. It takes several days for warfarin to develop its full anticoagulant effect. Therefore, acute therapy with heparin is tapered.
Elevate head of bed.	Head elevation may relieve dyspnea
Administer fibrinolytics as prescribed (streptokinase, urokinase, and recombinant t-PA) and monitor for adverse effects (bleeding).	Thrombolytics actively dissolve previously formed clots and thereby relieve the obstruction to the pulmonary artery blood flow, improving right ventricular function and pulmonary perfusion. Thrombolytics can be administered up to 14 days after the embolus. Heparin therapy is usually discontinued during this treatment.

Nursing Interventions	Rationales
Administer antiplatelet substances (aspirin, dextran, persantine) as prescribed and monitor effects.	Antiplatelet substances prevent platelet aggregation and can prevent deep-vein thrombosis.
Provide postoperative care to patient with vena caval filter implantation.	The filter traps emboli before they reach pulmonary vessels.
Administer stool softeners.	Defecation-triggered pulmonary embolism has been reported and therefore Valsalva maneuvers should be minimized.
Document characteristics of sputum.	Hemoptysis is evidence of partial or complete pulmonary infarction.
Identify high-risk patients for deep-vein thrombosis and consider preventive measures: graduated compression stockings, intermittent pneumatic compression, low-dose heparin, isometric exercises, and limb elevation.	Intermittent pneumatic compression devices increase femoral vein flow and prevent venous stasis and thrombosis. Isometric exercise prevents venous stasis and limb elevation improves venous return.

NURSING DIAGNOSIS: ACUTE PAIN

Related To decreased perfusion to pulmonary tissue from congestive atelectasis and/or pulmonary infarction

Defining Characteristics
Subjective report of chest pain: deep substernal crushing pain with radiation to arms and shoulders (massive emboli) or pleuritic chest pain
Subjective report of back pain
Tachycardia   Chest wall splinting

Patient Outcomes
Pain controlled to tolerable levels, as evidenced by
- patient's subjective report of pain control using pain rating scale
- heart rate 60–100 bpm

Nursing Interventions	Rationales
Perform comprehensive assessment of pain, including location, characteristics, and precipitating factors. Use pain-rating scale if possible.	Pain assessment establishes a baseline for evaluation of outcomes.
Observe for nonverbal cues of discomfort.	
Provide optimal pain relief with prescribed analgesics. Assure pretreatment analgesia prior to painful procedures.	
Modify pain control measures based on patient's response.	
Use therapeutic communication strategies to acknowledge pain experience.	This conveys acceptance of the pain experience.
Administer nonsteroidal anti-inflammatory drugs as prescribed and monitor effects.	Anti-inflammatory drugs decrease the pleuritic pain of pulmonary embolism due to inflammation.
Consider administration of sedatives.	Anxiety and fear can increase the pain experience.
Provide information about the pain, such as the causes of pain, anticipated discomforts from procedures, and the interventions that will be used to relieve it.	Lack of knowledge increases the pain experience.

NURSING DIAGNOSIS: HIGH RISK FOR DECREASED CARDIAC OUTPUT

Risk Factors
- Increased pulmonary artery resistance
- Increased pulmonary artery pressure
- Increased right ventricular work

Patient Outcomes
Cardiac output remains stable, as evidenced by
- blood pressure return to baseline with MAP > 60 mmHg
- CO 4–8 L/min; CI 2.5–4 L/min/m^2
- CVP 2–10 mmHg

- pulmonary artery systolic pressure 25–30 mmHg
- pulmonary artery diastolic pressure 8–12 mmHg
- absence of jugular vein distention
- normal liver size
- peripheral pulses that are palpable to patient baseline
- warm, dry skin

Nursing Interventions	Rationales
Monitor blood pressure, respiratory rate, and heart rate.	Heart rate and respiratory rate will be elevated as long as tissue perfusion is low. Blood pressure will be low until volume is corrected or if left failure following right failure occurs.
Monitor CVP. Observe for jugular vein distention and hepatic enlargement.	Elevated CVP, jugular vein distention, and hepatomegaly are associated with right ventricular failure.
Monitor cardiac output/cardiac index.	Cardiac output may drop due to right ventricular failure from increased pulmonary artery resistance.
Monitor peripheral circulation: Inspect skin color and temperature and check quality of peripheral pulses and capillary refill time (CRT).	Cool, clammy, pale skin, weak peripheral pulses, or increased CRT may indicate inadequate peripheral perfusion.
Balance fluid intake with fluid loss.	Loss of surfactant with pulmonary embolus causes regional pulmonary edema.
Note hourly changes in urine output.	Decreased urine output is an early indicator of inadequate kidney perfusion.

DISCHARGE PLANNING/CONTINUITY OF CARE

- Assess need for/type of long-term care and follow-up.
- If the discharge destination is home, assess existing supports and the need for assistance.
- Determine coping deficits/support needs and institute assistance measures.

- Determine knowledge deficits/teaching needs and document and institute a teaching plan.
- Refer patient to social services as appropriate.
- Communicate coping deficits/support needs and knowledge deficits/teaching needs to unit accepting patient on transfer.

REFERENCES

Currie, D. L. (1990). Pulmonary embolism: Diagnosis and management. *Critical Care Nurse Quarterly*, *13*(2), 41–49.

Dickinson, S. P. & Bury, G. M. (1989). Pulmonary embolism. *Nursing*, *8919*(4), 34–41.

Goldhaber, S. Z. (1991). Managing pulmonary embolism. *Hospital Practice*, 37–48.

Handerhan, B. (1991). Recognizing pulmonary embolism. *Nursing*, *91*(2), 107–109.

Holcomb, S. (1991). Pulmonary embolism: Preventing a disaster. *RN*, *54*(8), 52–58.

Hull, R., Mosser, K. M., & Salzman, E. (1989). Preventing pulmonary embolism. *Patient Care*, *1*, 63–81.

Kollef, M. & Neelon-Kollef, R. A. (1991). Pulmonary embolism associated with the act of defecation. *Heart & Lung*, *20*(5), 451–453.

Lancaster, S. & Dinwiddie, J. (1991). Filters that trap emboli. *RN*, *54*(9), 56–60.

PIOPED investigators. (1990). Tissue plasminogen activator for the treatment of acute pulmonary embolism. *Chest*, *97*(3), 528–532.

Polak, J. F. (1991). Doppler ultrasound of the deep leg veins. *Chest*, *99*(4), 165S–172S.

Prewitt, R. M. (1991). Principles of thrombolysis in pulmonary embolism. *Chest*, *99*(4), 157S–164S.

Sherman, S. (1991). Pulmonary embolism update. *Postgraduate Medicine*, *89*(8), 195–202.

Stratton, M. B. (1990). Ventilation-perfusion scintigraphy in diagnosis of pulmonary thromboembolism. *Focus on Critical Care*, *17*(4), 287–293.

▼

RESPIRATORY ACIDOSIS

The respiratory system is responsible for alveolar ventilation or inhalation of oxygen and diffusion across the alveolar-capillary membrane and exhalation of carbon dioxide and water. The $PaCO_2$ is a measure of the partial pressure of carbon dioxide dissolved in arterial blood plasma. It reflects the effectiveness of ventilation in relation to metabolic rate.

Respiratory acidosis represents an elevation of $PaCO_2$ (>45 mmHg) with resultant increase in carbonic acid due to changes in respiratory ventilation. Compensatory mechanisms to buffer the carbonic acid include the hemoglobin buffer system forming bicarbonate ions and deoxygenated hemoglobin and an increase in metabolic (renal) formation of ammonia acid excretions with reabsorption of bicarbonate.

ETIOLOGIES

- Primary mechanisms: hypoventilation with retention of carbon dioxide with lung disease secondary to
  - chronic obstructive pulmonary disease
  - restrictive pulmonary disease
  - asthma
  - airway obstructions
  - pulmonary edema
  - pnumothorax/hemothorax
  - mechanical ventilation
  - pneumonia
  - atelectasis
  - chest trauma
- Depressed function of the respiratory center of the brain secondary to
  - head trauma
  - general anesthesia
  - metabolic alkalosis
  - oversedation
  - barbiturate poisoning
- Neuromuscular disorders secondary to
  - spinal cord injury (hemiplegia/quadriplegia)
  - extrapyramidal disorders
  - amyotrophic lateral sclerosis
  - Guillain-Barré syndrome
  - myasthenia gravis
  - poliomyelitis
  - muscular dystrophy

CLINICAL MANIFESTATIONS

- Neurological: Carbon dioxide retention produces subjective symptoms, including
  - headache
  - visual disturbances
  - dizziness
  - fatigue

  Carbon dioxide retention produces objective symptoms, including
  - confusion, restlessness, somnolence, coma
  - weakness
  - loss of coordination
  - depressed reflexes
- Pulmonary: Carbon dioxide retention produces
  - initially increased respiratory rate (compensatory)
  - later decreased respiratory rate
  - increased respiratory effort
- Cardiovascular: Carbon dioxide retention produces
  - tachycardia
  - dysrhythmias

CLINICAL/DIAGNOSTIC FINDINGS

- Arterial pH < 7.35
- $PaCO_2$ > 45 torr or elevated above baseline
- Increased HCO_3 (compensatory in chronic respiratory acidosis)

NURSING DIAGNOSIS: INEFFECTIVE BREATHING PATTERN

Related To
- Primary lung disorders resulting in hypoventilation (see etiologies above)
- Depressed respiratory center in brain resulting in hypoventilation (see etiologies above)
- Neuromuscular disorders resulting in hypoventilation

Defining Characteristics
pH < 7.35
$PaCO_2$ > 45 torr or elevated above baseline

Clinical Clip

Acute hypoventilation will not result in changes in the metabolic system, that is, serum bicarbonate, renal electrolytes, or serum electrolytes. With chronic hypoventilation states, serum HCO_3 may be elevated (>28 mEq/L), urine pH decreased (<6.0), and serum potassium increased (>5 mEq/L).

Patient Outcomes
Acid-base balance is restored, as evidenced by
- pH 7.35–7.45
- $Paco_2$ 35–45 torr or return to baseline
- potassium 3.5–5.0 mEq/L

Nursing Interventions	Rationales
Identify and treat underlying etiology of carbon dioxide retention.	
Auscultate breath sounds.	Decreased breath sounds indicate decreased ventilation and may be causing CO_2 retention and respiratory acidosis.
Monitor respiratory rate and depth and work of breathing.	Hypoxemia associated with respiratory acidosis results in respiratory distress/failure.
Monitor for physiological signs of hypercapnia, including headache, drowsiness, change in level of consciousness, papilledema, blurred vision, confusion, seizures, sleep disturbances, flushing of skin, and clammy skin.	
Monitor for physiolgical signs of associated hypoxemia, including tachycardia, bounding pulse, hypertension, dysrhythmias, palpitations, chest pain, pallor, and cyanosis.	
Monitor for physiological signs associated with acidosis, including drowsiness, confusion, decreased level of consciousness, hypotension, bradycardia, and cool, clammy, pale skin.	
Monitor serial ABGs. Monitor capnography if available.	Capnography can track trending in CO_2 levels. Values need to be correlated with arterial pH, $Paco_2$ and clinical assessment findings.
Monitor for dysrhythmias and document and treat according to protocols.	As pH falls, cardiac dysrhythmias can occur.

Nursing Interventions	Rationales
Monitor GI functioning and distention.	Reduced diaphragmatic movement can produce CO_2 retention and respiratory acidosis.
Encourage turning, coughing, and deep breathing. Position in semi-Fowler's position.	This promotes ventilation.
Maintain airway clearance, that is, suction, chest physiotherapy, cough, and deep breath.	Airway obstruction or decreased alveolar diffusion can contribute to CO_2 retention.
Support on mechanical ventilation as necessary.	
Administer oxygen as indicated.	Prevents/corrects hypoxemia associated with hypoventilation.
Administer bronchodilators as prescribed and monitor effects.	Bronchodilators increase lung expansion and alveolar opening to improve ventilation.
Provide low-carbohydrate, high-fat diet if indicated.	High-carbohydrate, low-fat foods can increase CO_2 production.
Limit use of sedatives or tranquilizers.	Sedation can further depress ventilation and contribute to CO_2 retention.

NURSING DIAGNOSIS: DECREASED CARDIAC OUTPUT

Related To decreased contractility secondary to acidosis

Defining Characteristics
Hypotension
Warm, flushed skin
CO < 4 L/min
Cardiovascular collapse

Decreased heart rate
Dysrhythmias
CI < 2.5 L/min/m^2

Patient Outcomes
Cardiac output will be maintained/restored, as evidenced by
- blood pressure within 10 mmHg of patient baseline
- heart rate 60–100 bpm
- absence of dysrhythmias
- CO 4–8 L/min; CI 2.5–4 L/min/m^2
- absence of cardiovascular collapse

Nursing Interventions	Rationales
Assess for underlying cause of respiratory acidosis and institute treatment.	As long as the underlying cause persists, treatment of respiratory acidosis will be unsuccessful.
Assess/document cardiovascular status: heart rate, respiratory rate, blood pressure, hemodynamic parameters, mean arterial pressure, and peripheral pulses.	
Assess for signs of cardiovascular collapse: bradycardia, hypotension, increased CVP/PCWP, decreased CO/CI, decreased MAP, and weak peripheral pulses.	When pH falls to 7.0, the heart becomes unresponsive to catecholamines (epinephrine and norepinephrine) and heart rate and cardiac output decrease.
Monitor for signs of increased potassium: restlessness, irritability, lethargy, tall peaked T waves, and prolonged P-R interval.	Extracellular potassium may be high because the body exchanges intracellular potassium for extracellular hydrogen ions in an attempt to normalize pH.
Monitor for dysrhythmias and document and treat per protocols.	When the pH falls, cardiac dysrhythmias can occur.
Monitor serum calcium levels.	Calcium shifts out of the cells to assist in buffering extracellular hydrogen ions. As the acidosis is treated, decreased ionized calcium can produce signs of hypocalcemia (paresthesias, irritability, confusion, muscle weakness, and prolonged Q-T interval).

DISCHARGE PLANNING/CONTINUITY OF CARE

- Based on underlying pathology/etiology, assess need for/type of long-term care and follow-up.
- If the discharge destination is home, assess existing supports and the need for assistance.
- Determine coping deficits/support needs and institute assistance measures.
- Determine knowledge deficits/teaching needs and document and institute teaching plan.
- Refer patient to social services as appropriate.

- Communicate coping deficits/support needs and knowledge deficits/learning needs to unit accepting the patient on transfer.

REFERENCES

Kelly, B. J. (1991). The diagnosis and management of neuromuscular diseases causing respiratory failure. *Chest, 99*(6), 1485–1494.

Klahr, S. & Weiner, D. (1990). Disorders of acid-base metabolism. In J. Chen & J. Gill (Eds.), *Kidney and electrolyte disorders* (pp. 1–58). New York, NY: Churchill Livingtone.

Shapiro, B., Harrison, R. A., & Walton, J. R. (1989). *Clinical Application of Blood Gases* (4th ed.). Chicago, IL: Year Book Medical.

Szaflarski, N. L. & Cohen, N. H. (1991). Use of capnography in critically ill adults. *Heart & Lung, 20*(4), 363–374.

RESPIRATORY ALKALOSIS

The respiratory system is responsible for alveolar ventilation or inhalation of oxygen and diffusion across the alveolar-capillary membrane and exchange of carbon dioxide and water. The $PaCO_2$ is a measure of the partial pressure of carbon dioxide dissolved in arterial blood plasma. It reflects the effectiveness of ventilation in relation to metabolic rate.

Respiratory alkalosis is defined as an elevated blood pH (>7.45) in response to respiratory hyperventilation ($PaCO_2$ < 35 torr) with a deficit of carbonic acid. Compensatory mechanisms include increased renal excretion of bicarbonate and retention of hydrogen ions.

ETIOLOGIES

Hyperventilation caused by
- anxiety
- extreme emotions
- severe pain
- mechanical ventilation
- restrictive pulmonary disorders (asthma, pulmonary fibrosis, pregnancy)
- lack of oxygen (hypoxemia, severe anemia)
- congestive heart failure
- cirrhosis
- drug intoxication (paraldehyde, salicylate, methanol)
- rapid correction of metabolic acidosis (renal dialysis)
- nervousness
- sepsis
- brain trauma/lesions
- alcohol intoxication
- thyrotoxicosis

CLINICAL MANIFESTATIONS

- Neurological: Cerebral vasoconstriction produces
  - dizziness
  - faintness
  - light headedness
  - blurred vision

- Decreased calcium (nerves more irritable) produces
  - tingling of extremities and lips
  - carpopedal spasm
  - increased reflexes
  - seizures
- Gastrointestinal: Irritation of the emetic center produces
  - nausea
  - vomiting

CLINICAL/DIAGNOSTIC FINDINGS

- pH > 7.45
- Pa_{CO_2} < 35 torr
- Bicarbonate < 21 mEq/L (compensation)
- Decreased potassium (<3.5 mEq/L)
- Decreased chloride (<95 mEq/L)

NURSING DIAGNOSIS: ACID-BASE IMBALANCE

Related To carbon dioxide deficit

Defining Characteristics

Dizziness
Pa_{CO_2} < 45 torr
Carpopedal spasm
Increased reflexes
Blurred vision
pH > 7.45

Patient Outcomes

Acid-base balance will be maintained/restored, as evidenced by
- absence of neurological manifestations
- pH 7.35–7.45
- Pa_{CO_2} 35–45 torr

Nursing Interventions	Rationales
Assess underlying cause of respiratory alkalosis and institute treatment.	As long as the underlying cause persists, treatment of respiratory alkalosis will be unsuccessful.
Monitor serum potassium for signs of hypokalemia: flat/inverted T waves, dysrhythmias, fatigue, paresthesias, and drowsiness.	In alkalosis, potassium will move into the cells in exchange for hydrogen ions, producing hypokalemia.
Monitor for dysrhythmias.	Cardiac dysrhythmias are associated with hypokalemia.

Nursing Interventions	Rationales
Monitor serum calcium and for signs of hypocalcemia (paresthesias, numbness/tingling, muscle weakness, and prolonged Q-T interval).	Levels of ionized calcium decrease as pH increases.
Monitor for hypophosphatemia (dysrhythmias, confusion, lethargy, weakness, tremors).	In alkalosis, phosphate will move into cells as hydrogen moves out.

NURSING DIAGNOSIS: INEFFECTIVE BREATHING PATTERN

Related To central stimulation of respiration

Defining Characteristics
Increased respiratory rate
Dyspnea
$PaCO_2 < 35$ torr
Deep respirations
$pH > 7.45$

Patient Outcomes
An effective breathing pattern is restored, as evidenced by
- normal rate and depth of respiration
- $PaCO_2$ 35–45 torr
- pH 7.35–7.45
- $PaO_2 > 60$ torr or return to baseline

Nursing Interventions	Rationales
Assess for etiology of hyperventilation, that is, hypoxemia, CNS injury, hypermetabolic states, GI distention, pain, and stress.	
Assess/document ventilation: rate, depth, and rhythm of respiration; airway and breathing effort and use of accessory muscles; breath sounds; subjective complaints of SOB; and dyspnea.	
Assess ABGs and pulse oximetry as prescribed. Obtain tidal volume, vital capacity, and forced expiratory volume in 1 s.	

Nursing Interventions	Rationales
Monitor for indications of respiratory failure: low PaO_2, respiratory muscle fatigue, and low SaO_2.	Increased work of breathing may lead to respiratory failure.
Monitor for neuromuscular manifestations of respiratory alkalosis: paresthesia, tetany, and seizures.	Alkalosis may lead to hypocalcemia and irritability of nerve endings.
Monitor for cardiovascular manifestations of respiratory alkalosis: dysrhythmias and decreased cardiac output.	
Use rebreathing mask as indicated.	A rebreathing mask increases carbon dioxide retention to correct pH.
If on mechanical ventilation, reduce respiratory rate/tidal volume or add additional dead space to mechanical ventilation.	Decreasing rate/tidal volume or adding dead space increases carbon dioxide retention to correct pH.
Provide oxygen therapy if necessary.	Improve arterial oxygen content and prevent hypoxemic stimulus for hyperventilation.
Provide measures to promote comfort, control fever, and reduce anxiety.	Discomfort, increased temperature, and anxiety can increase oxygen consumption.
Provide mechanical ventilatory support if necessary.	Mechanical ventilation may be necessary to control pH and $PaCO_2$ levels.
Administer sedatives, pain relief, and neuromuscular blocking agents as prescribed and monitor patient response.	Drugs may be required to interrupt the hyperventilation breathing pattern.

DISCHARGE PLANNING/CONTINUITY OF CARE

- Based on underlying pathology/etiology, assess need for/type of long-term care and follow-up.
- If the discharge destination is home, assess existing supports and the need for assistance.
- Determine coping deficits/support needs and institute assistance measures.

- Determine knowledge deficits/teaching needs and document and institute a teaching plan.
- Refer patient to social services as appropriate.
- Communicate coping deficits/support needs and knowledge deficits/teaching needs to unit accepting patient on transfer.

REFERENCES

Horne, M., & Swearingen, P. (1989). *Pocket guide to fluid and electrolytes.* St. Louis, MO: Mosby-Yearbook.

Klahr, S. & Weiner, D. (1990). Disorders of acid-base metabolism. In J. Chen, & J. Gill (Eds), *Kidney electrolyte disorders* (pp. 1–58). New York, NY: Churchill Livingstone.

Shapiro, B., Harrison, R. A., & Walton, J. R. (1989). *Clinical application of blood gases* (4th ed.). Chicago, IL: Year Book Medical.

STATUS ASTHMATICUS

Status asthmaticus is considered an acute exacerbation of bronchial asthma. It is characterized by severe obstruction of the airways not relieved by conventional therapies. Dense exudate in the bronchial lumen and hyperinflation of alveoli are characteristic pathophysiological changes. Muscle spasm, inflammation, and mucous plugging contribute to the development of airway narrowing or obstruction and increased airway resistance.

In the asthmatic patient, the smooth muscle of the airway is hyperresponsive to many stimuli, including viral infection, dry air, cold, allergens, dust or pollutants, precipitous withdrawal of corticosteroids, medications, particularly aspirin and beta blockers, and foods. As a result, increased vital capacity, decreased forced expiratory volume in 1 min, and increased functional residual capacity predominate. Increased inspiratory muscle forces are required to open airways and promote adequate ventilation. The basic physiological abnormality in asthma is expiratory airflow obstruction.

ETIOLOGIES

- Bronchospasm
- Edema of bronchial wall
- Mucous plugging

CLINICAL MANIFESTATIONS

- Pulmonary: Acute airway obstruction produces
    - severe dyspnea
    - chest tightness
    - absent breath sounds
    - use of accessory muscles
    - cough (productive or nonproductive)
    - prolonged expiration (prolonged inspiratory-expiratory ratio)
    - anxiety
    - wheezing
    - inspiratory retractions
    - changes in speech

- Cardiovascular: Sympathetic nervous system activation and/or hypoxemia produce
  - tachycardia
  - EKG abnormalities
  - hypertension
  - decreased contractility
  - pulsus paradoxus (associated with forced expiratory volume in 1 s less than 1 L)
- Neurological: Impaired ventilation and oxygenation produce altered level of consciousness.
- Renal: Hypoxemia produces inadequate renal perfusion.

CLINICAL/DIAGNOSTIC FINDINGS

- Decreased forced expiratory volume in 1 s (FEV_1)
- Decreased peak expiratory flow rate
- Severe hypoxemia (PaO_2 < 60 torr)
- Increased $PaCO_2$ (> 45 torr) or elevated above baseline
- Vital capacity equals tidal volume
- Alveolar hyperinflation on chest x-ray
- Pneumothorax or pneumomediastinum on chest x-ray
- Acidosis (pH < 7.35)
- Eosinophils in sputum

NURSING DIAGNOSIS: INEFFECTIVE BREATHING PATTERN
Related To airway obstruction

Defining Characteristics
Tachypnea
PaO_2 > 45 mmHg
Respiratory distress
PaO_2 < 60 torr

Patient Outcomes
An adequate breathing pattern is restored, as evidenced by
- increased FEV_1
- resting respiratory rate 12–20
- $PaCO_2$ 35–45 torr or return to baseline
- PaO_2 > 60 torr

Nursing Interventions	Rationales
Monitor breath sounds.	Localized wheezing or crackles on chest auscultation may represent mucous plugging or atelectasis.

Nursing Interventions	Rationales
Monitor for signs of respiratory failure: severe dyspnea, use of accessory muscles, $PaO_2 < 60$ torr, $PaCO_2 > 45$ torr, pH < 7.35, and extreme fatigue. Assist with intubation and mechanical ventilation as required.	Asthmatic patients with severe bronchoconstriction and airway inflammation are at risk for development of respiratory failure. Carbon dioxide retention and other signs of deterioration may warrant more aggressive therapy. Volume-controlled ventilation with low tidal volumes and inspiratory flow rates are recommended.
Monitor for pulsus paradoxus.	Pulsus paradoxus means the patient is trying to take very deep breaths, usually using accessory muscles and therefore has markedly hyperinflated the lungs and dropped pleural pressure. Right ventricular strain is also common.
Administer oxygen as prescribed and titrate according to PaO_2 and SaO_2.	Higher oxygen concentrations may be needed during administration of bronchodilating drugs as pulmonary vasodilation causes significant ventilation/perfusion mismatching.
Assist with inspiratory maneuvers with continuous positive airway pressure (CPAP) or mechanical ventilation.	Continuous positive airway pressure or mechanical ventilation may be necessary to overcome the high distending pressures, reduce the inspiratory work of breathing, and relieve dyspnea.
Administer bronchial smooth-muscle dilators as prescribed and monitor patient response: epinephrine and sympathomimetics (beta-agonist bronchodilators) every 20 min for first hour, then every 1–3 hr; theophylline; parasympathetic blockers (atropine); and aminophylline.	Bronchodilators decrease airway resistance. Epinephrine is usually the first beta agonist administered. Patients with asthma find it difficult to use a metered-dose inhaler so initial treatments are often given by a nebulizer. Intravenous aminophylline may also be given as it may prolong the effects of nebulized beta agonists.

Nursing Interventions	Rationales
Administer mucolytics as prescribed and monitor patient response.	Patients with severe asthma usually have tremendous mucous impaction and require mucolytics to loosen secretions.
Administer glucocorticoids, that is, methylprednisolone, as prescribed and monitor patient response.	Glucocorticoids are used for their anti-inflammatory effects.
Promote adequate hydration.	Dehydration can thicken secretions. Patients with asthma are dehydrated from hyperventilation, diaphoresis, and inadequate fluid intake. Careful titration of intravenous fluids is important to prevent pulmonary edema.
Administer pulmonary physical therapy: chest clapping, coughing, and deep breathing.	Pulmonary physical therapy aids in removing secretions.
Suction patient as necessary.	Suctioning prevents/eliminates mucous plugging contributing to airway obstruction.
Administer muscle relaxants and sedatives as prescribed and monitor patient response.	Drugs may be required to prevent tachypnea and promote adequate ventilation.
Administer anesthesia as prescribed and monitor response.	Anesthetics may be used to relax smooth muscles of the chest. This increases respiratory compliance and decreases pulmonary artery pressures. Anesthetics also decrease bronchospasm associated with suctioning.
Administer intravenous magnesium as prescribed and monitor serum levels.	Magnesium may be beneficial to asthmatic patients who have refractory bronchospasm. Magnesium is a bronchodilator.
Administer antibiotics as prescribed for purulent bronchitis	
Determine peak expiratory flow rate and forced expiratory volume.	Inability to perform these tests indicates severe exacerbation.

NURSING DIAGNOSIS: IMPAIRED GAS EXCHANGE

Related To airway obstruction

Defining Characteristics
Restlessness
Irritability
Hypoxia (PaO_2 < 60 torr, SaO_2 < 90%)
Confusion
Cyanosis

Patient Outcomes
Gas exchange and oxygen balance are restored, as evidenced by
- PaO_2 > 80 torr or return to baseline
- SaO_2 > 90%
- absence of cyanosis
- absence of restlessness, confusion, irritability
- heart rate 60–100 bpm
- airways clear of mucous

Nursing Interventions	Rationales
Assess respiratory rate and depth and use of accessory muscles.	
Assess breath sounds. Monitor for sudden change or absence of breath sounds, fine or coarse crackles, wheezing, stridor, or pleural rubs.	
Assess for changes in level of consciousness and anxiety.	Anxiety and changes in level of consciousness may indicate oxygen desaturation.
Monitor hemoglobin, PaO_2 and SaO_2.	Hemoglobin is the major oxygen-carrying compound. The PaO_2 reflects how much oxygen is in the blood. The saturation of hemoglobin is reflected by SaO_2. Oxygen transport is compromised with oxygen saturation less than 90%.
Monitor arterial pH and blood lactate levels.	These levels reflect overall acid-base balance.

Nursing Interventions	Rationales
Monitor for symptoms of dyspnea, fatigue, drowsiness, headache, and apathy.	
Monitor for sudden changes in temperature and heart rate.	Increased temperature may indicate infection or retained secretions which may represent problems with airway clearance or atelectasis. Tachycardia may occur with problems of airway clearance or oxygenation.
Determine cardiac output.	Cardiac output is the most important determinant of oxygen delivery.
Encourage patient to turn, cough, and deep breathe.	Position changes, coughing, and breathing deeply maximize alveolar ventilation.
Limit patient activities. Provide an environment conducive to rest and provide uninterrupted rest periods.	Rest and limited activity decrease oxygen consumption.
Administer oxygen therapy as prescribed and monitor patient response.	Oxygen therapy improves oxygen delivery to peripheral tissues, reverses hypoxic pulmonary vasoconstriction, and acts as a bronchodilator.
Provide hydration therapy.	Asthmatic patients are often hypovolemic from increased insensible water losses and decreased oral intake.

NURSING DIAGNOSIS: ANXIETY

Related To
- Fear of dying
- Dyspnea

Defining Characteristics
Verbalizations of anxiety
Restlessness
Decreased attention span
Tachycardia

Patient Outcomes
The patient verbalizes a decreased level of anxiety.

Nursing Interventions	Rationales
Assess level and cause of anxiety.	Baseline assessment is necessary for the development of appropriate interventions.
Monitor oxygenation status. Provide oxygen therapy as prescribed.	Hypoxia is a physiological trigger which promotes restlessness and anxiety.
Use therapeutic use of self to reassure patient of proximity of the nursing staff.	Provision of emotional support during periods of dyspnea can decrease associated anxiety.
Encourage verbalization of anxiety associated with dyspnea. Provide a caring concerned attitude in interacting with the patient.	
Encourage participation in care as tolerated.	
Administer sedatives judiciously.	
Promote comfort measures.	
Explain ongoing assessment, procedures, and treatments.	

Clinical Clip

Acid-Base Imbalance

Early in status asthmaticus, the patient will present with respiratory alkalosis (carbonic acid deficit) in response to airway obstruction, dyspnea, and decreasing arterial oxygen content. As the disease becomes more severe and more lung units are obstructed, there is progressive decrease in the PaO_2 and in the normalization of $PaCO_2$ and pH. In a severe life-threatening attack, the PaO_2 is less than 50 torr and the $PaCO_2$ is greater than 45 torr. Metabolic acidosis can be superimposed on respiratory acidosis, which can be very dangerous.

DISCHARGE PLANNING/CONTINUITY OF CARE

- Assess need for/type of long-term care and follow-up.
- If the discharge destination is home, assess existing supports and the need for assistance.

- Determine coping deficits/support needs and institute assistance measures.
- Determine knowledge deficits/teaching needs and document and institute a teaching plan.
- Refer patient to social services as appropriate.
- Communicate coping deficits/support needs and knowledge deficits/learning needs to unit accepting patient on transfer.

REFERENCES

Cobridge, T. & Hall, J. B. (1991). Status asthmaticus in the adult: Assessment, drug therapy and mechanical ventilation. *Respiratory Management*, 21(5), 119–126.

Grunger, G., Cohen, J. D., Keslin, J., Gassner, S. (1991). Facilitation of mechanical ventilation in status asthmaticus with continuous intravenous tiopental. *Chest*, 99(5), 1216–1219.

Harmon, E. J. (1992). Status asthmaticus: The need for early intervention, aggressive management. *Consultant*, 32(1), 54–61.

Janson-Bjerklie, S. (1990). Status asthmaticus. *American Journal of Nursing*, 90(9), 52–55.

Summer, W. R. (1985). Status asthmaticus. *Chest*, 87(1), 87S–97S.

▼

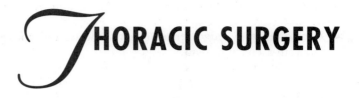

THORACIC SURGERY

Thoracic surgery may be indicated in any situation where there is evidence of intrathoracic damage or disease and chest wall deformities. The effects of surgery on lung function include a decrease in tidal volume, vital capacity, and functional residual capacity. The decreased vital capacity affects coughing and adequate clearance of secretions. Chest wall and diaphragm dysfunction and decreased functional residual capacity result in an altered distribution of gas in relation to perfusion. When functional residual capacity is reduced, airway closure occurs during normal tidal breathing, predisposing the patient to atelectasis. Anesthesia affects normal lung defense mechanisms resulting in impaired mucociliary clearance. Adjuncts to thoracic surgery in cases of cancer include fiberoptic instrumentation, laser therapy, photodynamic therapy, chemotherapy, and radiation therapy.

Postoperative care is focused on providing adequate ventilation and oxygenation. Lung expansion and maintaining airway clearance are nursing priorities.

ETIOLOGIES

- Blunt or penetrating injuries to the chest, resulting in
  - massive hemothorax
  - pericardial tamponade
  - esophageal, bronchial, tracheal, great-vessel injury
  - air embolism
  - pulmonary contusion
  - contamination of the pleural space
  - cardiac rupture
  - chest wall injuries
- Lung cancer
- Lung infection
  - empyema
  - bronchiectasis
  - bullous formations
- Chest wall deformities

CLINICAL MANIFESTATIONS

- Pulmonary: Impaired ventilation and gas exchange produce
  - dyspnea
  - tachycardia
  - paradoxic breathing pattern
  - tachypnea
  - use of accessory muscles
  - intercostal retractions
- Oncologic processes with local complications in the thorax produce
  - cough
  - hemoptysis
  - chest pain
  - sputum
  - dyspnea
- Cardiovascular: Impaired gas exchange and postoperative interstitial pulmonary edema produce
  - atrial dysrhythmias
  - hypertension
  - palpitations
  - activity intolerance
  - tachycardia
- Skin: Impaired ventilation and gas exchange produce
  - pallor
  - clammy skin
  - flushed skin
  - cyanosis
  - cool skin

CLINICAL/DIAGNOSTIC FINDINGS

- Chest x-ray findings suggestive of hemothorax, thoracic injury, injury to the great vessels, lung tumor
- Positive sputum cytology
- $SaO_2 < 90\%$
- $PaO_2 < 60$ torr
- Acidosis (pH < 7.35)
- $PaCO_2 > 45$ torr

▼

NURSING DIAGNOSIS: INEFFECTIVE BREATHING PATTERN

Related To
- Chest wall dysfunction
- Pleural space leaks
- Mediastinal shift
- Inadequate chest tube drainage
- Acute pain
- Underlying disease process
- Collapse of lung

Defining Characteristics
$PaCO_2 > 45$ torr with pH < 7.35
Decreasing PaO_2
Use of accessory muscles
Atelectatic crackles
Paradoxic breathing pattern/asymmetrical chest expansion
Respiratory rate > 30
Diminished breath sounds
Subcutaneous emphysema

Patient Outcomes

The breathing pattern is restored/returned to baseline, as evidenced by
- respiratory rate 12–20 at rest
- $PaCO_2$ return to baseline
- pH 7.35–7.45
- equal, full breath sounds
- symmetric chest expansion
- absence of signs and symptoms of air collection in chest
- absence of air or blood collection in the operative area
- resting spontaneous minute ventilation < 10 L/min

Nursing Interventions	Rationales
Observe for characteristics of respiration: inspiratory-expiratory ratio, use of accessory muscles, and unequal chest movements	
Assess/monitor ventilation and oxygenation by use of arterial blood gas analysis, capnography and/or pulse oximetry.	$PaCO_2$ is the assessment parameter used to evaluate ventilation. Capnography can track trending in CO_2 levels. It needs to be correlated with arterial pH, $PaCO_2$ and clinical assessment findings. The PaO_2 and SaO_2 are the assessment parameters used to evaluate oxygenation.
Auscultate breath sounds for degree of lung expansion.	
Observe for mediastinal shift (trachea off midline).	A mediastinal shift indicates a tension pneumothorax.
Monitor chest x-rays for degree of chest expansion.	
Palpate for subcutaneous emphysema.	Subcutaneous emphysema is associated with collection of air and/or blood in the operative area.
Administer ventilation to patient via endotracheal intubation with mechanical ventilation.	Assisted ventilation will improve the ventilatory pattern, returning the pH and $PaCO_2$ to within normal limits. The use of mechanical ventilation also allows internal stabilization of the chest wall, maintenance of an airway, optimal lung expansion, and improved airway clearance.

Nursing Interventions	Rationales
Position patient with head of bed elevated.	Elevation of the head of the bed facilitates diaphragmatic descent for best use of the ventilatory muscles.
Assist with removal of fluid (shift of mediastinum away from operated site) or injection of air (shift of mediastinum toward operated site).	
Assure patent drainage of chest tube system: ensure proper level of suction; milk chest tube to move thick drainage; and keep tubing free of clots and kinks.	
Administer bronchodilators as prescribed and monitor patient response.	Aminophylline has been proven to improve diaphragmatic function.
Provide for maximal diaphragmatic excursion: semi-Fowler's position, frequent repositioning from side to side, and support chest around chest tube.	
Suction with a measured catheter.	Suctioning too deeply can cause disruption of the bronchial stump.

NURSING DIAGNOSIS: IMPAIRED GAS EXCHANGE

Related To
- Effects of anesthesia and one-lung ventilation
- Positioning during surgery
- Atelectasis associated with hypoventilation or decreased functional lung tissue

Defining Characteristics
Restlessness
Irritability
Hypoxia ($PaO_2 < 60$ torr; $SaO_2 < 90\%$)
Adventitious breath sounds
Confusion
Cyanosis

Patient Outcomes
Gas exchange and oxygen balance will be restored, as evidenced by
- PaO_2 > 80 torr or return to baseline
- SaO_2 > 90%
- clear breath sounds
- absence of cyanosis
- absence of restlessness, confusion, irritability, dizziness
- airways clear of mucus

Nursing Interventions	Rationales
Assess respiratory system: respiratory rate and depth and use of accessory muscles. Assess for symptoms of dyspnea, fatigue, drowsiness, headache, and apathy.	
Assess for sudden change or absence of breath sounds, fine or coarse crackles, wheezing, and stridor or pleural rubs.	
Assess for changes in level of consciousness and anxiety.	Anxiety and changes in level of consciousness may indicate oxygen desaturation.
Monitor hemoglobin, PaO_2 and SaO_2.	Hemoglobin is the major oxygen-carrying compound. The PaO_2 reflects how much oxygen is in the plasma. The saturation of hemoglobin is reflected by SaO_2. Oxygen transport is compromised with oxygen saturations less than 90%.
Monitor pH and blood lactate levels.	These levels reflect overall acid-base balance.
Maintain chest tube system as appropriate.	Chest tubes are used to obliterate an abnormal pleural space and restore negative atmospheric pressure. Chest tubes may remove fluid and/or air from the pleural cavity.
Increase patient activity as tolerated. Ambulate as soon as possible.	
Position patient with good lung down.	Positioning the good lung down maximizes gas exchange by improving perfusion.

NURSING DIAGNOSIS: INEFFECTIVE AIRWAY CLEARANCE

Related To
- Weak/ineffective cough
- Anesthesia effects on normal lung defense mechanisms
- Oxygen therapy
- Sedation
- Pain
- Bronchospasm/bronchial edema
- Excessive tenacious secretions
- Immobility
- Chest wall restrictions

Defining Characteristics
Verbal statements by patient of inability to clear airway
Adventitious breath sounds
Dyspnea
Weak/ineffectual cough
Lung fields congested on chest x-ray

Patient Outcomes
The patient will maintain a patent airway, as evidenced by
- clear breath sounds or return to baseline
- absence of respiratory distress
- normal ABGs (pH 7.35–7.45, PaO_2 > 80 torr, $PaCO_2$ 35–45 torr, SaO_2 > 90%) or return to baseline
- cough or suctioning that produces thin mucus
- absence of clinical manifestations of infection
- clear lung fields on chest x-ray

Nursing Interventions	Rationales
Consider endotracheal intubation of patient.	Intubation will protect the airway from occlusion by accumulation of secretions, aspiration, or airway edema.
Provide chest physiotherapy.	Physiotherapy is used to loosen dry thick secretions and mucous plugs. When combined with postural drainage, the secretions are brought to the larger airways where they can be coughed up.
Tracheal suction with red rubber catheter as required.	

Nursing Interventions	Rationales
Implement measures to minimize sputum production.	Antibiotics and steroids may be administered to treat the underlying inflammatory process.
Apply humidified oxygen. Maintain hydration, replacing insensible loss plus 30 mL/hr (in the absence of renal or cardiac disease).	Humidification and hydration prevent thickening of retained secretions and increase the water content of mucous and reduce its viscosity. This allows easier clearance from the respiratory tract. Artificial airways bypass the body's normal humidification system.
Teach "huffing" cough after maximal inspiration.	Three short coughs use less energy than one large cough and produce less wheezing and airway collapse. Series coughing can enhance the effectiveness over a greater length of the airway.
Teach voluntary maximal inhalation after any expiratory maneuver.	This assists in reinflating the collapsed alveoli and prevents complications of pooled mucous, decreased oxygenation, and increased risk of infection.

NURSING DIAGNOSIS: ACUTE PAIN

Related To
- Thoracotomy incision
- Nerve plexus damage
- Tissue trauma from surgery
- Shoulder immobility
- Pleural inflammation
- Chest tube irritation
- Wound infection
- Anxiety

Defining Characteristics
Patient report of acute pain
Restlessness
"Beaten look"
Alteration in muscle tone
Hypertension
Increased or decreased respiratory rate

Eyes lack luster
Grimace
Diaphoresis
Tachycardia
Pupillary dilation

Patient Outcomes

Acute pain is relieved or reduced to tolerable levels, as evidenced by
- patient's subjective report that acute pain is relieved or tolerable (0–3 on a 0–10 scale)
- absence of nonverbal signs of acute pain

Nursing Interventions	Rationales
Assess for pain using a pain-rating scale.	
Assess for nonverbal cues of acute pain.	Multiple injuries may prevent the patient from providing verbal cues of acute pain.
Assess for anxiety and provide relief measures.	Anxiety may heighten pain perception.
Provide pain relief as prescribed: epidural pain medication, intravenous or intramuscular narcotics, cryoanalgesia, and transcutaneous electrical nerve stimulation.	Epidural medication blocks opiate nocioceptive pathways. Cryoanalgesia relieves pain by freezing intercostal muscles.
Position patient for comfort. Provide arm and shoulder support. Provide range-of-motion exercises.	
Splint incision during repositioning and respiratory maneuvers.	
Provide for general comfort measures: mouth care and hygiene.	

NURSING DIAGNOSIS: HIGH RISK FOR INJURY—HEMORRHAGE

Risk Factors
- Hemothorax
- Intraoperative blood loss
- Disruption of suture line

Patient Outcomes
The patient will be free of injury related to hemorrhage.

Nursing Interventions	Rationales
Assess indices of peripheral circulation and mentation: skin cool and pale, weak peripheral pulses, increased capillary refill time, and decreased mentation.	
Monitor for hemorrhage: chest tube output > 100 mL/hr, decreasing hemoglobin and hematocrit, hypotension, tachycardia, and urine output < 30 mL/hr.	
Monitor preload indicators with chest tube output and clinical signs of hypovolemia.	With resection of lung tissue, inflation of the pulmonary artery catheter balloon may obstruct a considerable portion of the remaining cross-sectional area of the pulmonary vasculature, reducing venous return to the left side of the heart and decreasing pressure. This falsely low value for left ventricular filling pressure is misleading and may result in fluid management that could aggravate pulmonary edema.
Provide for patent chest drainage system.	
Administer fluids carefully, monitoring hemodynamic parameters closely.	

NURSING DIAGNOSIS: ALTERED NUTRITION—LESS THAN BODY REQUIREMENTS

Related To
- Preoperative anorexia, malignancy
- Catabolism associated with surgery
- Increased metabolic demand (fever, blood loss, tissue damage)

See Appendix A

DISCHARGE PLANNING/CONTINUITY OF CARE

- Assess need for/type of long-term care and follow-up.
- If the discharge destination is home, assess existing supports and the need for assistance.
- Determine coping deficits/support needs and institute assistance measures.
- Determine knowledge deficits/teaching needs and document and institute a teaching plan.
- Refer patient to social services as appropriate.
- Communicate coping deficits/support needs and knowledge deficits/teaching needs to unit accepting patient on transfer.

REFERENCES

Bishop, M. (1991). Evaluation of a comprehensive algorithm for blunt and penetrating thoracic and abdominal trauma. *American Surgeon, 57*(12), 737–746.

Carroll, P. (1992). Nursing the thoracotomy patient. *RN, 55*(6), 34–43.

Entwistle, M. D., Roe, D. G., & Sapsford, D. J. (1991). Patterns of oxygenation after thoracotomy. *British Journal of Anesthesia, 67*(6), 704–711.

Ferrante, F. M. (1991). Interpleural analgesia after thoracotomy. *Anesthesia, 72*(1), 105–109.

Fisherman, R. S. (1991). Preoperative cardiopulmonary exercise testing: Determining the limit to exercise and predicting outcome after thoracotomy. *Journal of Cardiothoracic Vascular Anesthesia, 5*(6), 614–626.

Hammond, S. G. (1990). Chest injuries in the trauma patient. *Nursing Clinics of North America, 25*(1), 35–43.

Ivatury, R. R., Kazigo, J., Rohman, M., Gaudino, J., Simon, R., Stahl, W. H. (1991). Directed emergency room thoracotomy: A prognostic prerequisite for survival. *Journal of Trauma, 8,* 1076–1081.

Litwack, K. (1992). Practical points in the care of the thoracotomy surgery patient. *Journal of Postanesthesia Nursing, 5*(4), 276–278.

Murphy, D. F. (1991). Nurse-controlled intravenous analgesia: Effective control of pain after thoracotomy. *Anesthesia, 46*(9), 772.

Simpson, T., Want, G., DeTraglia, M., Speck, E., Taylor, D. (1992). The effects of epidural versus parenteral opiod analgesia on postoperative pain and pulmonary function in adults who have undergone thoracic and abdominal surgery. *Heart & Lung, 21*(2), 125–138.

Skinner, D. B. (1990). Technical and scientific advances in general thoracic surgery. *Annals of Thoracic Surgery, 49*(1), 14–25.

Renal Care

▼

ACUTE RENAL DIALYSIS

Acute renal dialysis is a process utilized to manage renal failure and/or edematous states. The three major principles governing dialysis are (1) diffusion or the movement of particles across a semipermeable membrane from an area of higher concentration to an area of lower concentration; (2) osmosis or movement of water across a semipermeable membrane from an area of lower concentration to an area of higher concentration; and (3) ultrafiltration or water exposed to hydrostatic pressure moves across a membrane from an area of higher pressure to an area of lower pressure. Three major modes of dialysis are currently available for use: hemodialysis, peritoneal dialysis, and continuous renal replacement therapy. All three of these modes utilize the above principles to some degree to remove solutes and water from the body.

Hemodialysis primarily utilizes the principles of ultrafiltration and diffusion for rapid removal of water and solutes, respectively. Vascular access is via a subclavian or femoral catheter, arteriovenous shunt, arteriovenous fistula, graft, or hemasite. Treatment is intermittent (3–4 hr three times a week) based on patient laboratory values and signs and symptoms. Major complications include hypotension, hypervolemia, electrolyte imbalance, dysrhythmias, disequilibrium syndrome (restlessness, headache, nausea, muscle twitching, disorientation, seizures), hypoxemia, mild thrombocytopenia and leukopenia, and thrombosis.

Peritoneal dialysis, the slowest mode of dialysis, utilizes the principles of diffusion and osmosis. Access is directly into the peritoneal cavity where a high glucose dialysate is infused and dwells while diffusion of solutes and osmosis of water occur across the peritoneal membrane. Peritoneal dialysis provides better clearance of large molecular weight substances than hemodialysis and lower clearance of smaller solutes. Treatment is usually continuous but may be intermittent (10–24 hr, three to four times a week). Major complications include peritonitis, loss of body protein, hyperglycemic hyperosmotic nonketotic coma (HHNC), pleural effusion, electrolyte imbalance, and dysrhythmias.

Three forms of continuous renal replacement therapy (CRRT) are currently available: (1) slow continuous ultrafiltration (SCUF), which uses the principle of ultrafiltration to remove primarily fluid; (2) continuous arteriovenous hemofiltration (CAVH), which uses the principle of ultrafiltration for both fluid and solute removal; and (3) continuous arteriovenous hemodialysis (CAVHD), which adds a diffusion compartment allowing for greater removal of solutes. Vascular access is obtained through cannulation of a large artery and vein, frequently the femoral. Treatment is continuous but slower than hemodialysis.

INDICATIONS

- Hemodialysis
  - uremia
  - electrolyte imbalance
  - volume overload
  - symptomatic metabolic acidosis
  - acute renal failure with volume overload, acidosis and hyperkalemia unable to manage medically
  - chronic renal failure
  - pericarditis
  - uremic encephalopathy
  - nueropathy
  - pulmonary edema refractory to diuretics
  - neuropathy
  - contraindications to other forms of dialysis
  - availability of trained staff and equipment
- Peritoneal dialysis
  - uremia
  - electrolyte imbalance
  - acute renal failure
  - chronic renal failure
  - refractory CHF
  - intraperitoneal chemical
  - volume overload
  - contraindications for hemodialysis
- Continual renal replacement therapy
  - hypervolemic or edematous patients unresponsive to diuretics
  - hemodynamically unstable in acute or chronic renal failure
  - oliguric patients requiring large quantities of fluid replacement
  - multisystem failure or multiple trauma, which require aggressive fluid removal
  - contraindication to hemo or peritoneal dialysis
  - inability to aggressively anticoagulate
  - lack of staff trained in other modes

CONTRAINDICATIONS

- Hemodialysis
  - hemodynamic instability
  - acute bleeding
  - lack of access to circulation
  - inability to anticoagulate
  - lack of trained staff and/or equipment
  - advanced cardiovascular disease
  - removal of high molecular weight toxins

- Peritoneal dialysis
  - need for rapid removal of fluid or solute
  - presence of abdominal adhesions or recurrent peritonitis, ostomies
  - traumatized abdomen
  - consider postoperative abdomen or peritonitis
  - sepsis
  - extreme obesity
  - history of ineffective clearances
- Continual renal replacement therapy
  - hematocrit > 45%
  - inability to anticoagulate

NURSING DIAGNOSIS: FLUID VOLUME DEFICIT
Related To removal of too much fluid

Defining Characteristics
Weight loss
CVP < 2 mmHg
Hypotension
Tachycardia
PCWP < 8 mmHg
Postural blood pressure

Patient Outcomes
Adequate fluid balance is maintained/restored, as evidenced by
- blood pressure within 10 mmHg of patient baseline without postural changes
- heart rate 60–100 bpm
- CVP 2–10 mmHg; PCWP 8–12 mmHg
- weight return to patient baseline

Nursing Interventions	Rationales
Monitor and document fluid balance: intake and output, daily weight, weight before and after dialysis, and fluid added/lost via dialysis.	
Monitor for cardiovascular signs of fluid deficit: decreased blood pressure, tachycadia, tachypnea, and decreased CVP/PCWP.	
Monitor for peripheral signs of fluid deficit: weak peripheral pulses, poor skin turgor, and dry mucous membranes.	

Nursing Interventions	Rationales
Monitor for signs of inadequate cerebral perfusion: dizziness, syncope, confusion, and weakness.	If fluid volume deficit and/or hypotension is severe, cerebral perfusion may be affected.
Monitor for signs of fluid overload: hypertension, increased PCWP/CVP, and edema.	If too much fluid is replaced or too little is removed, the patient may develop signs and symptoms of hypervolemia.
Monitor serum BUN and creatinine.	
Replace fluids as prescribed and monitor patient response.	

NURSING DIAGNOSIS: HIGH RISK FOR INJURY (PERITONEAL DIALYSIS)

Risk Factors
- Catheter insertion into peritoneal cavity
- Disruption of skin integrity
- Administration of fluids into peritoneal cavity
- Exchange/removal of electrolytes

Patient Outcome
The patient will remain free from injury.

Nursing Interventions	Rationales
Prevent injury during catheter insertion. Have patient empty bladder. Administer enema or cathartic to clear colon. Explain procedure to patient. Have dialysate set up and ready to infuse prior to insertion.	Emptying the bladder decreases the risk of bladder perforation during catheter insertion. Clearing the colon decreases the risk of colon perforation. Soliciting patient cooperation ensures a smoother procedure. The physician will want to infuse the dialysate as early as possible to facilitate catheter threading.
Use sterile technique when doing site care. Inspect site for purulence, redness, tenderness, or induration.	Infection at exit site must be treated quickly to prevent peritonitis.

Acute Renal Dialysis

Nursing Interventions	Rationales
Check composition of dialysate with physician order.	Administration of the wrong dialysate can cause fluid and/or electrolyte imbalances.
Ensure temperature of dialysate close to body temperature.	This minimizes loss of body heat and maximizes urea clearance.
Obtain baseline weight and vital signs.	
During inflow, ensure fluid flows freely. If not, assess for and correct cause.	Kinks in the tubing, air in the tubing, fibrin clots, constipation, and a dialysate bag hung below the abdomen can decrease inflow.
During dwell time, monitor patient for discomfort or respiratory distress and assess catheter for leakage or bleeding.	The addition of fluid to the abdomen may interfere with diaphragmatic excursion and cause respiratory distress. Leakage of dialysate is not uncommon, especially with infusion of large volumes of dialysate, but should decrease as the catheter insertion site matures and tissue seal occurs.
During drainage phase, ensure fluid flows freely, record patient complaints of discomfort, and record appearance of fluid drained.	Slow drainage may indicate air in tubing and need for patient repositioning or blockage of drainage tube. Pain may be caused by suction during drainage. Cloudy drainage fluid suggests infection.
Keep accurate intake and output records with each cycle.	
Monitor patient for insulin reaction after dialysis is discontinued.	The high glucose concentration of the dialysate causes increased insulin secretion. Rapid discontinuation of dialysis can cause an insulin reaction.
Assess patient for signs of fluid deficit/excess (see acute renal failure).	Fluid overload can occur if the tonicity of the fluid is too low. Fluid depletion can occur if the tonicity of the fluid is too high.
Monitor for signs of peritonitis: abdominal pain, cloudy outflow, nausea and vomiting, and increased temperature. Notify physician immediately.	Peritonitis is the major complication of peritoneal dialysis.

Nursing Interventions	Rationales
Assess for atelectasis: decreased breath sounds.	Abdominal distention and discomfort can cause hypoventilation.
Monitor serum electrolytes, BUN, creatinine, and albumin.	Hypertonic solutions used to remove excess fluid can cause hypernatremia. Using solutions with a sodium concentration of less than 130 mEq/L can prevent this. Potassium is removed or added to dialysate to control potassium levels.
Monitor serum glucose.	High glucose solutions can cause hyperglycemia.
Evaluate, monitor, and assess for abdominal pain and evaluate for possible etiology.	Pain can occur related to too rapid inflow, poor outflow, and overdistention from large volume or catheter pressure.

NURSING DIAGNOSIS: HIGH RISK FOR INJURY (HEMODIALYSIS/CONTINUOUS RENAL REPLACEMENT THERAPY)

Risk Factors
- Disruption of skin integrity (dialysis access site)
- Exchange/removal of fluid
- Exchange/removal of electrolytes

Patient Outcome
The patient will remain free from injury.

Nursing Interventions	Rationales
Assess arteriovenous shunt, if present, for palpable pulsation, warm, bruit, and red blood without separation. Monitor for separation and bleeding; have bulldog clamps attached to dressing. There should be no blood pressures or needle sticks in the arm with the shunt.	Although rarely used anymore, if present, an arteriovenous shunt must be checked for patency. If clotting is diagnosed early, the shunt can usually be declotted. If the arteriovenous shunt comes apart undetected, the patient can rapidly exsanguinate.

Acute Renal Dialysis

Nursing Interventions	Rationales
Assess arteriovenous fistula, if present, and prevent complications. Palpate and/or auscultate pulsation. Avoid constrictive clothing; there should be no blood pressures, tourniquets, or needle sticks. Patient should not sleep on that side. Assess extremity for cool skin or pain.	Steal syndrome can result when flow to the extremity distal to the fistula is decreased.
Assess subclavian catheter, if present, for access site. Assess for complications secondary to insertion: pneumothorax. Assess for site infection. Keep catheter flushed with heparin. Do not use site for anything else.	
Assess femoral catheter, if present, for access site. Assess for complications: retroperitoneal hemorrhage, femoral vein phlebitis, and thrombosis or site infection. Keep catheter flushed with heparin. Do not use site for anything else.	
Prevent/assess for infection. Utilize sterile technique for site care and handling of catheters. Assess for redness, inflammation, or exudate.	
Check composition of dialysate with physician order.	
Weigh patient before and after dialysis.	A weight gain of 1 kg/day is acceptable. The target is the patient's dry weight.
Monitor fluid balance for signs of hyper- or hypovolemia.	
Monitor ACT (normal 70–120 s)	
Monitor vital signs every 15–30 min depending on patient stability.	Hypotension is a frequent complication due to rapid fluid loss and increased temperature of dialysate.

Nursing Interventions	Rationales
Monitor for cardiac dysrhythmias.	Dysrhythmias may occur due to electrolyte disoders (especially potassium), hypoxia, or hypotension.
Hold drugs as ordered before dialysis.	Antihypertensives, long-acting nitrates, and narcotics can potentiate hypotension and should be held 4 hr before dialysis.
Monitor for leg cramps. Administer quinine sulfate as prescribed and monitor response.	Leg cramps occur when large amounts of fluid are removed and due to hypotension.
Monitor for signs of pericarditis and tamponade: chest pain (frequently pleuritic), dyspnea, friction rub, increased temperature, and manifestations of fluid overload.	Pericarditis and tamponade can develop as the result of volume overload, malnutrition, and/or inadequate dialysis.
Monitor electrolytes and acid-base balance.	Dialysis can cause electrolyte and/or acid-base imbalance.

DISCHARGE PLANNING/CONTINUITY OF CARE

See Acute Renal Failure

REFERENCES

Coloski, D., Mastrianni, J., Dube, R., & Brown, L. H. (1990). Continuous arteriovenous hemofiltration patient: Nursing care plan. *Dimensions of Critical Care Nursing, 9*(3), 130–142.

Ismail, N. & Hakim, R. (1991). Hemodialysis. In D. Z. Levine (Ed.), *Care of the renal patient* (2nd ed., pp. 220–246). Philadelphia, PA: Saunders.

Khanna, R. & Oreopoulos, D. G. (1991). Peritoneal dialysis. In D. Z. Levine (Ed.), *Care of the renal patient* (2nd ed., pp. 187–219). Philadelphia, PA: Saunders.

Lawyer, L. A. & Velasco, A. (1989). Continuous arteriovenous hemodialysis in the ICU. *Critical Care Nurse, 9*(1), 29–41.

Parker, J. & Ulrich, B. T. (1989). Peritoneal dialysis therapy. In B. T. Ulrich (Ed.), *Nephrology nursing* (pp. 153–171), Norwalk, CT: Appleton.

Price, C. A. (1989). Continuous arteriovenous ultrafiltration: A monitoring guide for ICU nurses. *Critical Care Nurse, 9*(1), 12–19.

Ulrich, B. T. (1989a). Principles of dialysis. In B. T. Ulrich (Ed.), *Nephrology nursing* (pp. 107–111). Norwalk, CT: Appleton.
Ulrich, B. T. (1989b). Hemodialysis and associated therapies. In B. T. Ulrich (Ed.), *Nephrology nursing* (pp. 113–151). Norwalk, CT: Appleton.

▼

ACUTE RENAL FAILURE

Acute renal failure is a potentially reversible decrease in renal function usually manifested by an accumulation of metabolic waste products and water and a decrease in urine output. It results from prerenal, intrarenal, or postrenal pathology, that is, decreased perfusion, ischemic or nephrotoxic injury, or obstruction. The prolonged and/or untreated presence of these conditions can lead to chronic renal failure.

Prerenal pathology causes decreased glomerular perfusion via vasoconstriction, decreased mean arterial pressure (from decreased blood volume, peripheral vasodilation or pump failure), or increased renal vascular resistance. When blood flow to the kidney is severely compromised, it causes retention of sodium and water and decreased secretion of metabolic waste products such as urea nitrogen. If the causative factor is corrected and glomerular perfusion reestablished, kidney function returns to normal and there is no actual damage to the kidneys.

Intrarenal pathology [most commonly acute tubular necrosis (ATN)] causes actual damage to the kidneys as a result of prolonged ischemia or nephrotoxins. The result is necrotic areas within the renal tubules and decreased glomerular filtration rate causing abnormal handling of sodium, water, and to a varying degree electrolytes and metabolic waste products. Even after correction of the original problem, recovery from ATN is more prolonged than prerenal failure. There are three stages of ATN: (1) the oliguric state (urine output < 400 mL/24 hr) lasting 6–8 weeks with retention of sodium, water, and waste products (some patients have nonoliguric ATN); (2) the diuretic stage (urine output > 400 mL/24 hr) lasting 2–3 weeks when azotemia (increased BUN and creatinine) gradually disappears heralding tubular recovery; and (3) the recovery state, which may require 6 months to a year to return to normal urine output and excretion. Of those patients with ATN, 50–60% will return to normal renal function, 25–30% will have permanent damage, and 15–20% will die. Death generally occurs as the result of failure to seek medical attention early enough, complications, or clinical mismanagement.

Postrenal pathology results in partial or complete obstruction of the urinary collecting system at any point. The interference with urine outflow can result in retrograde pressure involving both kidneys and predisposes to dysfunction of the nephrons.

ETIOLOGIES

Prerenal
- Arterial/venous problems
  - acute renal arteritis
  - aortic dissection
  - renal artery stenosis/thrombosis/occlusion
  - renal vein thrombosis
- Decreased volume
  - hemorrhage
  - third spacing
  - diarrhea
  - burns
  - vomiting
  - diabetes insipidus
- Vasodilation
  - sepsis
  - anesthesia
  - anaphylaxis
  - ganglionic blockade
- Pump failure
  - myocardial infarction
  - congestive heart failure
  - pulmonary embolus
- Increased renal vascular resistance
  - anesthesia
  - hepatorenal syndrome
  - surgery

Intrarenal
- Acute tubular necrosis (ATN)

Ischemic injury: any cause that decreases blood flow to the kidneys for more than 40 min
  - hypovolemia
  - renal vasoconstriction
  - burns
  - sepsis
  - myocardial ischemia
  - hypotension
  - hemorrhage
  - peritonitis
  - CHF
  - surgery

Nephrotoxins
  - heavy metals: mercury, arsenic, gold, lead
  - antibiotics: sulfonamides, amphotericin, aminoglycosides, cephalosporins
  - contrast media/dye
  - myoglobinuria: crush injuries, strenuous exercise, grand mal seizures, carbon monoxide poisoning, mismatched blood transfusion
  - nonsteroidal anti-inflammatory agents
  - organic solvents: carbon tetrachloride, ethylene glycol
  - diuretics: furosemide, thiazides
  - miscellaneous: cisplatinum, cyclosporine, cimetidine, diphenylhydantoin, allopurinol, captopril
- Glomerular disease
  - acute glomerulonephritis
  - lupus nephritis

- Vascular disease
  - vasculitis
  - atheroembolism
  - scleroderma
  - hemolytic uremic syndrome
- Interstitial disease
  - infections
  - allergic (drug induced)
  - hypercalcemia
- Tubular obstruction
  - myeloma protein
  - drugs (acyclovir, methotrexate)
  - uric acid
  - oxalate
- High-risk states
  - hemodynamic instability
  - severe multiple trauma
  - nephrotoxic drugs
  - prolonged surgery
  - burns
  - rhabdomyolysis

Postrenal
- Ureteral
  - stones
  - tumor
  - fibrosis
  - thrombus
  - necrotic papilla
- Lower genitourinary (GU) tract
  - bladder stone
  - benign prostatic hypertrophy or neoplasm
  - strictures
  - bladder neoplasm

CLINICAL MANIFESTATIONS

Prerenal
- Manifestations of primary/causative disorder

Intrarenal
- Secondary to uremia
  - lethargy
  - weakness
  - edema
  - seizures
  - uremic frost
  - nausea
  - somnolence
  - anorexia
  - pericardial rub
  - decreased wound healing
  - increased susceptibility to infection
- Secondary to electrolyte disorders
  - hyperkalemia: dysrhythmias, tall peaked T waves, restlessness, muscle weakness, numbness and tingling
  - hypocalcemia: muscle weakness, numbness and tingling, prolonged QT, dysrhythmias, heart failure
  - hyperphosphatemia: decreased CO, numbness and tingling, muscle cramps
  - metabolic acidosis: headaches, confusion, increased respiratory rate, fatigue, anorexia
- Secondary to stage
  - oliguric: signs and symptoms of hypervolemia (jugular venous distention [JVD], peripheral edema, S_3 or S_4, fine crackles)

- diuretic: signs and symptoms of hypovolemia (poor skin turgor, hypotension, dry mucous membranes)

Postrenal
- Prostatic obstruction: difficulty in initiating or maintaining urinary stream
- Stones: excruciating, colicky pain radiating to genital area

CLINICAL/DIAGNOSTIC FINDINGS

Prerenal
- Oliguria
- Urine osmolality > serum
- Specific gravity > 1.020
- Urea nitrogen > 600 mg/100 mL
- Urine sediment normal
- Urine Na < 20 mEq/L
- BUN > 20 mg/dL
- Creatinine > 1.2 mg/dL
- Urea-creatinine ratio > 15:1
- Urine creatinine normal

Intrarenal
- Degree of disturbance depends on severity of damage:
  - urine Na > 20 mEq/L
  - urine osmolality ≤ serum
  - creatinine > 1.2 mg/dL
  - urea-creatinine ratio < 10:1
  - urine creatinine low
  - metabolic acidosis (pH < 7.35, HCO_3 < 21 mEq/L)
  - hyponatremia (<135 mEq/L)
  - anemia (Hgb < 13 g/dL)
  - serum calcium <8.5 mg/dL
  - oliguria
  - BUN > 20 mg/dL
  - specific gravity 1.010
  - urine urea 200–300 mg/dL
  - urine sediment present
  - hyperkalemia (>5 mEq/L)
  - serum phosphate > 4.5 mg/dL

Postrenal
- Anuria

NURSING DIAGNOSIS: ALTERED URINARY ELIMINATION

Related To abnormal excretion of water, electrolytes, and waste products

Defining Characteristics
Oliguria
Hyperkalemia (>5 mEq/L)
Hypocalcemia (<8.5 mg/dL)
Metabolic acidosis (pH < 7.35, HCO_3 < 21 mEq/L)
BUN > 20 mg/dL
Creatinine > 1.2 mg/dL
Hyperphosphatemia (>4.5 mg/dL)

Patient Outcomes

The patient's urine elimination pattern will return to normal, as evidenced by
- urine output > 400 mL/24 hr
- electrolytes within normal range
- normal acid-base balance

Nursing Interventions	**Rationales**
Monitor serum electrolytes daily or more often if necessary.	
Monitor for signs/symptoms of hyperkalemia and document: tall peaked T waves, widened QRS, prolonged PR, muscle weakness, dysrhythmias, nausea, and restlessness.	In intrarenal failure the kidneys are unable to excrete potassium.
Monitor for signs/symptoms of hypocalcemia and document: prolonged QR, paresthesias, numbness and tingling, muscle cramps, dysrhythmias, and nausea and vomiting.	In intrarenal failure the kidneys retain phosphate, causing hyperphosphatemia and a decrease in serum calcium.
Monitor for signs and symptoms of uremia: increased BUN, increased creatinine, lethargy, anorexia, nausea, weakness, and somnolence.	Worsening of uremic symptoms may indicate the need for dialysis and determine the frequency of dialysis.
Watch for increased side effects or more dramatic response to drugs. Question orders for nephrotoxic drugs.	Since many drugs are excreted via the kidneys, a decrease in kidney function will require changes in dosage and/or frequency of administration.
Monitor for signs and symptoms that indicate the need for dialysis: severe uremia (BUN > 100 mg/dL, serum creatinine > 10 mg/dL), pericarditis, GI bleeding, and mental changes), uncontrolled hyperkalemia and severe catabolism, fluid overload, and uncontrolled metabolic acidosis.	
Institute measures to maintain normal potassium (see Hyperkalemia) and evaluate effects.	

Nursing Interventions	Rationales
Institute measures to maintain normal calcium (see Hypocalcemia) and evaluate effects.	
Provide high-carbohydrate, low-protein, controlled sodium, potassium, and phosphate diet.	High carbohydrates and low protein will promote protein sparing and provide adequate calories and amino acids for cellular healing.
Administer oral alkali and monitor results.	Metabolic acidosis may occur in ATN as the result of impaired renal excretion of hydrogen. Oral alkali are used to treat chronic metabolic alkalosis.

NURSING DIAGNOSIS: FLUID VOLUME EXCESS

Related To impaired water excretion in prerenal failure or the oliguric phase of intrarenal failure

Defining Characteristics
Increased weight
Increased blood pressure
CVP > 10 mmHg
Peripheral edema

Puffy eyelids
Bounding pulses
Ascites

Patient Outcomes
Fluid volume will be maintained/restored, as evidenced by
- weight that returns to patient baseline
- blood pressure within 10 mmHg of patient baseline
- absence of tissue fluid accumulation
- CVP 2–10 mmHg

Nursing Interventions	Rationales
Identify patients at high risk for acute renal failure (see etiologies).	Preventive measures can be instituted and the occurrence of prerenal failure or ATN possibly avoided by identifying patients at high risk.
Identify and institute correction of the cause.	Correction of the cause must be made to prevent more extensive or permanent kidney damage.

Nursing Interventions	Rationales
Monitor/record fluid balance: intake and output and daily weight.	
Monitor/record cardiovascular status: vital signs, hemodynamic parameters, peripheral pulses, and neck veins. Monitor for signs of overhydration: fine crackles, c/o shortness of breath, jugular venous distention, peripheral edema, tachycardia, and increased weight.	During the oliguric stage of ATN patients are at high risk for overhydration, resulting in heart failure. This is particularly true if the patient has underlying cardiac problems. Hemodynamic assessment can also assist in differentiating between pre- and intra-renal failure.
Maintain water and sodium restriction as prescribed.	
Administer diuretics as prescribed and document effect.	

NURSING DIAGNOSIS: FLUID VOLUME DEFICIT

Related To
- Diuretic phase of intrarenal failure
- Use of diuretics in prerenal failure

Defining Characteristics
Weight loss
CVP < 2 mmHg
Increased urine output
Tachycardia
Hypotension/postural blood pressure

Patient Outcomes
Fluid balance is maintained/restored, as evidenced by
- blood pressure return to patient baseline without postural changes
- heart rate 60–100 bpm
- CVP 2–10 mmHg
- weight return to patient baseline

Nursing Interventions	Rationales
Monitor for signs of continuing fluid deficit: tachycardia, hypotension, orthostatic changes, low hemodynamic parameters, weak peripheral pulses, poor skin turgor, and dry mucous membranes.	

Nursing Interventions	Rationales
Monitor for signs of fluid overload: increased CVP/PCWP, increased or decreased CO/CI, increased heart rate, bounding pulses, and adventitious lung sounds.	
Monitor BUN, creatinine, serum sodium, and serum potassium.	During the diuretic stage of ATN, BUN and creatinine should gradually decrease.
Monitor for signs and symptoms of hypokalemia: dysrhythmias, fatigue, muscle weakness, confusion, anorexia, flat T waves, and depressed ST segment.	Diuresis from diuretics or the diuretic phase of ATN can result in hypokalemia.
Monitor for signs and symptoms of sodium imbalance. Hyponatremia: anorexia, weakness, confusion, muscle twitching. Hypernatremia: thirst, lethargy, stupor, dry mucous membranes, tachycardia, increased deep-tendon reflexes.	Sodium can be lost due to renal wasting and/or diuresis resulting in hyponatremia. During diuresis water can be lost in excess of sodium, producing dehydration and hypernatremia.
Provide adequate fluids.	
Record intake and output and daily weight.	
Institute measures to maintain normal potassium (see Hypokalemia) and evaluate effects.	
Institute measures to maintain normal sodium levels (see Disturbances of Sodium) and evaluate effects.	

NURSING DIAGNOSIS: HIGH RISK FOR INFECTION

Risk Factors
- Impaired immune system secondary to uremia and stress
- Presence of invasive catheters

Patient Outcomes
The patient will remain free of infection.

Nursing Interventions	Rationales
Minimize use of invasive catheters, especially Foley catheters. Utilize aseptic technique when inserting IV or Foley catheters. Follow hospital procedures for care of sites (IV and Foley catheter).	Patients with ATN are particularly prone to infection due to effects on the immune system, making infection one of the primary causes of death.
Maintain dry skin surface; avoid damage to skin surface.	
Keep urinary drainage devices below bladder or clamp during transport.	This reduces the risk for backflow and infection.
Maintain acidic pH of urine.	An acidic urine decreases bacterial growth and the chance for infection.
Maintain adequate caloric and protein intake.	Adequate nutrition is necessary for proper healing and function of the immune system.
Administer prescribed antimicrobial therapy within 15 min of scheduled time.	
Observe for clinical manifestations of infection: increased temperature, malaise, cloudy, foul-smelling urine, and inflammation at IV site.	
Provide frequent mouth and skin care.	

NURSING DIAGNOSIS: ACTIVITY INTOLERANCE

Related To
- Uremia
- Anemia

Defining Characteristics
Patient complaints of weakness and fatigue
Dyspnea on exertion
Increased blood pressure, respiratory rate, and/or heart rate with activity

Patient Outcomes
The patient will return to baseline activity level.

Nursing Interventions	Rationales
Assess/record the patient's response to activity. Monitor heart rate, blood pressure, and respiratory rate before, during, and immediately after activity.	Vital signs should return to resting rate within 3–4 min.
Assess strength of gait and need for assistance.	
Assess subjective complaints during activity: fatigue, dizziness, and dyspnea.	
Monitor Hgb and Hct and transfuse if patient is symptomatic.	Hemolysis (dialysis and uremic effects on RBCs) and suppression of erythropoiesis can produce anemia and increase fatigue.
Allow for adequate rest/sleep periods. Minimize or group interruptions. Assess patient's normal sleep patterns/habits and try to accommodate them. Maintain quiet, calm environment.	
Provide adequate nutrition.	
Increase activity gradually when patient is able.	
Assist patient with ADLs as needed.	

NURSING DIAGNOSIS: IMPAIRED SKIN INTEGRITY

Related To
- Uremia
- Malnutrition

Defining Characteristics
Itching
Bruising
Edema

Dryness
Uremic frost

Patient Outcomes
The patient's skin integrity will be maintained.

Nursing Interventions	Rationales
Bathe daily.	
Apply creams/ointments to skin; use oil in bath.	
Administer medications to relieve itching.	
Cleanse bruises/open areas.	
Monitor edema.	
Avoid tight sheets and slippers.	
Reposition patient at least every 2 hr.	
Inspect for areas of breakdown or redness.	

DISCHARGE PLANNING/CONTINUITY OF CARE

- Based on underlying pathology/etiology, assess need for/type of long-term care and follow-up.
- If the discharge destination is home, assess existing supports and the need for assistance.
- Determine coping deficits/support needs and institute assistance measures.
- Determine knowledge deficits/teaching needs and document and institute teaching plan.
- Refer patient to social services as appropriate.
- Communicate coping deficits/support needs and knowledge deficits/teaching needs to unit accepting the patient on transfer.

REFERENCES

Baer, C. L. (1992). Acute renal failure. *Critical Care Nursing Quarterly*, 14(4), 1–21.

Burke, T. J. & Schrier, R. W. (1990). Acute renal failure. In H. C. Gonick, (Ed.), *Current nephrology* (Vol. 13, (pp. 245–261). Chicago, IL: Year Book Medical.

Clive, D. M. & Cohen, A. J. (1991). Acute renal failure. In J. M. Rippe, R. S. Irwin, J. S. Alpert, & M. P. Fink (Eds.), *Intensive care medicine* (2nd ed., pp. 764–774). Boston, MA: Little, Brown.

Crandall, B. I. (1989). Acute renal failure. In B. T. Ulrich (Ed.), *Nephrology nursing* (pp. 45–59). Norwalk, CT: Appleton.

Douglas, S. (1992). Acute tubular necrosis: Diagnosis, treatment and nursing implications. *AACN Clinical Issues in Critical Care Nursing, 3*(3), 688–697.

Innerarity, S. A. (1990). Electrolyte emergencies in the critically ill renal patient. *Critical Care Nursing Clinics of North America, 2*(1), 89–99.

Norris, M. K. (1989). Acute tubular necrosis: Preventing complications. *Dimensions of Critical Care Nursing, 8*(1), 16–26.

Stark, J. L. (1992). Acute tubular necrosis: Differences between oliguria and nonoliguria. *Critical Care Nursing Quarterly, 14*(4), 22–27.

▼

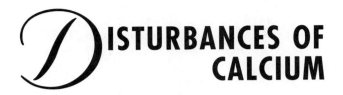

DISTURBANCES OF CALCIUM

Calcium, the body's most abundant ion, combines with phosphorus to form the mineral salts of bones and teeth. Calcium also is an important constituent of biological membranes affecting permeability and electrical properties, muscle contraction, blood coagulation, and enzyme activity. Calcium is regulated by parathyroid hormone (increases serum calcium), calcitonin (decreases serum calcium), and vitamin D (promotes GI absorption and bone release). Its biologically active form is the 50% of calcium which is ionized and non–protein bound. Protein levels thus can affect levels of biologically active calcium. Normal serum calcium is 8.5–10.5 mg/dL. Normal ionized calcium levels are 3.9–4.5 mg/dL.

Hypercalcemia

Hypercalcemia (serum levels above 10.5 mg/dL) occurs when calcium enters the vascular space more rapidly than it can be excreted or absorbed in bone. It is the result of increased mobilization of calcium from bone, increased intestinal reabsorption of calcium, or altered renal tubular reabsorption. It is most commonly seen in critically ill patients as the result of malignancy, hyperparathyroidism, immobilization, calcium administration, or renal failure. Hypercalcemia causes decreased membrane permeability, making depolarization more difficult and causing decreased neuromuscular excitability. Symptomatic hypercalcemia is associated with a high mortality rate, usually due to cardiac dysrhythmias, renal failure, or CNS impairment.

ETIOLOGIES

- Increased mobilization of calcium from bone
    - hyperparathyroidism
    - vitamin A/D administration
    - multiple fractures
    - pheochromocytoma
    - hyperthyroidism
    - immobilization
    - sarcoidosis
    - AIDS
    - malignancies: leukemia, lymphoma, multiple myeloma

- metastatic malignancy involving bone
- ectopic parathyroid secretion: bronchial cancer, liver cancer, squamous cell cancer
- posthypocalcemic hypercalcemia
• Increased intestinal reabsorption of calcium
  - vitamin D intoxication
  - excessive dietary intake
• Altered renal tubular reabsorption
  - hypophosphatemia
  - milk-alkali syndrome
  - chronic thiazide diuretic therapy
  - renal failure

CLINICAL MANIFESTATIONS

- Primary: deep bone pain, excessive thirst, anorexia, lethargy, weakened muscles
- Cardiovascular: Increased myocardial contractility and depressant effect can produce
  - AV block
  - hypertension
  - increased sensitivity to digoxin (> 17 mg/dL)
  - ventricular dysrhythmias
  - catecholamine resistance
- Neurological: depressant effects can produce
  - lethargy
  - muscle weakness
  - depression
  - stupor
  - decreased attention span
  - confusion
  - personality changes
  - coma (> 17 mg/dL)
- Musculoskeletal: Removal of calcium from bone (with increased parathyroid hormone) can produce
  - long-bone deformity
  - pathological fractures
  - calcium deposits: skin, cornea, kidney
  - bone pain
- Renal: Excess calcium load produces precipitation of calcium and inability to concentrate urine, resulting in
  - polyuria
  - flank pain
  - kidney stones
- Gastrointestinal: Depressed smooth-muscle contractility and decreased peristalsis can produce
  - anorexia
  - weight loss
  - duodenal ulcers
  - nausea and vomiting
  - constipation
  - abdominal pain

CLINICAL/DIAGNOSTIC FINDINGS

- Serum calcium > 10.5 mg/dL
- Serum phosphate < 2.5 mg/dL
- Serum potassium < 3.5 mEq/L

- EKG changes: shortened QT interval; shortened ST segment
- X-ray
  - decreased bone density
  - bone cysts
  - decalcification

NURSING DIAGNOSIS: ELECTROLYTE IMBALANCE—HYPERCALCEMIA

Related To
- Increased mobilization of calcium
- Increased intestinal reabsorption of calcium
- Altered renal tubular reabsorption
- Increased ionized calcium

Defining Characteristics
Calcium > 10.5 mg/dL
Deep-bone pain
Lethargy
Mental status changes

Phosphate < 2.5 mg/dL
Anorexia
Weakened muscles

Patient Outcomes
The patient's electrolyte balance will be restored, as evidenced by
- serum calcium level 8.5–10.5 mg/dL
- neurological status and sensorium return to patient baseline

Nursing Interventions	Rationales
Assess for etiology of hypercalcemia.	Hypercalcemia occurs as the result of some underlying disorder. Identification and treatment of the underlying disorder is essential in correcting hypercalcemia.
Identify patients at risk (see etiologies) and assess for clinical manifestations of hypercalcemia.	

Nursing Interventions	Rationales
Monitor serum calcium and phosphate levels.	Phosphate levels are measured because hypophosphatemia can precipitate hypercalcemia and if abnormal must be corrected to effectively treat hypercalcemia. In order to monitor the effectiveness of treatment, calcium and phosphate levels should be measured after each treatment and before further therapy is instituted to prevent overcorrection.
Monitor serum potassium and magnesium levels and watch for signs of depletion.	Potassium and magnesium levels may drop with therapeutic diuresis.
Administer intravenous normal saline and diuretics as prescribed and monitor response.	Rapid administration of normal saline will dilute serum calcium, enhance glomerular filtration rate, and increase renal excretion of calcium. Diuretics block reabsorption of sodium and chloride in the renal tubules, promoting diuresis and preventing fluid overload.
If patient is exhibiting toxic cardiovascular effects, administer verapamil or nifedipine as prescribed and monitor response.	These calcium blockers will antagonize hypercalcemia's toxic cardiovascular effects.
Administer calcium chelators as prescribed and monitor response: oral, rectal, or intravenous phosphates; ethylenediaminetetraacetic acid (EDTA) via a central line with adequate hydration.	Calcium chelators are effective in treating hypercalcemic emergencies because they lower calcium levels rapidly. Phosphates bind and precipitate calcium, inhibit bone release, and decrease the activation of vitamin D. The IV route is effective in 6–24 hr, oral in several days. Their major disadvantage is the potential for extraskeletal calcification, especially kidney stones. The EDTA binds with calcium and is excreted in the urine. Adequate hydration is essential during its administration to prevent renal toxicity.

Nursing Interventions	Rationales
Administer plicamycin (mithramycin) or indomethacin as prescribed and monitor response.	Plicamycin acts directly on bone to reduce decalcification and is usually used to treat hypercalcemia caused by neoplastic disease. It takes 12–24 hr to produce an effect and can cause renal, hepatic, and hematologic toxicity. In some malignancies indomethacin reduces bone release of calcium.
Administer calcitonin as prescribed and monitor response and for side effects (nausea, vomiting, abdominal cramps, skin rash, flushing and diarrhea).	Calcitonin will reduce bone release, increase deposit of calcium and phosphorus in bone, and increase renal excretion of calcium and phosphate. It should reduce serum calcium in 6–10 hr.
Administer sodium bicarbonate as prescribed and monitor response.	Sodium bicarbonate reduces the percentage of calcium that is ionized or biologically active.
Administer glucocorticoids as prescribed and monitor response.	Glucocorticoids such as prednisone inhibit the actions of vitamin D and inhibit GI absorption of calcium. They are most effective with vitamin D excess, sarcoidosis, multiple myeloma, and lymphoma and are not effective with hyperparathyroidism.
Encourage increased mobility.	Weight bearing stimulates deposit of calcium in bone and decreases bone release.
Control dietary intake of calcium. Avoid meats, leafy green vegetables, and dairy products.	

Nursing Interventions	Rationales
Institute preventive measures and assess for signs of duodenal ulcers. Document appearance and consistency of stools; hematest stools, emesis, or NG drainage. Assess for abdominal pain, tenderness, GI upset, or nausea and vomiting. Administer antacids, histamine H_2 receptor antagonists, and/or sucralfate as prescribed and monitor results. Monitor Hgb and Hct for occult bleeding.	Hypercalcemia stimulates gastric secretion, making patients prone to the development of duodenal ulcers.

NURSING DIAGNOSIS: ALTERED URINARY ELIMINATION

Related To polyuria and kidney stones secondary to hypercalcemia

Defining Characteristics
Increased urine output
Pain
Hematuria
Frequency
Urgency

Patient Outcomes
The patient will exhibit normal urinary elimination, as evidenced by
- absence of pain, frequency, or urgency
- normal urine output
- absence of hematuria

Nursing Interventions	Rationales
Monitor for signs of hypovolemia: decreased blood pressure, increased heart rate, and decreased CVP/PCWP.	
Monitor hourly urine output, daily weight, and intake and output.	
Moniter serum BUN and creatinine.	Hypercalcemia can impair kidney function, causing retention of waste products.

Nursing Interventions	Rationales
Assess for signs of kidney stones: acute pain, hematuria, fever, chills, pyuria, and abdominal distention.	Hypercalcemia can produce calcium deposits in the kidney, resulting in kidney stones.

Hypocalcemia
Hypocalcemia (serum levels below 8.5 mg/dL) results when calcium leaves the vascular space faster than it can be replaced. It results from impaired parathyroid hormone secretion, impaired vitamin D synthesis, removal of calcium from the circulation, or decreased bone turnover. In critically ill patients it most frequently is the result of parathyroid hormone or vitamin D deficiency. Increased phosphorous and decreased magnesium levels can also precipitate hypocalcemia. Hypocalcemia causes an increase in membrane permeability, causing spontaneous depolarization and hyperirritability of both smooth and skeletal muscle. Ionized levels of calcium less than 3 mg/dL can produce life-threatening dysrhythmias.

ETIOLOGIES

- Decreased parathyroid hormone secretion/action
  - hypoparathyroidism
  - vitamin D deficiency
  - cimetidine
  - hypomagnesemia
  - acute pancreatitis
- Impaired vitamin D synthesis/action
  - decreased intake
  - liver disease
  - malabsorption: biliary tract disease, inflammatory bowel disease, pancreatic insufficiency
  - sepsis
  - hypomagnesemia
- Removal of calcium from the circulation
  - hyperphosphatemia
  - rhabdomyolysis
  - blood administration
  - drugs: protamine, radiocontrast dye, albumin
  - pancreatitis
  - fat embolism
  - sepsis
- Decreased bone turnover
  - toxic shock syndrome
  - drugs: heparin, plicamycin, phenytoin, phosphates, protamine, calcitonin, cisplatin
  - hypothyroidism

CLINICAL MANIFESTATIONS

- Neuromuscular: Increased neuromuscular irritability can produce
  - paresthesias
  - fibrillary twitching
  - dysphagia
  - laryngeal spasm

- hyperactive reflexes
- seizures
- stiffness of hands, feet, and lips
- numbness and tingling of extremities
- spasms of smooth/skeletal muscle (face and limbs)
- Chovstek's or Trousseau's sign
- anxiety, dementia, depression, irritability, confusion
- Musculoskeletal: Increased neuromuscular irritability can produce
  - muscle weakness
  - joint pain
  - muscle cramps
- Cardiovascular: Decreased myocardial contractility, vasodilatation, and electrical changes can produce
  - CO < 4 L/min
  - CI < 2.5 L/min/m^2
  - SVR < 800 dyn/s/cm^{-5}
  - bradycardia
  - hypotension
  - cardiac failure
  - dysrhythmias
  - decreased sensitivity to digoxin and catecholamines
- Gastrointestinal: Spasm of smooth muscle can produce
  - diarrhea
  - nausea and vomiting

CLINICAL/DIAGNOSTIC FINDINGS

- Serum calcium < 8.5 mg/dL
- Serum phosphate > 4.5 mg/dL
- Hypo- or hypermagnesemia
- EKG changes: prolonged QT interval, prolonged ST segment
- X-ray: increased bone density

NURSING DIAGNOSIS: ELECTROLYTE IMBALANCE— HYPOCALCEMIA

Related To
- Decreased parathyroid hormone secretion/action
- Impaired vitamin D synthesis/action
- Removal of calcium from circulation
- Decreased bone turnover of calcium

Defining Characteristics
Paresthesias
Muscle spasms
Mental status changes
Phosphate > 4.5 mg/dL

Joint pain
Dysphagia
Calcium < 8.5 mg/dL

Patient Outcomes
The patient's electrolyte balance will be restored, as evidenced by
- serum calcium level 8.5–10.5 mg/dL
- serum phosphate 2.5–4.5 mg/dL
- absence of neuromuscular or musculoskeletal signs

Nursing Interventions	Rationales
Assess for the etiology of hypocalcemia.	Hypocalcemia occurs as the result of some underlying disorder. Identification and treatment of this underlying disorder is essential to treatment of hypocalcemia.
Identify patients at risk and assess for clinical manifestations of hypocalcemia.	
Monitor serum calcium and phosphate levels.	Hyperphosphatemia causes calcium precipitation, inhibits bone release, and suppresses vitamin D. Administration of calcium to a patient with hyperphosphatemia may cause calcium precipitation. To monitor the effectiveness of treatment, calcium and phosphate levels should be measured after each treatment and before further therapy to prevent overcorrection.
Monitor serum magnesium levels and correct imbalances.	Severe hypo- or hypermagnesemia inhibits parathyroid hormone (PTH) secretion, impairs PTH action, and causes vitamin D resistance. Hypocalcemia in the presence of hypomagnesemia is corrected by magnesium, not calcium.
Administer intravenous calcium gluconate cautiously and according to guidelines.	Intravenous administration of calcium will increase serum levels within 30 min. Too rapid administration of calcium can precipitate hypotension. Infusion of calcium into an infiltrated IV can cause tissue sloughing. Mixing calcium with sodium bicarbonate or sodium phosphate can cause precipitation.

Disturbances of Calcium

Nursing Interventions	Rationales
Administer oral calcium supplements and vitamin D as prescribed at least 1 hr after meals and monitor for constipation.	Concomitant administration of vitamin D increases absorption of calcium. Constipation is a major side effect of oral calcium administration.
Administer phosphate binding gels (aluminum hydroxide antacids) as prescribed, immediately after meals, and monitor for constipation.	In patients with elevated phosphorous levels, phosphate binding gels bind phosphorus in the GI tract, removing it from the body. As long as phosphate levels are high, treatment for hypocalcemia will be ineffective.
Encourage foods high in calcium: meats, leafy green vegetables, and milk products.	

NURSING DIAGNOSIS: DECREASED CARDIAC OUTPUT

Related To decreased cardiac contractility secondary to hypocalcemia and/or digoxin toxicity

Defining Characteristics
CO < 4 L/min
Tachycardia
Signs of heart failure
CI < 2.5 L/min/m^2
CVP > 10 mmHg
PCWP > 12 mmHg

Patient Outcomes
Cardiac output will be maintained/restored, as evidenced by
- CO 4–8 L/min; CI 2.5–4 L/min/m^2
- heart rate 60–100 bpm
- CVP 2–10 mmHg; PCWP 8–12 mmHg
- absence of signs of heart failure

Nursing Interventions	Rationales
Monitor for and document signs and symptoms of decreased cardiac output/heart failure: hypotension, tachycardia, tachypnea, CVP > 10 mmHg, PCWP > 12 mm Hg, jugular venous distention, fine crackles, c/o shortness of breath, thready pulses, edema, and urine output < 30 mL/hr.	Hypocalcemia and/or digoxin toxicity can cause decreased cardiac contractility, decreasing cardiac output.
Monitor the EKG for signs of digoxin toxicity [premature ventricular contractions (PVCs), paroxysmal atrial tachycardia (PAT), Mobtiz I] and document.	Digoxin toxicity can develop in patients on digoxin receiving calcium supplements because calcium potentiates digoxin's effects.
Monitor the EKG for signs of hypocalcemia and document: prolonged QT interval and prolonged ST segment.	
Monitor magnesium levels and treat as appropriate.	Hypomagnesemia may occur with hypocalcemia and contribute to decreased cardiac output.

NURSING DIAGNOSIS: HIGH RISK FOR IMPAIRED GAS EXCHANGE

Risk Factors
- Severe hypocalcemia
- Laryngeal spasm

Patient Outcomes
The patient exhibits
- adequate oxygenation via ABGs or pulse oximetry
- the absence of laryngeal spasm
- a serum calcium of 8.5–10.5 mg/dL

Nursing Interventions	Rationales
Assess and monitor patient's respiratory status: rate, depth, and quality of respirations; subjective complaints of dyspnea or SOB; constrictive feeling in throat; and breath sounds.	
Maintain oxygen and suction equipment at bedside.	In the presence of laryngeal spasm or respiratory distress the patient may need supplementary oxygen and assistance with removal of secretions.
Measure and record pulse oximetry if patient is in distress and/or at least every 8 hr.	Pulse oximetry is a noninvasive estimate of SaO_2 and thus of the adequacy of oxygenation.
Position patient for ease of respiratory effort, that is, head of bed elevated.	
Minimize activity to decrease oxygen need.	
Reposition patient every 2 hr.	Repositioning will enhance ventilation and prevent stasis of secretions.

DISCHARGE PLANNING/CONTINUITY OF CARE

- Based on underlying pathology/etiology, assess need for/type of long-term care and follow-up.
- If the discharge destination is home, assess existing supports and the need for assistance.
- Determine coping deficits/support needs and institute assistance measures.
- Determine knowledge deficits/teaching needs and document and institute a teaching plan.
- Refer patient to social services as appropriate.
- Communicate coping deficits/support needs and knowledge deficits/teaching needs to unit accepting the patient on transfer.

REFERENCES

Cullen, L. (1992). Interventions related to fluid and electrolyte balance. *Nursing Clinics of North America, 27*(2), 569–598.

Graves, L. (1990). Disorders of calcium, phosphorus and magnesium. *Critical Care Nursing Quarterly, 13*(3), 3–13.

Huether, S. E. (1990). The cellular environment: Fluids and electrolytes, acids and bases. In K. L. McCance & S. E. Huether (Eds.), *Pathophysiology: The biologic basis for disease in adults and children* (pp. 97–99). St. Louis, MO: Mosby.

Stark, J. L. (1991). The renal system. In J. G. Alspach (Ed.), *Core curriculum in critical care nursing* (4th ed., pp. 585–591). Philadelphia, PA: Saunders.

Terry, J. (1991). The other electrolytes: Magnesium, calcium and phosphorus. *Journal of Intravenous Nursing, 14*(3), 167–176.

Zaloga, G. P. (1990). Calcium disorders. *Problems in Critical Care, 4*(3), 382–401.

Zaloga, G. P. & Chernow, B. (1989). Divalent ions: Calcium, magnesium and phosphorus. In B. Chernow (Ed.), *Essentials of critical care pharmacology* (pp. 348–366). Baltimore, MD: Williams & Wilkins.

▼

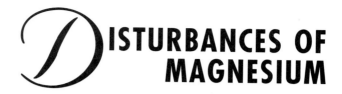ISTURBANCES OF MAGNESIUM

Magnesium is essential for normal metabolic activity affecting numerous enzymes throughout the body. It is important for normal neuromuscular transmission, muscle contraction, normal growth, wound healing, temperature regulation, myocardial function, and immunocompetence. Variations in its levels are associated with potassium and calcium disorders. The normal serum level is 1.5–2.5 mg/dL.

Hypermagnesemia
Hypermagnesemia (serum level above 2.5 mg/dL) results from decreased renal excretion of magnesium, increased intake of magnesium, or acidosis. Since magnesium acts as a sedative on nerves and muscles, it reduces neuromuscular excitability, causing central nervous system depression and vasodilation. Signs and symptoms usually do not appear until the serum level is greater than 4 mg/dL.

ETIOLOGIES

- Decreased excretion
  - renal failure
  - untreated DKA or adrenal insufficiency
  - hypothyroidism
- Excess intake
  - antacids, laxatives
  - lithium intoxication
  - treatment of eclampsia

CLINICAL MANIFESTATIONS

- Only occur when levels exceed 4 mg/dL
- Neurological: Sedation of nervous system results in
  - lethargy
  - muscle weakness
  - obtundation
  - confusion

- respiratory paralysis
- depressed tendon reflexes
- coma
- seizures
- Cardiovascular: Vasodilatation, decreased contractility, and conduction abnormalities can produce
  - hypotension
  - dysrhythmias
  - tachycardia or bradycardia
  - SVR < 800 dyn/s/cm^{-5}
  - cardiac failure

CLINICAL/DIAGNOSTIC FINDINGS

- Magnesium > 2.5 mg/dL
- Hyperkalemia (>5 mEq/L)
- EKG: peaked T wave, increased PR interval, widened QRS

NURSING DIAGNOSIS: DECREASED CARDIAC OUTPUT

Related To
- Vasodilation (hypermagnesemia)
- Decreased cardiac contractility
- Conduction abnormalities

Defining Characteristics
Hypotension
Dysrhythmias
SVR < 800 dyn/s/cm^{-5}
Cardiac failure

Patient Outcomes
Cardiac output will be maintained/restored, as evidenced by
- CO 4–8 L/min; CI 2.5–4 L/min/m^2
- blood pressure return to patient baseline
- SVR 800–1200 dyn/s/cm^{-5}
- absence of dysrhythmias
- absence of signs of cardiac failure

Nursing Interventions	Rationales
Assess for cause of hypermagnesemia	Since magnesium imbalances occur as the result of some other disorder, the identification and treatment of the underlying cause is a key factor in resolution.

Nursing Interventions	Rationales
Identify and monitor serum magnesium levels of patients at risk. Monitor for signs and symptoms of excess.	Identifying patients at risk enables preventive measures to be taken and identifies those patients whose magnesium levels need to be periodically monitored. Normal serum magnesium levels do not always rule out a deficit because serum levels do not always reflect tissue reserves.
Monitor and document cardiovascular status: heart rate, respiratory rate, blood pressure, and hemodynamic parameters.	
Monitor for signs of heart failure: jugular venous distention, fine crackles, shortness of breath, decreased blood pressure, increased heart rate, increased CVP, increased PCWP, and peripheral edema.	
Monitor the EKG for signs of rhythm problems and document and treat per protocols.	
Discontinue any preparations containing magnesium (antacids, laxatives).	
Administer intravenous calcium cautiously as prescribed and monitor effects.	Calcium antagonizes the neurological and cardiovascular effects of hypermagnesemia. Administered too rapidly, calcium can cause hypotension. Administered via an infiltrated IV can cause tissue sloughing.
Initiate saline and diuretic diuresis and monitor for fluid deficit.	Saline and diuretic diuresis enhance the excretion of magnesium.
Initiate peritoneal or hemodialysis if renal function is compromised (see Acute Renal Failure).	

NURSING DIAGNOSIS: INEFFECTIVE BREATHING PATTERN

Related To respiratory muscle weakness secondary to hypermagnesemia

Defining Characteristics
Increased respiratory rate
Tidal volume 5 mL/kg
$SaO_2 < 90\%$
pH < 7.35
$PaO_2 < 80$ torr
$PaCO_2 > 45$ torr
$SvO_2 < 60\%$

Patient Outcomes
The patient will exhibit adequate oxygenation/ventilation, as demonstrated by
- ABGs: pH 7.35–7.45, $PaCO_2$ 35–45 torr, $PaO_2 > 80$ torr, $SaO_2 > 90\%$
- SvO_2 60–80%
- tidal volume 5–7 mL/kg
- serum magnesium is 1.5–2.5 mg/dL

Nursing Interventions	Rationales
Monitor patient's respiratory status: rate, depth, and quality of respirations; c/o dyspnea or SOB; and breath sounds.	
Monitor ABGs, SvO_2 and/or pulse oximetry as prescribed and prn respiratory distress.	The $PaCO_2$ is the assessment parameter used to evaluate ventilation. The PaO_2 and SaO_2 are the assessment parameters used to evaluate oxygenation. Pulse oximetry provides a noninvasive method to estimate SaO_2. The SvO_2 reflects oxygen transport and tissue utilization.
Maintain oxygen and suction equipment at the bedside. Provide supplementary oxygen as required. Suction as needed.	Oxygen may be required to maintain adequate oxygenation. Due to respiratory muscle weakness, the patient may need assistance in removing secretions.
Position patient for ease of respiratory effort, that is, head of bed elevated.	Elevation of the head of the bed facilitates diaphragmatic excursion and ventilation.

Nursing Interventions	Rationales
Assess for tolerance to activity. Provide adequate rest.	Adequate rest and controlled activity decrease oxygen requirements.
Reposition patient every 2 hr.	

NURSING DIAGNOSIS: ACTIVITY INTOLERANCE

Related To neurological and musculoskeletal changes resulting from hypermagnesemia

Defining Characteristics
Muscle weakness
Muscle cramps
Lethargy
Seizures
Paresthesias

Patient Outcomes
The patient's activity level will return to baseline.

Nursing Interventions	Rationales
Assess muscle strength and need for assistance.	
Monitor patient response to activity: blood pressure, heart rate and rhythm, and respiratory rate before, during, and after activity. Note tachycardia, dysrhythmias, dyspnea, diaphoresis, dizziness, or fatigue.	Blood pressure, heart rate, and respiratory rate should return to baseline levels within 4 min after exercise.
Minimize physical activity during acute imbalance: provide all daily cares for patient and maintain on bedrest.	
Allow for adequate rest/sleep periods: minimize or group interruptions and assess patient's normal sleep patterns/habits and try to accommodate them	Inadequate rest increases oxygen demands and may decrease exercise tolerance.

Nursing Interventions	Rationales
Provide passive/active range-of-motion (ROM) exercises to patient if bedridden	Range-of-motion exercises help to maintain muscle strength and tone.
Increase activity gradually. Terminate if there are signs or symptoms of intolerance.	
Provide supplemental oxygen during activity.	Oxygen administration can increase exercise tolerance.

Hypomagnesemia

Hypomagnesemia (serum level below 1.5 mg/dL) occurs with decreased intake, excess intestinal loss, excess renal loss, or redistribution. Low magesium levels increase neuromuscular excitability. Signs and symptoms do not usually appear until serum levels are below 1.0 mg/dL.

ETIOLOGIES

- Intestinal loss
  - malabsorption: chronic diarrhea, inflammatory bowel disease, pancreatic insufficiency
  - enterostomy drainage
  - vomiting, prolonged NG suction
- Decreased intake
  - alcoholism, malnutrition
  - parenteral nutrition with inadequate magnesium
- Renal loss
  - renal disease: acute or chronic renal failure, interstitial nephritis
  - diuresis: diuretics (furosemide, hydrochlorothiazide, ethacrynic acid), mannitol, saline, syndrome of inappropriate antidiuretic hormone (SIADH), primary aldosteronism, diabetes
  - drugs: amphotericin, cyclosporin, aminoglycosides, ethanol, digoxin, carbenicillin, pentamidine
  - electrolyte disorders: acidosis, hypokalemia, hypophosphatemia
- Redistribution
  - parenteral hyperalimentation
  - pancreatitis
  - sepsis
  - skin loss: diaphoresis, burns
  - insulin
  - refeeding after starvation

CLINICAL MANIFESTATIONS

- Musculoskeletal: Hyperirritability of muscles can produce
  - increased reflexes
  - muscle cramps
  - paresthesias (feet and legs)
  - coarse tremors
  - seizures
- Cardiovascular: Decreased contractility and accompanying electrolyte disorders can produce
  - dysrhythmias
  - CI < 2.5 L/min/m^2
  - increased blood pressure
  - potentiate action of digoxin (digoxin toxicity)
  - CO < 4 L/min
  - SVR > 1200 dyn/s/cm^{-5}
- Neurological: Hyperirritability of the central nervous system can produce
  - disorientation
  - hallucinations
  - positive Chvostek's sign
  - confusion
  - coma
- Effects exaggerated by presence of hypokalemia, hypocalcemia, or metabolic acidosis

CLINICAL/DIAGNOSTIC FINDINGS

- Magnesium < 1.5 mg/dL
- Hypokalemia (<3.5 mEq/L)
- Hypocalcemia (<8.5 mg/dL)
- Hypophosphatemia (<2.5 mg/dL)
- EKG: flat broad T wave, widened QRS, prolonged QT interval

NURSING DIAGNOSIS: DECREASED CARDIAC OUTPUT

Related To
- Vasoconstriction
- Conduction abnormalities
- Decreased contractility

Defining Characteristics
Hypertension
Dysrhythmias
CI < 2.5 L/min/m^2
SVR > 1200 dyn/s/cm^{-5}
CO < 4 L/min

Patient Outcomes
Cardiac output will be maintained/restored, as evidenced by
- CO 4–8 L/min; CI 2.5–4 L/min/m^2
- blood pressure return to patient baseline
- SVR 800–1200 dyn/s/cm^{-5}
- absence of dysrhythmias

Nursing Interventions	Rationales
Assess for cause of hypomagnesemia.	Since magnesium imbalances occur as the result of some other disorder, the identification and treatment of the underlying cause is a key factor in resolution.
Identify and monitor serum magnesium levels of patients at risk. Monitor for signs and symptoms of deficit.	Identifying patients at risk enables preventive measures to be taken and identifies those patients whose magnesium levels need to be periodically monitored. Normal serum magnesium levels do not always rule out a deficit because serum levels do not always reflect tissue reserves.
Monitor and document cardiovascular status: heart rate, blood pressure, respiratory rate, and hemodynamic parameters (CO/CI, CVP/PCWP, SVR).	
Monitor for signs of heart failure: jugular venous distention, fine crackles, c/o shortness of breath, decreased blood pressure, increased heart rate, increased PCWP, increased CVP, and peripheral edema.	
Monitor the EKG for signs of rhythm problems and document and treat per protocols.	
If patient is on digoxin, monitor for signs of digoxin toxicity (abdominal pain, anorexia, nausea and vomiting, bradycardia, dysrhythmias, and visual disturbances).	Hypomagnesemia potentiates the action of digoxin.
Administer oral magnesium as prescribed if depletion is mild.	

Nursing Interventions	Rationales
Administer intravenous magnesium replacement as prescribed if patient symptomatic or oral administration is not possible. Monitor for side effects: diarrhea, flushing, sweating, and drowsiness.	
Monitor heart rate, blood pressure, respiratory rate, CO, and EKG closely during intravenous magnesium administration.	Magnesium has calcium antagonistic properties and can cause a drop in cardiac output, blood pressure, and heart rate.
Monitor serum potassium and for signs and symptoms of hypokalemia (dysrhythmias, fatigue, drowsiness, anorexia, nausea and vomiting).	Low magnesium levels interfere with the kidney's ability to reabsorb potassium. Patients with hypomagnesemia develop hypokalemia that does not respond to traditional therapy, that is, potassium replacement.
Monitor serum calcium and for signs and symptoms of hypocalcemia (paresthesias, irritability, muscle weakness, bradycardia, dysrhythmias, nausea and vomiting).	Hypomagnesemia suppresses secretion of parathyroid hormone, producing a hypocalcemia unresponsive to calcium supplements.
Encourage foods rich in magnesium: green leafy vegetables, nuts, legumes, whole wheat bread, and brown rice (avoid processed food).	
Identify patients on diuretics that waste magnesium; hold and contact physician.	Thiazide diuretics can cause hypomagnesemia. The patient should be placed on diuretics that do not waste magnesium, such as amiloride, triamterene, or spironolactone.

NURSING DIAGNOSIS: ACTIVITY INTOLERANCE

Related To musculoskeletal changes resulting from hypomagnesemia

Defining Characteristics
Coarse tremors
Muscle cramps
Seizures
Paresthesias

Patient Outcomes
The patient's activity level will return to baseline.

Nursing Interventions	Rationales
Assess muscle strength and need for assistance.	
Monitor patient response to activity: blood pressure, heart rate and rhythm, and respiratory rate before, during, and after activity. Note tachycardia, dysrhythmias, dyspnea, diaphoresis, dizziness, or fatigue.	Blood pressure, heart rate, and respiratory rate should return to baseline levels within 4 min after exercise.
Minimize physical activity during acute imbalance: Provide all daily cares for patient and maintain on bedrest.	
Allow for adequate rest/sleep periods: Minimize or group interruptions and assess patient's normal sleep patterns/habits and try to accommodate them.	Inadequate rest increases oxygen demands and may decrease exercise tolerance.
Provide passive/active ROM exercises to patient if bedridden.	Range-of-motion exercises help to maintain muscle strength and tone.
Increase activity gradually. Terminate if there are signs or symptoms of intolerance.	
Provide supplemental oxygen during activity.	Oxygen administration can increase exercise tolerance.

DISCHARGE PLANNING/CONTINUITY OF CARE

- Based on underlying pathology/etiology, assess need for/type of long-term care and follow-up.
- If the discharge destination is home, assess existing supports and need for assistance.
- Determine coping deficits/support needs and institute assistance measures.
- Determine knowledge deficit/teaching needs and document and institute a teaching plan.

- Refer patient to social services as appropriate.
- Communicate coping deficits/support needs and knowledge deficits/teaching needs to unit accepting the patient on transfer.

REFERENCES

Cerrato, P. L. (1992). Don't overlook this mineral deficiency. *RN, 55*(7), 61–62.

Cullen, L. (1992). Interventions related to fluid and electrolyte balance. *Nursing Clinics of North America, 27*(2), 569–598.

Friday, B. A. & Reinhart, R. A. (1991). Magnesium metabolism: A case report and literature review. *Critical Care Nurse, 11*(5), 62–73.

Graves, L. (1990). Disorders of calcium, phosphorus and magnesium. *Critical Care Nursing Quarterly, 13*(3), 3–13.

Stark, J. L. (1991). The renal system. In J. G. Alspach (Ed.), *Core curriculum in critical care nursing* (4th ed., pp. 595–599). Philadelphia, PA: Saunders.

Terry, J. (1991). The other electrolytes: Magnesium, calcium and phosphate. *Journal of Intravenous Nursing, 14*(3), 167–176.

Workman, M. L. (1992). Magnesium and phosphorus: The neglected electrolytes. *AACN Clinical Issues in Critical Care Nursing, 3*(3), 655–663.

Zaloga, G. P. & Roberts, J. E. (1990). Magnesium disorders. *Problems in Critical Care, 4*(3):425–436.

▼

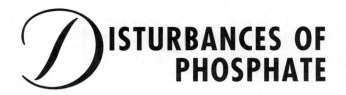ISTURBANCES OF PHOSPHATE

Phosphate, the major intracellular anion, is essential for cell structure, division and growth, energy metabolism, muscle contraction and nerve transmission. It acts as a buffer of hydrogen and participates in delivery of oxygen by red blood cells. Most of phosphate is found in bone. Normal serum levels are 2.5–4.5 mg/dl.

Hyperphosphatemia
Hyperphosphatemia (serum levels above 4.5 mg/dL) occurs as a result of decreased renal excretion, a shift into extracellular tissue, or excessive intake of phosphate. It most commonly results from renal insufficiency and its major clinical features are the result of concomitant hypocalcemia.

ETIOLOGIES

- Decreased renal excretion
  - chronic renal failure
  - hypoparathyroidism
- Shift into ECF/excessive intake
  - chemotherapy: usually for leukemia or lymphoma
  - cathartic abuse; phosphate-containing laxatives
  - excess intravenous/oral administration of phosphate
  - massive tissue necrosis: rhabdomyolysis
  - hemolytic reactions

CLINICAL MANIFESTATIONS

- Cardiovascular: Decreased myocardial contractility from concomitant hypocalcemia can produce
  - tachycardia
  - CI < 2.5 L/min/m^2
  - CO < 4 L/min

- Gastrointestinal: Spasm of smooth muscle can produce
  - nausea
  - abdominal cramps
  - diarrhea
- Neuromuscular: Increased neuromuscular irritability from concomitant hypocalcemia can produce
  - increased reflexes
  - paresthesia
  - tetany
  - numbness and tingling
- Musculoskeletal: Increased musculoskeletal irritability from concomitant hypocalcemia can produce
  - joint pain
  - muscle spasms
  - muscle cramps

CLINICAL/DIAGNOSTIC FINDINGS

- Serum phosphate > 4.5 mg/dL
- Serum calcium < 8.5 mg/dL

NURSING DIAGNOSIS: DECREASED CARDIAC OUTPUT

Related To decreased cardiac contractility secondary to hypocalcemia associated with hyperphosphatemia

Defining Characteristics
CO < 4 L/min
Tachycardia
Signs of heart failure
CI < 2.5 L/min/m^2
Calcium < 8.5 mg/dL
Phosphate > 4.5 mg/dL

Patient Outcomes
Cardiac output will be maintained/restored, as evidenced by
- CO 4–8 L/min; CI 2.5–4 L/min/m^2
- heart rate 60–100 bpm
- absence of signs of heart failure
- serum calcium 8.5–10.5 mg/dL
- serum phosphate 2.5–4.5 mg/dL

Nursing Interventions	Rationales
Assess for cause of hyperphosphatemia.	Since phosphate imbalances occur as the result of some other disorder, the identification and treatment of the underlying cause is a key factor in resolution.
Identify patients at risk (see Etiologic Factors) and institute preventive measures.	

Nursing Interventions	Rationales
Monitor serum phosphate and calcium levels.	As serum phosphate increases, it combines with free calcium and ionized calcium levels fall. As serum phosphate decreases, calcium levels will rise.
Monitor for and document signs and symptoms of decreased cardiac output: vital signs and hemodynamic parameters (CVP/PCWP, CO/CI).	Decreased contractility can cause decreased CO/CI. This in turn leads to an increase in CVP and/or PCWP, increased heart rate, decreased blood pressure, and left and/or right ventricular failure.
Monitor for signs of heart failure: jugular venous distention, fine crackles, c/o SOB, bounding pulses, peripheral edema, increased CVP/PCWP, increased heart rate, decreased blood pressure, and decreased urine output.	
Monitor the EKG for rhythm problems and document and treat according to protocols.	Concomitant hypocalcemia can cause EKG changes and rhythm disturbances.
Administer phosphate-binding medications as prescribed.	These medications (aluminum hydroxide) bind with phosphate in the GI tract and remove phosphate from the body.
Administer acetazolamide as prescribed and monitor response.	Acetazolamide prevents proximal tubule reabsorption of phosphate.
Administer saline and diuretics as prescribed and document response.	Saline and diuretics can increase urine excretion of phosphate.
Administer calcium supplements and vitamin D.	
Avoid giving foods rich in phosphate: whole grain cereals, hard cheese or cream, dried fruit, nuts, dried vegetables, and desserts made with milk.	
In patients with renal failure, institute hemo or peritoneal dialysis (see Acute Dialysis)	

NURSING DIAGNOSIS: ACTIVITY INTOLERANCE

Related To musculoskeletal changes with hyperphosphatemia

Defining Characteristics
Joint pain
Numbness and tingling
Muscle spasms
Muscle cramps
Paresthesias
Tetany

Patient Outcomes
The patient's activity level will return to baseline.

Nursing Interventions	Rationales
Assess for musculoskeletal signs of hyperphosphatemia/hypocalcemia: joint pain, muscle cramps, tonic spasms of muscles of face and limbs, paresthesias, and numbness and tingling.	
Assess muscle strength and steadiness.	
Assess need for assistance with ADLs or activity; provide as necessary.	
Assess heart rate, respiratory rate, and blood pressure before, during, and after activity.	Heart rate, respiratory rate, and blood pressure should return to baseline within 4 min after activity.
Minimize physical activity during acute imbalance. Allow for adequate rest/sleep periods.	Inadequate sleep or rest increases oxygen demand and may decrease activity tolerance.
Increase activity gradually. Terminate if there are signs or symptoms of intolerance.	
Provide supplemental oxygen during activity.	Supplementary oxygen can increase activity tolerance.

Hypophosphatemia

Hypophosphatemia (serum levels below 2.5 mg/dL) occurs as a result of intracellular shifts, increased renal or gastrointestinal loss, or decreased intake of phosphate. It causes alterations in neuromuscular (most common), cardiovascular, renal, hematological, and skeletal muscle function. Severe deficits (<1 mg/dL) can produce life-threatening respiratory arrest.

ETIOLOGIES

- Cellular shifts
  - carbohydrate administration with inadequate phosphate: TPN
  - respiratory and metabolic alkalosis
  - malignancies: leukemia, osteoblastic metastasis
  - anabolic state, malnutrition
  - insulin injection; DKA, HHNC
  - drugs: epinephrine, anabolic steroids, glucagon
  - gram-negative sepsis
- Gastrointestinal loss
  - antacids: aluminum hydroxide, aluminum carbonate, calcium carbonate
  - malabsorption, diarrhea, NG suction
  - malnutrition
  - vitamin D deficiency
- Renal wasting
  - vitamin D deficiency
  - hyperparathyroidism
  - hyperthermia
  - electrolyte disorders: hypokalemia, hypomagnesemia
  - volume expansion
  - drugs: glucocorticoids, thiazide diuretics, sodium bicarbonate
  - renal tubular disease, postrenal transplant, nephrotic syndrome
- Decreased intake
  - alcoholism
  - malnutrition

CLINICAL MANIFESTATIONS

- Cardiovascular: Decreased myocardial contractility and electrical dysfunction can produce
  - CO < 4 L/min
  - CI < 2.5 L/min/m^2
  - heart failure
  - dysrhythmias
  - impaired response to pressors
- Pulmonary: Diaphragm and respiratory muscle weakness can produce
  - rapid, shallow respirations
  - $PaCO_2$ > 45 torr
  - tidal volume < 5 mL/kg
  - vital capacity < 10 mL/kg
  - respiratory failure
  - PaO_2 < 80 torr

- Neuromuscular: Deranged cellular energy metabolism produces
  - paresthesia
  - ataxia
  - confusion
  - coma
  - weakness
  - disorientation
  - lethargy
  - tremors
  - hyporeflexia
  - stupor
  - seizures
  - paralysis
  - hallucinations
  - rhabdomyolysis
- Musculoskeletal: Impaired bone mineralization can produce
  - joint stiffness
  - pathological fractures
  - bone pain
- Hematologic: Red cell fragility and impaired platelet and leukocyte function can produce
  - bleeding
  - infection
  - easy bruising
- Gastrointestinal: Adenosine triphosphate (ATP) deficiency can produce
  - nausea and vomiting
  - liver dysfunction
  - anorexia
  - insulin resistance

CLINICAL/DIAGNOSTIC FINDINGS

- Serum phosphate < 2.5 mg/dL
- Thrombocytopenia (platelets < 150,000/mm^3)
- Anemia (hemoglobin < 13 g/dL)

NURSING DIAGNOSIS: DECREASED CARDIAC OUTPUT

Related To decreased cardiac contractility secondary to hypophosphatemia

Defining Characteristics
CO < 4 L/min
Increased heart rate
CVP > 10 mmHg
Phosphate < 2.5 mg/dL
CI < 2.5 L/min/m^2
Signs of heart failure
PCWP > 12 mmHg

Patient Outcomes
Cardiac output will be maintained/restored, as evidenced by
- CO 4–8 L/min; CI 2.5–4 L/min/m^2
- heart rate 60–100 bpm
- CVP 2–10 mmHg; PCWP 8–12 mmHg
- absence of signs of heart failure
- serum phosphate 2.5–4.5 mg/dL

Nursing Interventions	Rationales
Assess for cause of hypophosphatemia.	Since phosphate imbalances occur as the result of some other disorder, the identification and treatment of the underlying cause is a key factor in resolution.
Identify patients at risk (see Etiologic Factors) and institute preventive measures.	
Monitor serum phosphate and calcium levels.	As serum phosphate increases, it combines with free calcium and ionized calcium levels fall. As serum phosphate decreases, calcium levels will rise.
Monitor for and document signs and symptoms of decreased cardiac output: vital signs and hemodyanamic parameters (CVP/PCWP, CO/CI).	Decreased contractility can cause decreased CO/CI This in turn leads to an increase in CVP and/or PCWP, increased heart rate, decreased blood pressure, and left and/or right ventricular failure.
Monitor for signs of heart failure: jugular venous distention, fine crackles, c/o SOB, bounding pulses, peripheral edema, increased CVP/PCWP, increased heart rate, decreased blood pressure, and decreased urine output	
Monitor the EKG for rhythm problems and document and treat according to protocols.	Concomitant hypercalcemia can cause EKG changes and rhythm disturbances.
Administer intravenous phosphate as prescribed if level is below 2 mg/dL.	Severe hypophosphatemia can cause life-threatening respiratory arrest and requires immediate correction.
Administer oral preparations of phosphate when serum level exceeds 2 mg/dL.	Repletion is carried out over 5–7 days to replace intracellular phosphate stores; then a maintenance dose is established.

Nursing Interventions	Rationales
Monitor for side effects of phosphate administration: diarrhea, hyperphosphatemia, hypocalcemia, calcium precipitation, renal failure, and hypotension.	Monitor serum potassium, especially in patients with renal insufficiency and document any signs of hyperkalemia.
Most phosphate supplements also contain potassium and can cause hyperkalemia.	

NURSING DIAGNOSIS: INEFFECTIVE BREATHING PATTERN

Related To diaphragm and respiratory muscle weakness secondary to hypophosphatemia

Defining Characteristics
Increased respiratory rate
Tidal volume < 5 mL/kg
SaO_2 < 90%
pH < 7.35
PaO_2 < 80 torr
$PaCO_2$ > 45 torr
SvO_2 < 60%

Patient Outcomes
The patient exhibits adequate oxygenation/ventilation, as demonstrated by
- ABG's: pH 7.35–7.45, PaO_2 > 80 torr, $PaCO_2$ 35–45 torr, SaO_2 > 90%
- SvO_2 70–90%
- tidal volume 5–7 mL/kg
- serum phosphate 2.5–4.5 mg/dL

Nursing Interventions	Rationales
Monitor and document respiratory status: rate, depth, and quality of respirations; subjective complaints of dyspnea or SOB; and breath sounds (airway and breathing effort, use of accessory muscles)	Hypophosphatemia can cause weakness of the diaphragm and respiratory muscles resulting in ineffective breathing.

Nursing Interventions	Rationales
Monitor ABG's, SvO$_2$, and/or pulse oximetry as prescribed and if there are indications of respiratory difficulty.	PaCO$_2$ is the assessment parameter used to evaluate ventilation. PaO$_2$ and SaO$_2$ are the assessment parameters used to evaluate oxygenation. Pulse oximetry provides a noninvasive estimate of SaO$_2$. The SvO$_2$ is the assessment parameter used to evaluate oxygen transport and tissue extraction.
Maintain oxygen and suction equipment at bedside, and administer as needed.	
Position patient for ease of respiratory effort, that is, head of bed elevated.	
Minimize activity to decrease oxygen need.	
Reposition patient every 2 hr.	Regular repositioning enhances ventilation and prevents stasis of secretions.

NURSING DIAGNOSIS: ACTIVITY INTOLERANCE

Related To musculoskeletal changes with hypophosphatemia

Defining Characteristics
Joint stiffness
Paresthesias
Ataxia
Lethargy
Bone pain
Tremors
Weakness

Patient Outcomes
The patient's activity level will return to baseline.

Nursing Interventions	Rationales
Assess musculoskeletal signs of hypophosphatemia/hypercalcemia: paresthesias, tremors, ataxia, weakness, joint stiffness, and bone pain.	

Nursing Interventions	Rationales
Assess muscle strength and steadiness	
Assess need for assistance with ADLs or activity; provide as necessary.	
Assess heart rate, respiratory rate, and blood pressure before, during, and after activity.	Heart rate, respiratory rate, and blood pressure should return to baseline within 4 min after activity.
Minimize physical activity during acute imbalance. Allow for adequate rest/sleep periods.	Inadequate sleep or rest increases oxygen demand and may decrease activity tolerance.
Increase activity gradually. Terminate if there are signs or symptoms of intolerance.	
Provide supplemental oxygen during activity	Supplementary oxygen can increase activity tolerance.

DISCHARGE PLANNING/CONTINUITY OF CARE

- Based on underlying pathology/etiology, assess need for/type of long-term care and follow-up
- If the discharge destination is home, assess existing supports and the need for assistance.
- Determine coping deficits/support needs and institute assistance measures.
- Determine knowledge deficits/teaching needs and document and institute a teaching plan.
- Refer patient to social services as appropriate.
- Communicate coping deficits/support needs and knowledge deficits/teaching needs to unit accepting the patient on transfer.

REFERENCES

Cullen, L. (1992). Interventions related to fluid and electrolyte balance. *Nursing Clinics of North America, 27*(2), 569–598.

Graves, L. (1990). Disorders of calcium, phosphorus and magnesium. *Critical Care Nursing Quarterly, 13*(3), 3–13.

Huether, S. E. (1990). The cellular environment: Fluids and electrolytes, acids and bases. In K. L. McCance & S. E. Huether (Eds.), *Pathophy-

siology: The biologic basis for disease in adults and children (pp. 99–100). St. Louis, MO: Mosby.

Stark, J. L. (1991). The renal system. In J. G. Alspach (Ed.), *Core Curriculum for Critical Care Nursing* (4th ed., pp. 591–595). Philadelphia, PA: Saunders.

Terry, J. (1991). The other electrolytes: Magnesium, calcium and phosphorus. *Journal of Intravenous Nursing, 14*(3), 167–176.

Workman, M. L. (1992). Magnesium and phosphorus: The neglected electrolytes. *AACN Clinical Issues in Critical Care Nursing, 3*(3), 655–663.

Zaloga, G. P. (1990). Phosphate disorders. *Problems in Critical Care, 4*(3), 416–424.

▼

DISTURBANCES OF POTASSIUM

Potassium is the major intracellular cation and the primary determinant of resting transmembrane potential and cellular excitability. Abnormal serum potassium levels alter neuromuscular and cardiac function. The majority of the body's potassium is within cells, but altered levels of potassium only become dangerous when present in the extracellular fluid (ECF). Shifts of potassium between the cells and ECF are influenced by pH, insulin, catecholamines, and aldosterone. Normal serum potassium is 3.5–5.0 mEq/L.

Hyperkalemia
Hyperkalemia (serum levels above 5.0 mEq/L) usually results from impaired urinary excretion, salt depletion, increased potassium load, or movement out of cells. It is a life-threatening electrolyte imbalance that initially causes cells to fire more easily, but as it worsens and too many positive charges are inside the cell, decreased impulse formation results. Neuromuscular signs and symptoms usually appear when serum potassium reaches 6 mEq/L. The most serious result of hyperkalemia is cardiac arrest.

ETIOLOGIES

- Abnormal redistribution between ECF and cells
    - metabolic acidosis
    - hyperosmolality
    - insulin deficiency
    - $beta_2$-adrenergic blockade
    - cell lysis with chemotherapy
    - arginine infusion
    - succinylcholine
    - digoxin toxicity
    - rapid breakdown of tissues: crush injuries, burns, massive hemolysis, surgery, fever, sepsis, extreme infection, rhabdomyolysis, and extreme exercise
- Impaired renal excretion
    - renal failure
    - severe volume depletion
    - adrenal insufficiency

- Increased intake
  - salt substitute
  - potassium salts
  - penicillin G potassium
  - banked blood
- Antikaluretic diuretics
- Pseudohyperkalemia
  - traumatic hemolysis during blood drawing
  - severe leukocytosis
  - marked thrombocytosis

CLINICAL MANIFESTATIONS

- Most asymptomatic until > 6 mEq/L
- Neurological: Decreased cardiac output and impaired nerve transmission can produce
  - restlessness
  - lethargy
  - irritability
  - anxiety
- Musculoskeletal: Hypopolarization of nerves and muscles, impaired motor and sensory nerve impulse transmission, and irritation of local pain receptors can produce
  - reduced sensation
  - depressed reflexes
  - irritability to flaccid paralysis
  - numbness and tingling of extremities
  - muscle weakness (starts in legs and progresses)
- Cardiovascular: Myocardial depression can produce
  - bradycardia
  - CO < 4 L/min
  - dysrhythmias
  - CI < 2.5 L/min/m^2
- Gastrointestinal: Hyperactivity of smooth muscle can produce
  - nausea
  - abdominal cramps
  - diarrhea
  - hyperactive bowel sounds

CLINICAL/DIAGNOSTIC FINDINGS

- Potassium > 5 mEq/L
- Metabolic acidosis (pH < 7.35, HCO$_3$ < 21 mEq/L)
- EKG changes: tall peaked T waves, prolonged PR interval (K$^+$ > 6 mEq/L), widened QRS (K$^+$ > 6 mEq/L)

NURSING DIAGNOSIS: DECREASED CARDIAC OUTPUT

Related To
- Altered cardiac cell membrane excitability
- Cardiac dysrhythmias
- Myocardial depression

Defining Characteristics

Bradycardia
Dysrhythmias
Potassium > 5.0 mEq/L
EKG changes
CO < 4 L/min
CI < 2.5 L/min/m^2

Patient Outcomes

Cardiac output will be maintained/restored, as evidenced by
- CO 4–8 L/min; CI 2.5–4 L/min/m^2
- serum potassium 3.5–5.0 mEq/L
- heart rate 60–100 bpm
- EKG showing normal intervals and waveforms
- EKG showing absence of dysrhythmias

Nursing Interventions	Rationales
Assess for causes/sources of hyperkalemia, that is, patients at risk: renal failure, medications, salt substitute, GI bleeding, banked blood, and increased catabolism (infection, trauma).	Potassium imbalance is the result of some underlying disorder. This disorder must be corrected to successfully treat the potassium imbalance. In some cases, potassium imbalance can be anticipated and prevented.
Assess and document cardiovascular status: vital signs, hemodynamic parameters, and cardiac rhythm.	Electrical disturbances and dysrhythmias can cause decreased CO/CI This in turn leads to an increase in CVP and/or PCWP, increased heart rate, decreased blood pressure, and if prolonged, heart failure.
Monitor serum potassium levels and assess for signs of hyperkalemia	In order to monitor the effectiveness of treatment, potassium levels should be measured after each treatment before further therapy is instituted to prevent overcorrection.
Monitor the EKG for signs of hyperkalemia and document.	Patients who develop dysrhythmias should have their potassium levels checked as part of their treatment.
Monitor/control intake of foods high in potassium: bananas, melons, oranges, broccoli, meats, greens, tomatoes, dairy products, dried peas or beans, potatoes, and whole grain breads.	

Nursing Interventions	**Rationales**
Monitor and document urine output.	Since the kidneys are the primary regulator of potassium balance, a decreased urine output increases the risk for hyperkalemia. Potassium supplements should not be given or should be given cautiously to patients with decreased urine output.
Monitor acid-base balance.	Acidosis can precipitate hyperkalemia by causing potassium to move out of cells into the ECF. The acid-base disturbance must be corrected to adequately treat the potassium imbalance.
Administer cation exchange resins (Kayexalate) as prescribed. If given as enema, encourage patient to retain 30–60 min for full effect.	These resins exchange sodium for potassium in the GI tract, reducing serum levels of potassium. Oral Kayexalate may take from 2 to 12 hr to be effective. Rectal Kayexalate is usually effective within 30–90 min.
Give intravenous calcium gluconate cautiously, according to guidelines, and monitor effect.	Calcium counteracts the neuromuscular and cardiac effects of hyperkalemia but will not change the serum level. If the patient is digoxin toxic, calcium can cause cardiac standstill. Too rapid administration of calcium can cause hypotension. Infusion of calcium into an infiltrated IV can cause tissue sloughing.
Administer intravenous glucose and insulin as prescribed and monitor effect.	Glucose and insulin will shift potassium into the cells, temporarily reducing the serum level. Rebound hyperkalemia may occur in 4–6 hr if hyperkalemia is not corrected.

Nursing Interventions	Rationales
Administer sodium bicarbonate as prescribed and monitor effect.	Sodium bicarbonate shifts potassium into the cells, temporarily reducing the serum level. Onset of the effect is 5–10 min with effects lasting 1–2 hr. Note: Mixing sodium bicarbonate with calcium can cause precipitation.
If patient is not in renal failure, administer diuretics as prescribed and document response. If not correctable via other therapies, institute dialysis (see Acute Dialysis).	

NURSING DIAGNOSIS: ACTIVITY INTOLERANCE

Related To neurological and musculoskeletal changes resulting from hyperkalemia

Defining Characteristics
Decreased reflexes   Muscle weakness
Numbness and tingling in extremities

Patient Outcomes
The patient will return to baseline:
- neurological and musculoskeletal status
- activity level

Nursing Interventions	Rationales
Monitor for musculoskeletal signs: reduced sensation, depressed reflexes, muscle irritability/flaccidity, numbness/tingling of extremities, and muscle weakness. If present, monitor and/or assist with ADL and activity as needed.	

Nursing Interventions	Rationales
Monitor/record patient response to activity. Assess muscle strength and steadiness. Supervise/assist patient when ambulating. Monitor blood pressure, heart rate and rhythm, and respiratory rate before, during, and after activity. Note tachycardia, dysrhythmias, dyspnea, diaphoresis, dizziness, or fatigue.	Heart rate, blood pressure, and respiratory rate should return to baseline within 4 min after activity.
Minimize physical activity during acute imbalance. Provide all daily cares for patient. Maintain on bedrest. Place light, urinal, water, and so on, within reach.	
Allow for adequate rest/sleep periods: Minimize or group interruptions and assess patients normal sleep patterns/habits and try to accommodate them.	
Provide passive/active ROM exercises to patient if bedridden	
Increase activity gradually. Terminate if there are signs or symptoms of intolerance.	
Provide supplemental oxygen during activity.	Oxygen administration can increase exercise tolerance.

Hypokalemia
Hypokalemia (serum levels below 3.5 mEq/L) usually results from potassium loss exceeding intake or intracellular shifts of potassium. It is frequently associated with other fluid and electrolyte disturbances. Hypokalemia decreases membrane excitabity, making depolarization more difficult. Neuromuscular signs and symptoms appear when serum potassium is about 2.5 mEq/L. Cardiac dysrhythmias may occur earlier, especially in patients with cardiac problems.

ETIOLOGIES

- Gastrointestinal loss
  - vomiting
  - suction
  - excessive laxative/enema use
  - diarrhea
  - fistula

- Renal loss
  - renal tubular disorders
  - loop or thiazide diuretics
  - large-dose corticosteroids
  - stress reaction
  - osmotic diuresis
  - hypomagnesemia
  - low plasma renin activity: primary hyperaldosteronism
  - high/normal plasma renin activity: renal artery
  - stenosis, malignant hypertension, Cushing's disease
- Decreased intake (rare)
  - alcoholics
  - anorexia
- Extracellular fluid loss
  - sweating
  - extensive burns
- Shift into cells
  - metabolic alkalosis
  - theophylline toxicity
  - barium poisoning
  - hypothermia
  - administration of insulin and glucose
  - $beta_2$-adrenergic stimulation

CLINICAL MANIFESTATIONS

- Cardiovascular: Inhibition of smooth muscles and slowed repolarization (hyperpolarization) can produce
  - hypotension
  - increased sensitivity to digoxin
  - dysrhythmias (increased sensitivity to reentrant dysrhythmias)
- Musculoskeletal: Hyperpolarization, decreased impulse formation, and conduction cause nerves and cells to be less excitable and produce (<2.5 mEq/L)
  - fatigue
  - tender muscles
  - paresthesia
  - leg cramps
  - muscle weakness leading to paralysis (primarily legs)
- Renal: Stimulation of thirst center and resistance to ADH produce:
  - polyuria
  - polydipsia
- Neurological: Decreased nerve transmission and dysrhythmias can produce:
  - drowsiness
  - confusion
  - irritability
  - coma
- Gastrointestinal: Inhibition of smooth muscles can produce:
  - anorexia
  - abdominal distension
  - nausea and vomiting
  - paralytic ileus

CLINICAL/DIAGNOSTIC FINDINGS

- Potassium < 3.5 mEq/L
- Metabolic alkalosis (pH > 7.45, HCO_3 > 28 mEq/L)
- EKG changes: flat/inverted T waves, depressed ST segment, prominent U wave

NURSING DIAGNOSIS: DECREASED CARDIAC OUTPUT

Related To
- Altered cardiac cell membrane excitability
- Cardiac dysrhythmias
- Inhibition of smooth muscles

Defining Characteristics
Hypotension
Dysrhythmias
EKG changes
Potassium < 3.5 mEq/L

Patient Outcomes
Cardiac output will be maintained/restored, as evidenced by
- blood pressure return to patient baseline
- serum potassium 3.5–5.0 mEq/L
  - EKG showing normal intervals and waveforms
  - EKG showing absence of dysrhythmias

Nursing Interventions	Rationales
Assess for causes/sources of hypokalemia: diuretics, inadequate intake, GI loss, and alkalosis.	Potassium imbalance is the result of some underlying disorder. This disorder must be corrected to successfully treat the potassium imbalance. In some cases, potassium imbalance can be anticipated and prevented.
Assess and document cardiovascular status: vital signs, hemodynamic parameters, and cardiac rhythm.	Electrical disturbances and dysrhythmias can cause decreased CO/CI This in turn leads to an increase in CVP and/or PCWP, increased heart rate, decreased blood pressure, and if prolonged, heart failure.
Monitor serum potassium levels and assess for signs of hypokalemia	In order to monitor the effectiveness of treatment, potassium levels should be measured after each treatment and before further therapy is instituted to prevent overcorrection.

Nursing Interventions	Rationales
Monitor EKG for signs of hypokalemia and document.	The EKG changes in hypokalemia are not as level specific as in hyperkalemia. Patients who develop dysrhythmias should have their potassium levels checked as part of their treatment.
Monitor and document urine output.	Since the kidneys are the primary regulator of potassium balance, an increased urine output increases the risk for hypokalemia.
Monitor acid-base balance	Alkalosis can precipitate hypokalemia by causing potassium to move into cells. The acid-base disturbance must be corrected to adequately treat the potassium imbalance.
Administer intravenous potassium supplement as prescribed and monitor effect. Do not give at rate faster than 20 mEq/hr. Give at slower rates to patients on digoxin. Avoid use of peripheral vein. Assess IV site for erythema, heat, or pain.	Giving intravenous potassium at rates above 20 mEq/hr can precipitate life-threatening dysrhythmias and hyperkalemia. Digoxin slows the rate of uptake of potassium by cells and can predispose the patient to transient hyperkalemia. Peripheral administration of potassium can cause local irritation of veins, phlebitis, and pain. Irritation may be relieved by applying ice or adding an anesthetic such as xylocaine to the IV solution.
Administer oral potassium supplements as prescribed and monitor for GI upset.	Oral potassium supplements can cause nausea, vomiting, abdominal pain, and abdominal distention.
Monitor patients on digoxin for signs of increased digoxin effect: PVCs, PAT, and Mobitz I.	Hypokalemia can potentiate the effects of digoxin.

NURSING DIAGNOSIS: ACTIVITY INTOLERANCE

Related To neurological and musculoskeletal changes resulting from hypokalemia

Defining Characteristics
Fatigue
Tender muscles
Muscle weakness
Paresthesias
Leg cramps

Patient Outcomes
The patient will return to baseline:
- neurological and musculoskeletal status
- activity level

Nursing Interventions	Rationales
Monitor for musculoskeletal signs: paresthesia, tender muscles, leg cramps, and muscle weakness. If present, monitor and/or assist with ADL and activity as needed.	
Monitor/record patient response to activity. Assess muscle strength and steadiness. Supervise/assist patient when ambulating. Monitor blood pressure, heart rate and rhythm, and respiratory rate before, during, and after activity. Note tachycardia, dysrhythmias, dyspnea, diaphoresis, dizziness, or fatigue.	Heart rate, blood pressure, and respiratory rate should return to baseline within 4 min after activity.
Minimize physical activity during acute imbalance. Provide all daily cares for patient. Maintain on bedrest. Place light, urinal, water, and so on, within reach.	
Allow for adequate rest/sleep periods: Minimize or group interruptions and assess patient's normal sleep patterns/habits and try to accommodate them.	

Nursing Interventions	Rationales
Provide passive/active ROM exercises to patient if bedridden.	
Increase activity gradually. Terminate if there are signs or symptoms of intolerance.	
Provide supplemental oxygen during activity.	Oxygen administration can increase exercise tolerance.

NURSING DIAGNOSIS: HIGH RISK FOR INEFFECTIVE BREATHING PATTERN

Risk Factors
- Weakness of respiratory muscles
- Paralysis of respiratory muscles
- Potassium < 2–2.5 mEq/L

Patient Outcomes
The patient will exhibit an effective breathing pattern, as evidenced by
- normal respiratory depth and pattern
- respiratory rate 12–20 breaths per minute
- pH 7.35–7.45, PaO_2 > 80 torr, $PaCO_2$ 35–45 torr
- SaO_2 > 90%

Nursing Interventions	Rationales
Assess and document respiratory status every hour as long as patient is hypokalemic: airway and breathing effort; rate and depth of respiration; breath sounds; ABGs or pulse oximetry as indicated; and subjective complaints of SOB or DOE.	
Administer oxygen as prescribed.	
Keep manual ventilation bag at bedside.	
Position patient for ease of respiratory effort, that is, head of bed elevated.	

Nursing Interventions	Rationales
Reposition patient every 2 hours.	Regular repositioning will enhance ventilation and prevent stasis of secretions.
If necessary, utilize suction to assist patient in removal of secretions	

DISCHARGE PLANNING/CONTINUITY OF CARE

- Based on underlying pathology/etiology, assess need for/type of long-term care and follow-up.
- If the discharge destination is home, assess existing supports and the need for assistance.
- Determine coping deficits/support needs and institute assistance measures.
- Determine knowledge deficits/teaching needs and document and institute a teaching plan.
- Refer patient to social services as appropriate.
- Communicate coping deficits/support needs and knowledge deficits/teaching needs to unit accepting patient on transfer.

REFERENCES

Black, R. M. (1991). Disorders of plasma sodium and plasma potassium. In J. M Rippe, R. S. Irwin, J. S. Alpert, & M. P. Fink, (Eds.) *Intensive care medicine* (2nd ed., pp. 803–810). Boston, MA: Little, Brown.

Calhoun, K. A. (1990). Serum potassium concentration abnormalities. *Critical Care Nursing Quarterly, 13*(3); 34–38.

Cullen, L. (1992). Interventions related to fluid and electrolyte balance. *Nursing Clinics of North America, 27*(2), 569–598.

Huether, S. E. (1990). The cellular environment: Fluids and electrolytes, acids and bases. In K. L. McCance & S. E. Huether, (Eds.), *Pathophysiology: The biologic basis for disease in adults and children* (pp. 92–97). St. Louis, MO: Mosby.

Innerarity, S. A. (1992). Hyperkalemia emergencies. *Critical Care Nursing Quarterly, 14*(4), 32–39.

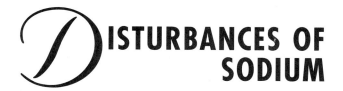

DISTURBANCES OF SODIUM

Sodium is the major cation in extracellular fluid (ECF). It maintains concentration and volume of ECF by determining serum osmolality and maintains membrane action potentials. This latter function influences conduction of nerve impulses, neuromuscular irritability, and muscle contraction. Serum concentration is controlled by regulation of water intake and excretion via ADH and sodium reabsorption and excretion via aldosterone. Normal serum sodium is 135–145 mEq/L.

Hypernatremia
Hypernatremia (serum level above 145 mEq/L) results from either a gain of sodium in excess of water or a loss of water in excess of sodium. This imbalance creates a hyperosmotic plasma, causing fluid to shift out of cells into the ECF. Cells become dehydrated and ECF volume increases. The shift of fluid out of cerebral cells increases central nervous system irritability. Hypernatremia is less common than hyponatremia but has a worse prognosis due to potentially severe neurological dysfunction.

ETIOLOGIES

- Gain of sodium
  - hypertonic tube feeding without water supplement
  - hypertonic saline solution administration
  - administration of sodium bicarbonate
  - salt water drowning
  - increased oral intake of sodium
  - primary aldosteronism
- Loss of water
  - watery diarrhea
  - decreased water intake
  - diabetes insipidus
  - increased insensible loss (diaphoresis)
  - osmotic diuresis (hyperglycemia)

CLINICAL MANIFESTATIONS

- Neurological: Central nervous system irritability can produce
  - restlessness
  - delirium
  - coma
  - decreased deep-tendon reflexes
  - nuchal rigidity
  - excitement
  - lethargy
  - seizures
- Vascular: Movement of water out of cells can produce
  - hypertension
  - dry, sticky mucous membranes
  - extreme thirst
  - fever

CLINICAL/DIAGNOSTIC FINDINGS

- Sodium > 145 mEq/L
- Urine specific gravity > 1.015 (indicates water deficit)
- Urine sodium low

NURSING DIAGNOSIS: FLUID VOLUME DEFICIT

Related To loss of water in excess of sodium

Defining Characteristics
Dry, sticky mucous membranes
CVP < 2 mmHg
Sodium > 145 mEq/L
Specific gravity > 1.015
Urine sodium low

Extreme thirst
PCWP < 8 mmHg
Fever
Hypotension

Patient Outcomes
Fluid volume will be maintained/restored, as evidenced by
- absence of thirst
- moist mucous membranes
- normal temperature
- serum sodium 135–145 mEq/L
- blood pressure return to patient baseline
- CVP 2–10 mmHg; PCWP 8–12 mmHg

Nursing Interventions	Rationales
Identify patients at risk (see etiologies) and monitor serum sodium.	Hypernatremia may be preventable by identifying patients at risk and instituting measures to replace water losses.

Nursing Interventions	Rationales
Assess for the cause of hypernatremia.	Since hypernatremia occurs as the result of some other disorder, the identification and treatment of the underlying cause is the key factor in its resolution.
Assess for and document peripheral indicators of fluid balance: mucous membranes, temperature, skin turgor, and thirst.	Weak, thready pulses, poor skin turgor, dry mucous membranes, and thirst indicate fluid volume deficit.
Monitor and document fluid balance: Intake and output and daily weight.	Decreased urine output (<30 mL/hr) reflects decreased renal perfusion due to inadequate fluid replacement. If decreased renal perfusion is prolonged, acute renal failure may develop. Hourly monitoring is required to evaluate the adequacy of fluid replacement. Daily weights and intake and output measurements also assist in evaluating fluid balance and adequacy of fluid replacement.
Monitor and document cardiovascular status: vital signs, including orthostatic changes, and hemodynamic parameters.	Increased respiratory rate, increased heart rate, decreased blood pressure, orthostatic changes, low CVP, PCWP, and CO/CI, and MAP indicate fluid volume deficit.
Monitor and document serum sodium during treatment.	Serum sodium should not be lowered more than 15 mEq/L over any 4–6 hr period because this can precipitate cerebral edema (see the next intervention).
Monitor for signs of neurological deterioration during treatment.	Patients with chronic hypernatremia may develop cerebral edema if sodium is corrected too rapidly. Water can shift into brain cells due to differences between the osmolality of ICF and ECF.

Nursing Interventions

Administer hypotonic fluid replacement orally or intravenously as prescribed and monitor for signs of fluid overload.

Administer diuretics as prescribed and document response.

Rationales

Fluid volume deficit may indicate a loss of water in excess of sodium. A hypotonic solution will replace fluid losses without increasing sodium concentration further.

Administration of diuretics may assist in removal of sodium.

NURSING DIAGNOSIS: ALTERED THOUGHT PROCESSES

Related To
- Fluid shift out of cerebral cells
- Central nervous system irritability

Defining Characteristics

Delirium
Excitement
Coma

Restlessness
Lethargy

Patient Outcomes

The patient will return to baseline mentation.

Nursing Interventions

Assess for degree of neurological/psychological dysfunction and document: orientation, confusion, delirium, restlessness, excitement, lethargy and coma.

Monitor serum sodium levels.

Assess patient for indicators of cerebral edema: lethargy, headache, nausea and vomiting, seizures, increased blood pressure, and decreased heart rate.

Rationales

Fluid and sodium imbalances can precipitate changes in neurological function. The severity of these derangements reflects the severity of the imbalances and should improve with treatment.

Sodium levels below 145 mEq/L can produce central nervous system irritability. Cerebral edema can occur if hypernatremia is corrected too rapidly.

Nursing Interventions	Rationales
Minimize effects of environment on mental status: reorient patient; maintain quiet environment, minimizing extraneous stimuli; provide simple, brief explanations of activities, procedures, and equipment; and provide meaningful, relaxing stimuli to patient.	The stresses of the critical care environment (sensory overload, sensory deprivation, and sleep deprivation) can aggravate mental status changes produced physiologically. Taking preventive measures may minimize these environmental effects.
Prevent patient injury (see Appendix C).	

Hyponatremia

Hyponatremia (serum level below 135 mEq/L) results from either an excess loss of sodium or an excess gain of water. This creates a hypo-osmotic plasma causing fluid to shift out of the ECF into cells. In cerebral tissue this produces brain swelling. The appearance of signs and symptoms in hyponatremia depends on the severity and rapidity of onset of the deficit (or water gain). If the condition develops slowly, signs and symptoms may not be apparent until serum sodium falls below 125 mEq/L.

ETIOLOGIES

- Loss of sodium
  - loss of GI secretions: vomiting, suction, and diarrhea
  - excessive sweating
  - use of diuretics
  - Addison's disease
  - excessive tap water enemas
- Gain of water
  - excess 5% dextrose intravenous solutions
  - excess plain water intake
  - fresh water drowning
  - SIADH
  - drugs: oral hypoglycemics, antineoplastics, tricyclics, phenothiazines

CLINICAL MANIFESTATIONS

- Neurological: brain swelling can produce
  - weakness
  - muscle twitching
  - seizures
  - confusion
  - hemiparesis
  - coma

- Gastrointestinal
  - anorexia
  - nausea and vomiting

CLINICAL/DIAGNOSTIC FINDINGS

- Sodium < 135 mEq/L
- Urine specific gravity low with loss of sodium; high with gain of water
- Urine sodium high

NURSING DIAGNOSIS: FLUID VOLUME EXCESS

Related To gain of water in excess of sodium

Defining Characteristics

Sodium < 135 mEq/L
PCWP > 12 mmHg
CVP > 10 mmHg
Elevated blood pressure

Patient Outcomes

Fluid balance will be maintained/restored, as evidenced by
- serum sodium 135–145 mEq/L
- CVP 2–10 mmHg; PCWP 8–12 mmHg
- blood pressure returns to patient baseline

Nursing Interventions	Rationales
Identify patients at risk and monitor serum sodium levels.	Serum sodium levels below 120 mEq/L can produce seizures and significant changes in mental status.
Assess for cause of hyponatremia.	Since hyponatremia occurs as the result of some other disturbance, identification and correction of the underlying cause is the key factor in its resolution. It will also help determine whether the patient is sodium depleted or water overloaded, assisting in guiding therapy.
Monitor and document fluid balance: intake and output and daily weight	

Nursing Interventions	Rationales
Monitor and document cardiovascular status: vital signs, hemodynamic parameters, and peripheral pulses	Increased respiratory rate, heart rate, blood pressure, CVP, PCWP and peripheral pulses are all indicators of fluid overload. If the fluid overload is severe, a drop in CO/CI may indicate impending cardiac failure.
Institute fluid restriction as prescribed and monitor response.	In the patient who has water in excess of sodium this may restore normal fluid balance.
Administer hypertonic saline as prescribed and monitor closely for signs of hypernatremia, worsening overload, and heart failure.	Hypertonic saline is used to replace serum sodium in patients with severe symptomatic hyponatremia but can produce hypernatremia, fluid overload, and heart failure.
Institute hemofiltration as prescribed and monitor response (see Acute Dialysis).	In patients with hyponatremia due to water overload with compromised renal function, hemofiltration may be necessary to remove excess water.

NURSING DIAGNOSIS: ALTERED THOUGHT PROCESSES

Related To
- Fluid shift into cerebral cells
- Brain swelling

Defining Characteristics
Confusion
Coma
Seizures

Patient Outcomes
The patient will return to baseline mentation.

Nursing Interventions	Rationales
Assess for degree of neurological/psychological dysfunction and document: orientation, confusion, muscle twitching, hemiparesis, coma, and seizures.	Fluid and sodium imbalances can precipitate changes in neurological function. The severity of these derangements reflects the severity of the imbalances and should improve with treatment.

Nursing Interventions	Rationales
Monitor serum sodium levels.	Sodium levels below 120 mEq/L can produce changes in level of consciousness and seizures.
Assess patient for indicators of cerebral edema: lethargy, headache, nausea and vomiting, seizures, increased blood pressure, and decreased heart rate.	
Minimize effects of environment on mental status: Reorient patient; maintain quiet environment, minimizing extraneous stimuli; provide simple, brief explanations of activities, procedures, and equipment; and provide meaningful, relaxing stimuli to patient.	The stresses of the critical care environment (sensory overload, sensory deprivation, and sleep deprivation) can aggravate mental status changes produced physiologically. Taking preventive measures may minimize these environmental effects.
Prevent patient injury (see Appendix C)	

DISCHARGE PLANNING/CONTINUITY OF CARE

- Based on underlying pathology/etiology, assess need for/type of long-term care and follow-up.
- If the discharge destination is home, assess existing supports and the need for assistance.
- Determine coping deficits/support needs and institute assistance measures.
- Determine knowledge deficits/teaching needs and document and institute a teaching plan.
- Refer patient to social services as appropriate.
- Communicate coping deficits/support needs and knowledge deficits/teaching needs to unit accepting the patient on transfer.

REFERENCES

Cullen, L. (1992). Interventions related to fluid and electrolyte balance. *Nursing Clinics of North America, 27*(2), 569–598.

Huether, S. E. (1990). The cellular environment: Fluids and electrolytes, acids and bases. In K. L. McCance & S. E. Huether (Eds.), *Pathophysiology: The biologic basis for disease in adults and children* (pp. 88–92). St. Louis, MO: Mosby.

Isley, W. L. (1990). Serum sodium concentration abnormalities. *Critical Care Nursing Quarterly, 13*(3), 82–88.

Oh, M. S. & Carroll, H. J. (1989). Electrolyte and acid-base disorders. In B. Chernow, (Ed.), *Essentials of critical care pharmacology* (pp. 303–317). Baltimore, MD: Williams & Wilkins.

Stark, J. L. (1991). The renal system. In J.G. Alspach, (Ed.), *Core curriculum for critical care nursing* (4th ed., pp. 578–585). Philadelphia, PA: Saunders.

DISTURBANCES OF WATER BALANCE

Water accounts for 50–60% of body weight in adults. The highest percentage of water is found within cells, but water will shift based on osmotic concentration differences between intracellular and extracellular fluid. Water balance is controlled directly by antidiuretic hormone (ADH) and indirectly by sodium balance. Generally speaking, when sodium is lost, water follows, and when sodium is retained, water is also retained. Disorders of water balance refer to the group of disorders in which both sodium and water are lost or gained in relatively equal amounts.

Primary Water Excess
Primary water excess is abnormal retention of both water and electrolytes in approximately the same proportion as normal. It results from the kidney's inability to rid the body of unneeded water and electrolytes. Severe water excess can lead to heart failure, particularly if the patient has underlying cardiovascular dysfunction.

ETIOLOGIES

- Usually iatrogenic, i.e., conditions that favor retention of both sodium and water, such as
  - cardiac insufficiency
  - cirrhosis, ascites
  - protein depletion: malnutrition
  - stress or steroid therapy
  - renal disease
- Rapid administration of intravenous saline
- Psychosis

CLINICAL MANIFESTATIONS

- Cardiovascular: Fluid excess can produce
  - CVP > 10 mmHg
  - distended neck veins
  - PCWP > 12 mmHg
  - increased blood pressure

- bounding pulses
- tachycardia
- increased temperature
- increased weight
- Pulmonary: Fluid excess can produce
  - increased respiratory rate
  - fine crackles
  - dyspnea
- Skin: Fluid excess can produce
  - peripheral edema
  - puffy eyelids
  - taut, shiny skin

CLINICAL/DIAGNOSTIC FINDINGS

Laboratory studies will generally be normal because water and electrolytes are gained in approximately the same proportion as normal.

NURSING DIAGNOSIS: FLUID VOLUME EXCESS

Related To retention of both sodium and water

Defining Characteristics

Increased weight
Increased blood pressure
CVP > 10 mmHg
Peripheral edema
Puffy eyelids
Bounding pulses
Ascites
Taut, shiny skin

Patient Outcomes

Fluid volume will be maintained/restored to normal, as evidenced by
- weight return to patient baseline
- blood pressure within 10 mmHg of patient baseline
- absence of tissue fluid accumulation
- CVP 2–10 mmHg

Nursing Interventions	Rationales
Assess for underlying etiology of fluid retention.	Primary water excess occurs as the result of some underlying disorder. Identification and treatment of this underlying disorder is essential in correcting primary water excess.
Identify patients at risk (see etiologies) and monitor their fluid balance closely: Record accurate intake and output and daily weight.	A consistent imbalance between intake and output and/or increase in weight will be the earliest sign of primary water excess.

Nursing Interventions	Rationales
Maintain water and sodium restriction as prescribed.	Water and sodium restriction will prevent worsening of the fluid retention. Diuretics will assist in removing excess fluid.
Administer diuretics as prescribed and document effect.	Diuretics may facilitate water loss.
Monitor potassium and observe for signs of potassium depletion: EKG changes, dysrhythmias, fatigue, leg cramps, drowsiness, and anorexia	Generally when the kidneys retain sodium and water, potassium is lost, producing hypokalemia. In addition, treatment with diuretics can lead to hypokalemia.
Monitor for cardiovascular signs of fluid volume excess: tachycardia, hypertension, tachypnea, and increased CVP/PCWP	
Monitor for peripheral indicators of fluid volume excess: bounding peripheral pulses, distended neck veins, and peripheral edema.	
Monitor for signs of heart failure: fine crackles, c/o SOB, jugular venous distention, tachycardia, urine output < 30 mL/hr, peripheral edema, and decreased CO/CI	If fluid volume excess is severe, it can lead to compromised cardiovascular status and possibly heart failure.
Monitor for signs of fluid volume deficit: decreased blood pressure, tachycardia, decreased CVP/PCWP, and weak pulses.	Treatment with diuretics and water/sodium restriction can lead to fluid volume deficit.

NURSING DIAGNOSIS: IMPAIRED GAS EXCHANGE

Related To pulmonary edema secondary to primary water excess

Defining Characteristics
Fine crackles
$CVP > 10$ mmHg
Dyspnea
$SaO_2 < 90\%$

Pink, frothy sputum
$PCWP > 20$ mmHg
$PaO_2 < 80$ torr

Patient Outcomes

The patient will demonstrate normal gas exchange, as evidenced by
- PaO_2 > 80 torr or return to patient baseline
- SaO_2 > 90%
- absence of adventitious breath sounds
- CVP 2–10 mmHg; PCWP 8–12 mmHg

Nursing Interventions	Rationales
Monitor and document patient's respiratory status: rate, depth, and quality of respirations; complaints of dyspnea or SOB; and breath sounds.	Primary water excess can cause fluid collection in the lungs, especially if the patient has underlying cardiac or pulmonary disease or is on bedrest.
Monitor ABGs as prescribed and prn respiratory distress.	$PaCO_2$ is the assessment parameter used to evaluate ventilation. The PaO_2 and SaO_2 are the assessment parameters used to evaluate oxygenation.
Monitor and document pulse oximetry at least once a shift and prn respiratory distress.	
Maintain oxygen and suction equipment at bedside.	
Provide supportive measures to facilitate respiratory effort: elevate HOB; reposition every 2 hr; provide oxygen as needed; and suction as needed.	

Primary Water Deficit

Primary water deficit is an abnormal loss of water and electrolytes in approximately the same proportions as normal. This occurs as the result of increased loss or decreased intake. Severe water deficit can lead to hypovolemic shock and, if prolonged, acute renal failure.

ETIOLOGIES

- Gastrointestinal loss (most common)
    - vomiting
    - fistulas
    - frequent tap water enemas
    - diarrhea
    - NG suction

- Trapped fluids (third spacing)
  - bowel obstruction
  - peritonitis
  - burns
  - crushing injuries
- Severe diaphoresis
- Overzealous use of diuretics
- Addison's disease

CLINICAL MANIFESTATIONS

- Cardiovascular: Fluid loss can produce
  - CVP < 2 mmHg
  - flat neck veins
  - weak, thready pulses
  - decreased temperature
  - PCWP < 8 mmHg
  - decreased blood pressure
  - tachycardia
- Pulmonary: Fluid loss can produce increased respirations.
- Renal: Fluid loss and decreased renal perfusion can produce:
  - urine output < 30 mL/hr
  - decreased weight
- Skin: Fluid loss can produce
  - dry mucous membranes
  - decreased skin turgor
- Neurological: Fluid loss and decreased blood pressure can produce
  - dizziness
  - syncope

CLINICAL/DIAGNOSTIC FINDINGS

Laboratory studies will generally be normal because water and electrolytes are lost in approximately the same proportion as normal.

NURSING DIAGNOSIS: FLUID VOLUME DEFICIT
Related To loss of water and sodium

Defining Characteristics
Weight loss
CVP < 2 mmHg
Hypotension
Postural blood pressure
Negative intake and output

Tachycardia
PCWP < 8 mmHg
Urine output < 30 mL/hr

Patient Outcomes
Fluid balance is maintained/restored, as evidenced by
- blood pressure within 10 mmHg of patient baseline without postural changes
- heart rate 60–100 bpm
- CVP 2–10 mmHg; PCWP 8–12 mmHg

- weight return to patient baseline
- urine output > 30 mL/hr
- balanced intake and output

Nursing Interventions	Rationales
Assess for etiology of primary water deficit.	Since primary water deficit occurs as the result of some underlying disorder, the identification and treatment of the underlying cause is a key factor in its resolution.
Identify patients at risk (see etiologies) and institute preventive measures.	Primary water deficit may be prevented in many instances by ensuring adequate replacement of fluid losses.
Monitor and document fluid balance: intake and output, and daily weight.	A urine output of less than 30 mL for 2 hr is an indicator of decreased renal perfusion and the earliest sign of fluid volume deficit.
Monitor for and document cardiovascular signs of continuing fluid deficit: decreased blood pressure, tachycardia, tachypnea, and increased CVP/PCWP.	
Monitor for/document peripheral signs of continuing fluid deficit: weak peripheral pulses, poor skin turgor, dry mucous membranes.	
Monitor for/document signs of decreased cerebral perfusion: dizziness, syncope, confusion, and weakness.	
Monitor for signs of hidden fluid losses: abdominal distension.	Third spacing of fluids such as can occur with bowel obstruction or peritonitis can be detected by measuring abdominal girth.
Administer fluid and electrolytes as prescribed and monitor for signs of fluid overload.	

▼

DISCHARGE PLANNING/CONTINUITY OF CARE

- Based on underlying pathology/etiology, assess need for/type of long-term care and follow-up.
- If the discharge destination is home, assess existing supports and need for assistance.
- Determine coping deficits/support needs and institute assistance measures.
- Determine knowledge deficits/teaching needs and document and institute teaching plan.
- Refer patient to social services as appropriate.
- Communicate coping deficits/support needs and knowledge deficits/teaching needs to unit accepting the patient on transfer.

REFERENCES

Cullen, L. (1992). Interventions related to fluid and electrolyte balance. *Nursing Clinics of North America, 27*(2), 569–598.

Davidhizar, R. (1991a). Understanding water intoxication. Part 1. *Advances in Clinical Care, 6*(2), 30–31.

Davidhizar, R. (1991b). Understanding water intoxication: Nursing care for the patient with self induced water intoxication. Part 2. *Advances in Clinical Care, 6*(3), 16–19.

Gershan, J. A., Freeman, C. M., Ross, M. C., Greenlees, K., Smejkal, C., Brukwitzki, G., Schneider, K., Jiricka, M. K., Johnson, D., & Anderson, C. (1990). Fluid volume deficit: Validating the indicators. *Heart & Lung. 19*(2), 152–156.

Huether, S. E. (1990). The cellular environment: Fluids and electrolytes, acids and bases. In K. L. McCance & S. E. Huether (Eds.), *Pathophysiology: The biologic basis for disease in adults and children* (pp. 89–92). St. Louis, MO: Mosby.

Porth, C.M. (1990). *Pathophysiology: Concepts of altered health states.* Philadelphia, PA: Lippincott.

▼

METABOLIC ACIDOSIS

Metabolic acidosis is an acid-base imbalance caused by either a gain in acid or a loss of base (bicarbonate). It results in an increase in hydrogen ion concentration, a pH below 7.35, and a bicarbonate (HCO_3) below 21 mEq/L or a base excess (BE) below -3. Measuring the anion gap helps identify the precipitating cause. A normal anion gap (6–16 mEq/L) in the presence of a metabolic acidosis indicates a HCO_3 loss with retention of chloride. An increased anion gap indicates an accumulation of anions (acids) other than chloride such as keto or lactic acids. Signs and symptoms appear when bicarbonate levels are 20 mEq/L or less. At pH levels of 7.0 or below, both heart rate and cardiac output decrease and fatal dysrhythmias can develop.

ETIOLOGIES

- Increased anion gap
  - Lactic acid production (anaerobic metabolism); the most common are shock, strenuous exercise, generalized seizures, heart failure, liver disease, and severe anemia.
  - Ketoacid formation: fasting, malabsorption, ethanol intoxication, starvation, diabetic ketoacidosis, renal failure, ketogenic diet (high fat, low carbohydrate)
  - Drug toxicity: salicylates, methanol, paraldehyde, ethylene glycol
  - Rhabdomyolysis
- Normal anion gap
  - Acid administration: administration of chloride containing acids (ammonium chloride, hydrochloric acid), anion exchange resins (cholestyramine chloride), carbonic anhydrase inhibitors (acetazolamide), hyperalimentation with HCl containing amino acid solutions
  - Bicarbonate losses: GI (diarrhea, pancreatic fistulas, urinary diversions, loss of small bowel secretions) and renal (renal tubular acidosis, postchronic hypocapnia)
- Impaired renal acid excretion with hyperkalemia

CLINICAL MANIFESTATIONS

- Neurological: Central nervous system depression and cerebral vasodilatation produce
  - headache
  - confusion
  - drowsiness
  - fatigue
  - stupor
  - coma
- Cardiovascular: Arterial vasodilatation and decreased contractility produce
  - hypotension
  - CO < 4 L/min
  - unresponsiveness to catecholamines
  - dysrhythmias
  - warm, flushed skin
- Gastrointestinal: Irritation of brain emetic center produces
  - anorexia
  - abdominal pain
  - vomiting
- Due to compensation: Increased rate and depth of respirations (Kussmaul respirations)
- Other clinical manifestations of primary disorder

CLINICAL/DIAGNOSTIC FINDINGS

- pH < 7.35
- HCO_3 < 21 mEq/L
- Base excess < -3
- Pa_{CO_2} < 35 torr (compensatory)
- Anion gap increased or normal depending on cause
- Acid urine
- Increased ammonia in urine
- Look for increased potassium and increased chloride

NURSING DIAGNOSIS: DECREASED CARDIAC OUTPUT

Related To decreased contractility secondary to acidosis

Defining Characteristics
Hypotension
Warm flushed skin
CI < 2.5 L/min/m^2
Cardiovascular collapse

Dysrhythmias
CO < 4 L/min
Decreased heart rate

Patient Outcomes
Cardiac output will be maintained/restored, as evidenced by
- blood pressure within 10 mmHg of patient baseline
- heart rate 60–100 bpm
- absence of dysrhythmias

- CO 4–8 L/min; CI 2.5–4 L/min/m^2
- absence of cardiovascular collapse

Nursing Interventions	Rationales
Assess for underlying cause of metabolic acidosis and institute treatment.	As long as the underlying cause persists, treatment of metabolic acidosis will be unsuccessful.
Assess and document cardiovascular status: vital signs, hemodynamic parameters, and peripheral pulses. Assess for signs of cardiovascular collapse: bradycardia, hypotension, increased CVP/PCWP, decreased CO/CI, decreased MAP, and weak peripheral pulses.	When pH falls to 7.0, the heart becomes unresponsive to catecholamines (epinephrine and norepinephrine) and heart rate and cardiac output decrease.
Monitor for signs of increased potassium	Extracellular potassium may be high because the body exchanges intracellular potassium for extracellular hydrogen ions in an attempt to normalize pH.
Monitor serum calcium levels.	Calcium shifts out of the cells to assist in buffering extracellular hydrogen ions. As the acidosis is treated, decreased ionized calcium can produce signs of hypocalcemia.
Monitor for dysrhythmias and document and treat per protocols.	Cardiac dysrhythmias may occur when the pH falls to 7.0.
Administer sodium bicarbonate as prescribed and monitor effects.	The administration of sodium bicarbonate will vary depending on the severity of the acidosis and the ability to correct the underlying cause. Sodium bicarbonate itself can potentially cause problems such as paradoxical acidosis from increased intracellular PaCO_2, hyperosmolality, alkalemia and sodium overload. Levels should be measured after each dose and prior to administration of an additional dose to prevent overcorrection.

Nursing Interventions	Rationales
In chronic metabolic acidosis administer oral alkali as prescribed and monitor results.	Chronic metabolic acidosis may occur in patients with chronic renal failure. If possible, this acidosis is controlled with the administration of oral alkali.

NURSING DIAGNOSIS: ALTERED THOUGHT PROCESSES

Related To
- CNS depression
- Increased calcium
- Cerebral vasodilation

Defining Characteristics

Confusion
Drowsiness
Coma
Stupor
Unconsciousness
Lethargy

Patient Outcomes
The patient's mentation will return to baseline.

Nursing Interventions	Rationales
Assess for degree of neurological/psychological dysfunction and document.	
Minimize effects of environment on mental status: 1. Reorient patient with each contact. 2. Maintain quiet environment, minimizing extraneous stimuli. 3. Provide simple, brief explanations of activities, procedures, or equipment. 4. Provide meaningful, relaxing stimuli.	The stresses of the critical care environment (sensory overload, sensory deprivation, and sleep deprivation) can aggravate mental status changes produced physiologically. Taking preventive measures may minimize these environmental effects.
Protect patient from injury (see Appendix C).	

DISCHARGE PLANNING/CONTINUITY OF CARE

- Based on underlying pathology/etiology assess need for/type of long-term care and follow-up.
- If the discharge destination is home, assess existing supports and the need for assistance.
- Determine coping deficits/support needs and institute assistance measures.
- Determine knowledge deficits/teaching needs, and document and institute a teaching plan.
- Refer patient/significant other to social services as appropriate.
- Communicate coping deficits/support needs and knowledge deficits/teaching needs to unit accepting the patient on transfer.

REFERENCES

Black, R. M. (1991). Metabolic acidosis and metabolic alkalosis. In J. M. Rippe, R. S. Irwin, J. S. Alpert, & M. P. Fink (Eds.), *Intensive care medicine* (2nd ed., pp. 779–793). Boston, MA: Little, Brown.

Lorenz, A. (1989). Lactic acidosis: A nursing challenge. *Critical Care Nurse, 9*(4), 64–73.

Pfister, S. M. & Bullas, J. B. (1989). Arterial blood gas evaluation: Metabolic acidemia. *Critical Care Nurse, 9*(1), 70–72.

Porth, C. M. (1990). *Pathophysiology: Concepts of altered health states*, (pp. 523–526.) Philadelphia, PA: Lippincott.

METABOLIC ALKALOSIS

Metabolic alkalosis is an acid-base imbalance caused by either a gain in base or a loss of acid resulting in a pH greater than 7.35 and a HCO_3 greater than 28 mEq/L or a base excess greater than +3. Metabolic alkalosis occurs in conditions that either increase bicarbonate or produce excess retention of bicarbonate via the kidneys. Signs and symptoms occur less frequently with metabolic alkalosis as compared to other acid-base disorders because bicarbonate ions cross the blood-brain barrier more slowly, producing less of a change in cerebrospinal fluid pH than in increases in hydrogen ions or CO_2. Symptoms related to cerebral vasoconstriction and decreased calcium are more likely with respiratory alkalosis where alkalosis develops more rapidly. Severe metabolic alkalosis (pH > 7.55) can lead to respiratory failure, dysrhythmias, seizures, and coma.

ETIOLOGIES

- Bicarbonate retention
  - excessive alkaline drugs: antacids, laxative abuse, baking soda, sodium bicarbonate
  - massive blood transfusion
  - renal retention
  - rapid correction of compensated respiratory acidosis
- Hydrogen and chloride loss
  - gastrointestinal: vomiting, gastric suctioning, diarrhea (if high in chloride content)
  - excessive aldosterone: hyperaldosteronism, Cushing's disease
  - excessive use of mercurial, thiazide, and loop diuretics
  - high-dose IV penicillins
  - postchronic hypercapnia
- Hydrogen movement into cells
  - hypokalemia
  - refeeding

CLINICAL MANIFESTATIONS

- Cerebral vasoconstriction produces
  - dizziness
  - lightheadedness
  - faintness
  - blurred vision
- Decreased calcium (nerves more irritable) produces
  - tingling of extremities and lips
  - carpopedal spasm
  - seizures
  - increased reflexes
- Irritation of emetic center: nausea, vomiting
- Compensatory hypoventilation

NOTE: Most patients have no clinical manifestations. Manifestations are usually associated with volume depletion (weakness, muscle cramps, postural dizziness) or hypokalemia (muscle weakness, polyuria, polydipsia).

CLINICAL/DIAGNOSTIC FINDINGS

- pH > 7.45
- Bicarbonate > 28 mEq/L
- Base excess > +3
- $Paco_2$ > 45 torr (compensation)
- Look for decreased serum potassium and decreased serum chloride
- EKG: atrial tachycardia

NURSING DIAGNOSIS: ACID-BASE IMBALANCE

Related To
- Bicarbonate retention
- Hydrogen and chloride loss
- Hydrogen movement into cells

Defining Characteristics

Dizziness
Increased reflexes
HCO_3 > 28 mEq/L

Blurred vision
Carpopedal spasm
pH > 7.45

Patient Outcomes

Acid-base balance will be maintained/restored, as evidenced by
- absence of neurological manifestations
- pH 7.35–7.45
- HCO_3 21–28 mEq/L

Nursing Interventions	Rationales
Assess for underlying cause of metabolic alkalosis and institute treatment.	As long as the underlying cause persists, treatment of metabolic alkalosis will be unsuccessful.
Monitor pH during diuretic use.	Diuretics can block chloride reabsorption in the kidney, producing bicarbonate retention via both volume and chloride loss.
Monitor pH during gastrointestinal loss.	Chloride is a major component of GI secretions. Chloride loss causes bicarbonate ions to be conserved and can cause metabolic alkalosis.
Monitor serum potassium and for signs of hypokalemia.	In hypokalemia, the kidneys conserve potassium and excrete hydrogen ions, producing metabolic alkalosis. In metabolic alkalosis, potassium will move into the cells in exchange for hydrogen ions, producing hypokalemia.
Monitor serum calcium and for signs of hypocalcemia.	Levels of ionized calcium decrease as pH increases.
If metabolic alkalosis is due to chloride loss, provide potassium chloride replacement as prescribed and monitor response.	The chloride anion replaces bicarbonate anions and the potassium allows the kidneys to conserve hydrogen ions. Potassium also can replace a concurrent potassium deficit.
Administer acetazolamide as prescribed and monitor for signs of hypokalemia.	Acetazolamide decreases bicarbonate reabsorption in the proximal tubules of the kidneys but can result in potassium loss.
If administering hydrochloric acid, monitor IV site closely.	Hydrochloric acid can increase pH, but when given intravenously can injure small veins, especially with infiltration. The solution can be buffered by administering it in an amino acid solution or with fat emulsions.

Nursing Interventions	Rationales
Administer normal saline or 0.45 normal saline as prescribed and monitor results.	Sudden decreases in extracellular fluid volume (such as can occur with diuretic therapy) can produce an increase in renal reabsorption of sodium and bicarbonate, producing metabolic alkalosis.

NURSING DIAGNOSIS: INEFFECTIVE BREATHING PATTERN

Related To central depression of respiration

Defining Characteristics
Decreased respiratory rate
PaO_2 < 80 torr
Diminished breath sounds
Shallow respirations
$PaCO_2$ > 45 torr

Patient Outcomes
An effective breathing pattern will be restored/maintained, as evidenced by
- normal rate and depth of ventilation
- $PaCO_2$ 35–45 torr
- PaO_2 > 80 torr or return to patient baseline

Nursing Interventions	Rationales
Assess and document ventilation: rate, depth, and rhythm of respiration; airway and breathing effort and use of accessory muscles; and breath sounds. Assess ABGs and pulse oximetry as ordered and prn respiratory distress. Assess pulmonary function parameters: tidal volume and vital capacity. Assess for subjective complaints of shortness of breath and dyspnea on exertion.	Metabolic alkalosis causes compensatory hypoventilation in an attempt to retain acid (CO_2) and normalize pH. Until corrected, ongoing assessment/evaluation of the patient's breathing pattern must be made.

Nursing Interventions	Rationales
Support airway as appropriate: airway, supplementary oxygen, suctioning, and intubation equipment/ventilator.	
Position patient for ease of respiratory effort, that is, head of bed elevated.	
Allow frequent rest periods during activity. Minimize activity to decrease oxygen need.	
Monitor for signs of respiratory infection: decreased breath sounds and increased temperature.	Hypoventilation can cause atelectasis and pooling of secretions precipitating pneumonia.

DISCHARGE PLANNING/CONTINUITY OF CARE

- Based on underlying pathology/etiology, assess need for/type of long-term care and follow-up.
- If the discharge destination is home, assess existing supports and the need for assistance.
- Determine coping deficits/support needs and institute assistance measures.
- Determine knowledge deficits/teaching needs and document and institute a teaching plan
- Refer patient to social services as appropriate.
- Communicate coping deficits/support needs and knowledge deficits/teaching needs to unit accepting the patient on transfer.

REFERENCES

Black, R. M. (1991). Metabolic acidosis and metabolic alkalosis. In J. M. Rippe, R. S. Irwin, J. S. Alpert, & M. P. Fink (Eds.), *Intensive Care Medicine* (2nd ed., pp. 779–793). Boston, MA: Little Brown.

Marik, P. E., Kussman, B. D., Lipman, J., & Kraus, P. (1991). Acetazolamide in the treatment of metabolic alkalosis in critically ill patients. *Heart & Lung, 20*(5), 455–459.

Porth, C. M. (1990). *Pathophysiology: Concepts of altered health states* (pp. 526–527). Philadelphia, PA: Lippincott.

Miscellaneous

▼

DRUG INTOXICATION

Drug overdose results from inadvertent or intentional self-administration of prescription and/or over-the-counter drugs. Signs and symptoms vary depending on the drug(s) ingested with primary concern relating to neurological, pulmonary, and/or cardiovascular depression. Prognosis varies depending on the type and amount of drug taken and the rapidity of treatment.

ETIOLOGIES

Stimulants
- Sympathomimetics
  - amphetamines: methylphenidate (Ritalin), pemoline (Cylert), phentermine (Fastin), mazindol (Sanorex), amphetamine
  - bronchodilators
  - cocaine
  - monoamine oxidase inhibitors: phenelzine (Nardil), isocarboxazid (Marplan), tranylcypromine (Parnate)
- Anticholinergics
  - antihistamines: diphenhydramine (Benadryl), chlorpheniramine (Chlor-Trimeton), hydoxyzine (Atarax), promethazine (Phenergen)
  - antipsychotics: trifluoperazine (Stelazine), thioridazine (Mellaril), prochlorperazine (Compazine), chlorpromazine (Thorazine), haloperidol (Haldol)
  - tricyclic antidepressants: amitriptyline (Elavil), doxepin (Sinequan), imipramine (Tofranil), maprotiline (Ludiomil), trazadone, amoxapine, nortriptyline
  - over-the-counter cough, cold, allergy, sleep, antimotion sickness, and antinausea medications
- Hallucinogens: LSD, marijuana, mescaline, phencyclidine (PCP)
- Withdrawal syndromes: beta blockers, clonidine, cyclic antidepressants, ethanol, narcotics, nitrates, sedative hypnotics

Depressants
- Sympatholytics: alpha blockers, angiotensin converting enzyme (ACE) inhibitors, antiarrhythmics, beta blockers, clonidine, cyclic antidepressants, digitalis
- Cholinergics: bethanechol, neostigmine, physostigmine
- Opiods: analgesics, antidiarrheal drugs, heroin, opium
- Sedative-hypnotics
  - alcohol
  - barbiturates: secobarbital (Seconal), pentobarbital Nembutal), butalbital (Fiorinal), thiopental (Pentothal), phenobarbital
  - benzodiazepines: midazolam (Versed), triazolam (Halcion), lorazepam (Ativan), diazepam (Valium), flurazepam (Dalmane), alprazolam (Xanax), oxazepam (Serax), temazepam (Restoril)
- Miscellaneous: calcium channel blockers, anticonvulsants, antiarrhythmics

Mixed
Lithium, salicylates, ethylene glycol, methanol, acetaminophen

CLINICAL MANIFESTATIONS

- Amphetamines
  - neurological: headache, dilated pupils, anxiety, restlessness, nervousness, agitation, confusion, delirium, tremors, seizures, coma
  - cardiovascular: hypertension, tachyarrhythmias, cardiovascular collapse
  - renal: urinary retention
- Cocaine
  - neurological: headache, agitation, anxiety, tremors, hyperreflexia, muscle twitching, seizures
  - cardiovascular: chest pain, tachycardia, hypertension, hyperthermia
  - pulmonary: tachypnea, abnormal respiratory pattern
  - gastrointestinal: nausea and vomiting
- Monoamine oxidase inhibitors
  - neurological: headache, agitation, rigidity, tremors, hyperreflexia, seizures, coma
  - cardiovascular: tachycardia, hypertension, diaphoresis, hyperpyrexia
  - pulmonary: respiratory depression
- Anticholinergics
  - neurological: excitement, delirium, anxiety, seizures, hallucinations
  - cardiovascular: tachycardia, warm flushed skin, atrial and ventricular tachycardia, AV blocks; mild hypertension; hyperpyrexia
  - pulmonary: tachypnea
  - gastrointestinal: ileus, constipation
  - renal: urinary retention
- Antipsychotics
  - neurological: ataxia, confusion, lethargy, slurred speech, hyperreflexia, coma

- cardiovascular: tachycardia, AV block, bundle branch block, prolonged PR and QT intervals, ST depression, T-wave abnormalities, widening QRS, tachyarrhythmias; hypotension
- pulmonary: respiratory depression, pulmonary edema
- gastrointestinal: nausea and vomiting, decreased bowel sounds
• Tricyclic antidepressants
  - neurological: decreased mental status, seizures
  - cardiovascular: hypotension, dysrhythmias, conduction abnormalities, hyperthermia
  - pulmonary: tachypnea
  - gastrointestinal: ileus
  - renal: urinary retention
• Hallucinogens
  - neurological: euphoria, lethargy, coma, violent behavior, agitation, hallucinations, generalized rigidity
  - cardiovascular: hypertension, tachycardia, hyperthermia
  - pulmonary: tachypnea
  - gastrointestinal: nausea and vomiting, diarrhea
• Benzodiazepines
  - neurological: slurred speech, lethargy, ataxia, nystagmus, coma
  - pulmonary: respiratory depression
• Barbiturates
  - neurological: sedation, coma
  - cardiovascular: hypotension, myocardial depression, vasodilation, cardiovascular collapse
  - pulmonary: respiratory depression, apnea
  - gastrointestinal: decreased bowel sounds, ileus
  - skin: bullous skin lesions over pressure points

CLINICAL/DIAGNOSTIC FINDINGS

- Increased anion gap metabolic acidosis (ethylene glycol, methanol and salicylate poisoning)
- Serum osmolality usually increased
- Serum ketones present
- Increased or decreased potassium
- Increased or decreased glucose
- Altered liver function tests (acetaminophen, ethanol, mushrooms, heavy metals)
- Altered renal function (ethylene glycol, isopropyl alcohol, amphetamines, cocaine, ethanol, heroin, phencyclidine)
- Myoglobinuria (PCP, cyclic antidepressants)
- EKG: SVT, bradycardia; ventricular tachyarrhythmias (sympathomimetics, digoxin, chloral hydrate); wide QRS and prolonged QT intervals (cyclic antidepressants, lithium, phenothiazines, quinine); AV block, bradycardia
- Positive urine toxicology

- Positive serum toxicology
- Positive gastric contents

NURSING DIAGNOSIS: INEFFECTIVE BREATHING PATTERN

Related To effects of drugs on respiratory center producing either stimulation or depression

Defining Characteristics
Hypercapnea ($PaCO_2$ > 45 torr)
Hypoventilation
Tachypnea/bradypnea
Ineffective cough
SaO_2 < 90%
Decreasing PaO_2

Patient Outcomes
An adequate breathing pattern will be maintained/restored, as evidenced by
- ABGs: pH 7.35–7.45, $PaCO_2$ 35–45 torr, PaO_2 > 80 torr
- respirations 12–20 per minute
- effective cough
- SaO_2 > 90%

Nursing Interventions	Rationales
Assess/record respiratory status: rate, depth, and rhythm of respiration; airway, breathing effort, and use of accessory muscles; breath sounds; ABGs and pulse oximetry; pulmonary function parameters (tidal volume, vital capacity); and strength of cough and ability to mobilize secretions.	The respiratory system may be depressed or stimulated related to drug effects on the central nervous system and must be monitored continuously.
Support airway as appropriate: airway, supplementary oxygen, suctioning, and intubation equipment/ventilator.	If the patient's level of consciousness is depressed, intubation may be done prophylactically to ensure an open airway and prevent aspiration.
Position patient for ease of respiratory effort, that is, HOB elevated.	
Provide adequate humidification with oxygen	Adequate humidification is necessary to loosen and allow elimination of secretions.

Nursing Interventions	Rationales
Assist removal of secretions via nasotracheal or orotracheal suctioning as needed.	Due to an altered level of consciousness, the patient may be unable to adequately mobilize secretions.
Reposition patient every 2 hr.	
Monitor fluid balance closely.	Large amounts of fluid are administered to help flush the system of drugs placing the patient at risk for fluid overload and possible pulmonary congestion.
Use sterile suctioning technique.	
Monitor swallowing closely. Insert NG tube if patient is unable to swallow and/or gag reflex is absent.	If the level of consciousness is altered, an NG tube is inserted to protect the airway and administer medication.

NURSING DIAGNOSIS: ALTERED THOUGHT PROCESSES

Related To drug effects on the central nervous system resulting in either stimulation or depression

Defining Characteristics
Confusion
Restlessness
Disorientation
Lethargy
Incoherent
Coma

Patient Outcomes
The patient's thought processes will return to patient baseline.

Nursing Interventions	Rationales
Obtain overdose history: time and amount, substance/s taken, current medications, observed signs and symptoms, recent significant events, psychiatric history, allergies, and chronic disease history.	The history is vital so that appropriate treatment can be initiated immediately. Drug toxicology reports may take several hours to obtain.

Nursing Interventions	Rationales
Assess/monitor neurological status and record and report changes to physician: alertness and orientation, clarity of speech, movement of extremities, sensation intactness, appropriateness of behavior, cranial nerve fuction, and seizure activity. Establish baseline normal if possible.	The severity of neurological deficits will depend on the type and amount of drug(s) taken and how promptly the patient receives treatment. Toxic effects may result in either CNS stimulation or depression.
Monitor fluid and electrolyte balance: serum electrolytes, intake and output, daily weight, and hourly urine output.	Electrolyte imbalances can occur as result of both the drugs taken and/or treatment. Fluids are administered in large amounts during treatment and can produce fluid overload and worsen neurological deficits.
Monitor patient's temperature and treat as appropriate.	Drug overdose can produce either hyper- or hypothermia. Antipyretics will generally be ineffective for drug-induced hyperthermia.
Minimize effects of environment on mental status: 1. Reorient patient as needed. 2. Maintain quiet environment, minimizing extraneous stimuli. 3. Provide simple, brief explanations of activities, procedures, and equipment. 4. Provide meaningful, relaxing stimuli to patient. 5. Provide consisent caregivers when possible.	The stresses of the critical care environment (sensory overload, sensory deprivation, and sleep deprivation) can aggravate mental status changes produced physiologically. Taking preventive measures may minimize these environmental effects.
Administer naloxone and 50% dextrose IV as prescribed and monitor and record effects.	If the cause of decreased mental status is unclear, the administration of 50% dextrose will protect the patient from possible damage due to hypoglycemic coma and naloxone will reverse the effects of narcotics.
Administer activated charcoal as prescribed and monitor and record effects.	Activated charcoal prevents absorption of the drug by binding the chemical with the gut lumen and eliminating it in the stool.

Nursing Interventions	Rationales
Perform gastric lavage as prescribed and note stomach contents.	Gastric lavage directly removes the injested chemical. It is most effective when administered in the left lateral decubitis position with Trendelenburg or the left side down.
Administer syrup of ipecac as prescribed only if patient is mentally intact.	Syrup of ipecac induces vomiting and will remove any drug left in the stomach. The patient must be sitting up and mentally intact to prevent aspiration. Do not use with activated charcoal.
Perform whole bowel irrigation as prescribed and monitor and record results.	Bowel irrigation prevents absorption of ingested chemicals by promoting rectal evacuation.
Administer diuretics as prescribed and record response.	Diuretics enhance excretion by keeping the urine dilute, thus decreasing passive distal tubular reabsorption of chemicals.
Monitor and record urine pH.	Urine pH (neutral is 6) may be increased or decreased via administration of alkaline or acidic fluids. This can enhance renal excretion of acidic or basic chemicals by ion trapping, making less drug available for absorption.
Administer 0.9 NS with $NaHCO_3$ added as prescribed at rate of desired urine output, monitoring closely for signs of fluid retention/overload.	This is used to either produce systemic alkalinization or force alkaline diuresis. Alkaline diuresis is used with salicylate and barbiturate poisoning. Systemic alkalinization is used with cyclic antidepressants.
Administer renal dopamine as prescribed and record response.	This will help maintain urine output the same as fluid administration.

Nursing Interventions	Rationales
Institute hemodialysis or hemoperfusion/hemofiltration as prescribed (see acute dialysis) and monitor and record response.	Hemoperfusion or hemodialysis may be necessary if the patient continues to deteriorate, has signs of severe intoxication, has taken a lethal dose, has impaired renal function, or a more rapid rate of removal is required.
Institute plasmaphoresis as prescribed and monitor and record response.	
Administer sedatives, anticonvulsants, and/or paralyzing agents if prescribed and monitor and record response.	Certain drugs (sympathomimetics, central stimulants, drug withdrawal) can produce neuromuscular hyperactivity, severe agitation, and/or seizures requiring pharmacological sedation.
Institute measures to protect patient from injury: Apply restraints as necessary; place siderails up and bed in low position; pad siderails; and keep patient in room close to nursing station.	Due to altered thought processes and level of consciousness, the patient is particularly prone to injury. If the drug ingestion was intentional, the patient also needs to be constantly monitored to prevent further self-inflicted harm.

NURSING DIAGNOSIS: DECREASED CARDIAC OUTPUT

Related To
- Vasomotor depression
- Myocardial depression
- Catecholamine depletion

Defining Characteristics
Hypotension or hypertension
Dysrhythmias
EKG abnormalities

Patient Outcomes
Cardiac output will be maintained/restored, as evidenced by
- blood pressure within 10 mmHg of patient baseline
- absence of dysrhythmias and EKG changes

Drug Intoxication 433

Nursing Interventions	Rationales
Assess/monitor drug effects on cardiovascular system: blood pressure, heart rate, respiratory rate, and temperature; hemodynamics (CVP/PCWP, CO/CI, SVR); and signs of cardiac stress (c/o chest pain, ischemia on EKG, dysrhythmias)	At toxic levels many drugs can cause myocardial depression, changes in vascular tone (vasoconstriction or vasodilatation), and/or interference with vasomotor center control of vital functions.
Monitor EKG continuously and document rhythm/dysrhythmias.	Dysrhythmias can be caused by toxic drug levels.
Administer fluids and/or vasopressors as prescribed to correct hypotension and monitor and record response.	Hypotension is most often due to loss of peripheral vascular tone. If unresponsive to fluids, hypotension may be due to myocardial depression and require vasopressors such as norepinephrine or high-dose dopamine for correction.
Administer medication to control hypertension as prescribed and monitor and record response	Hypertension is seen with cocaine, amphetamines, tricyclic antidepressants, and drug withdrawal. Vasodilators or beta blockers may be used if hypertension is severe.
Administer medications to correct dysrhythmias per protocols.	

NURSING DIAGNOSIS: INEFFECTIVE INDIVIDUAL COPING

Related To
- Situational crisis
- Loss of control/independence

Defining Characteristics
Destructive behavior toward self
Inability to problem solve
Verbalization of inability to cope

Patient Outcomes
The patient will display coping behaviors that are health promoting.

Nursing Interventions	Rationales
Assess for cause of drug overdose.	Long-term treatment and follow-up will be determined by whether the overdose was intentional or accidental and whether the patient currently has suicidal intentions.
Assess current emotional status, that is, remorseful and/or expresses regret at being unsuccessful.	
Assess support systems/coping mechanisms/current stresses.	
Assist patient in identifying and utilizing support systems.	
Encourage verbalization of feelings.	This promotes development of a trusting relationship with the caregiver.
Communicate nonjudgmental, caring attitude.	Same as for previous intervention.
Provide for psychiatric support and follow-up.	

NURSING DIAGNOSIS: HIGH RISK FOR INJURY

Risk Factors
- Toxic effects of drugs
- Altered level of consciousness
- Risk for aspiration
- Risk for seizures

Patient Outcomes
The patient will remain free of injury.

Nursing Interventions	Rationales
Assess for toxic effects of drugs.	
Administer appropriate treatment to reverse toxic effects and monitor and record response.	
See Appendix C.	

NURSING DIAGNOSIS: HIGH RISK FOR SELF-DIRECTED VIOLENCE

Risk Factors
- Self-destructive behavior
- Substance abuse withdrawal
- Low self-esteem
- Depression
- Expressions of hopelessness/wanting to die

Patient Outcomes
The patient will be protected from further self-directed violence.

NOTE: Serious suicide attempts and/or substance abuse problems require psychiatric follow-up and/or specialized treatment programs where behavior can be modified.

Nursing Interventions	Rationales
Assess for history of substance abuse/previous suicide attempts.	This will help determine the seriousness of the self-directed violence.
Assess events precipitating this hospitalization.	This helps determine the cause of the drug intoxication and facilitates the planning for further treatment.
Assess for intent of drug intoxication, that is, suicidal or accidental and continued expression/signs of suicidal intention.	This will help determine the seriousness of the self-directed violence and the type of follow-up treatment required.
Protect patient from further injury. Observe patient at least every 15 min and place in bed within sight of nurse's station. Explain precisely and simply the measures you are taking and why. Restrain as needed.	
Set limits on patient behavior using concise, easily understood language.	

Nursing Interventions	Rationales
Approach patient in calm manner.	The patient may be frightened and/or easily agitated, particularly while drug effects are present. A nonthreatening approach may help soothe the patient.
Acknowledge patient's feelings and allow patient to express feelings freely in nonjudgmental atmosphere.	This conveys empathy and helps to develop a therapeutic relationship.
Maintain quiet, calm environment: Miminize noise as much as possible and limit number of people present in room at one time.	Reducing sensory stimulation can help limit confusion and/or aggressive outbursts.
Maintain some level of light in room.	The patient may be confused and/or frightened on return to a normal level of consciousness due to the strange environment and stimuli. Some level of light will help self-orientation and facilitate visual observation.
Explain all procedures and cares.	
Orient/reorient frequently.	
Provide for psychiatric follow-up and care.	

DISCHARGE PLANNING/CONTINUITY OF CARE

- Assess need for/type of long-term care and follow-up.
- If the discharge destination is home, assess existing supports and the need for assistance.
- Determine coping deficits/support needs and institute assistance measures.
- Determine knowledge deficits/teaching needs and document and institute a teaching plan.
- Refer patient to social services as appropriate.
- Communicate coping deficits/support needs and knowledge deficits/learning needs to unit accepting patient on transfer.

REFERENCES

Freas, G. C. (1989). Poisoning. In B. Chernow (Ed.), *Essentials of critical care pharmacology* (pp. 274–302). Baltimore, MD: Williams & Wilkins.

Rippe, J. M., Irwin, R. S., Alpert, J. S., & Fink, M. P. (Eds.). (1991). *Intensive Care Medicine*. Boston, MA: Little, Brown.

Perrin, K. O. & Williams-Burgess, C. (1990). The suicidal patient in the CCU: Nursing approaches. *Critical Care Nurse*, *10*(7), 59–64.

HYPOVOLEMIC SHOCK

Severe hypovolemic shock results in a sudden loss of blood volume, thus decreasing venous return to the heart and decreasing cardiac output. If volume is not rapidly replaced, decreased tissue perfusion results. In response to the decreased cardiac output, the body initiates compensatory mechanisms to attempt to maintain perfusion. These mechanisms account for the major signs and symptoms seen in patients on initial assessment. Release of catecholamines triggers the blood vessels in the skin, lungs, intestines, liver, and kidneys to constrict, thereby increasing the volume of blood flow to the brain and heart. Because of the decreased flow of blood in the skin, the patient's skin will be cool to the touch. With decreased blood flow to the lungs, hyperventilation will occur to maintain adequate gas exchange. As blood flow to the liver decreases, metabolic waste products accumulate in the blood. As intravascular volume decreases, urine output decreases due to the reabsorption of water by the kidneys in response to the release of antidiuretic hormone (ADH) by the posterior lobe of the pituitary gland.

Decreased tissue perfusion results in cellular dysfunction. The cells shift to anaerobic metabolim and lactic acid is formed. Decreased blood flow affects all of the body systems, and they will begin to fail without sufficient oxygen supply.

ETIOLOGIES

- Trauma
  - thoracic injury with hemothoraxes
  - abdominal injuries
  - pelvic injuries
  - amputations
  - major blood vessel disruption
- Surgery
- Burns

- Severe dehydration
  - diarrhea
  - vomiting
  - diabetic ketoacidosis
  - diabetes insipidus
- Third spacing into peritoneum
- Intestinal obstruction

CLINICAL MANIFESTATIONS

- Cardiovascular: Loss of blood volume and decreased perfusion produce
  - flat neck veins (loss of venous return)
  - hypotension
  - decreased cardiac output (<4 L/min)
  - narrowed pulse pressure
  - decreased pulses (radial and carotid)
- Respiratory: Loss of blood volume, oxygen-carrying capacity, and impaired gas exhanges produce
  - rapid, shallow respirations
  - use of accessory muscles
- Neurological: Decreased tissue perfusion produces
  - anxiety
  - decreasing level of consciousness
- Skin: Decreased peripheral perfusion produces
  - cool, clammy, pale skin
  - diaphoresis
  - delay in capillary refill time

CLINICAL/DIAGNOSTIC FINDINGS

- Loss of blood volume produces
  - hemoglobin < 13 g/dL
  - hematocrit < 35% women; < 42% men
  - decreasing PaO_2
  - BUN > 20 mg/dL
  - creatinine > 1.2 mg/dL
  - sodium > 145 mEq/L
  - PT > 13 s
  - PTT > 45 s
  - platelet count < 150,000/mm^3
  - pH < 7.35
- Body stress response activation of the sympathetic nervous system produces
  - hyperglycemia (> 115 mg/dL)
  - white blood cell count > 10,000/mm^3

- respiratory alkalosis ($PaCO_2$ < 35 torr, pH > 7.45)
- temperature elevation
* Decreased tissue perfusion produces
  - metabolic acidosis (HCO_3 < 22 mEq/L, pH < 7.35)
  - ammonia > 45 μmol/L

NURSING DIAGNOSIS: FLUID VOLUME DEFICIT

Related To loss of effective circulating blood volume

Defining Characteristics
Hypotension
CO < 4 L/min; CI < 2.5 L/min/m^2
CVP < 2 mmHg; PCWP < 8 mmHg
Tachycardia
Cool, pale, dry skin mucous membranes
Urine output < 30 mL/hr

Patient Outcomes
Adequate fluid balance is maintained/restored, as evidenced by
* MAP > 60 mmHg
* CO 4–8 L/min; CI 2.5–4 L/min/m^2
* CVP 2–10 mmHg; PCWP 8–12 mmHg
* heart rate 60–100 bpm
* pink, moist mucous membranes
* warm, pink skin
* urine output > 30 mL/hr

Nursing Interventions	Rationales
Monitor cardiovascular status: blood pressure; heart rate, including orthostatic changes; hemodynamics (CVP, PCWP, CO, CI, MAP); peripheral pulses.	Increased heart rate, decreased blood pressure, and/or orthostatic changes; low CVP, PCWP, CO, CI and MAP; and weak peripheral pulses indicate persistent hypovolemia. Normalization of these measurements will reflect adequate fluid replacement.
Monitor fluid balance: intake and output, daily weight.	Intake and output and daily weight provide a means to trend and evaluate fluid balance.

Nursing Interventions	Rationales
Monitor renal function: BUN, creatinine, and hourly urine output.	BUN and creatinine reflect renal function and their increase indicate prolonged decreased renal perfusion. Decreased urine output is an early sign of decreased perfusion and inadequate fluid replacement.
Administer intravenous colloids, crystalloids, or blood products according to protocol until signs and symptoms of hypovolemia stabilize. Monitor for signs of fluid overload: increased CVP, PCWP, adventitious breath sounds, jugular vein distention, and respiratory distress. Instruct patient on the need for blood replacement as necessary.	Fluid volume replacement is necessary to fill the depleted vascular space.
Monitor coagulation studies and complete blood count.	These studies enable monitoring of the patient's response to treatments and prevention of complications related to coagulation defects.
Monitor for complications of massive transfusion therapy: acidosis, hyperammonemia, citrate intoxication, coagulopathies, and hypothermia.	
Consider intubation for airway control.	
Initiate transfusion resuscitation via large-bore intravenous lines as prescribed and monitor patient response and complications (see the intervention above relating to complications of massive transfusion therapy).	Blood loss greater than 1000 mL requires blood transfusions with red blood cells (RBCs) for replacement. Fresh frozen plasma, platelets, and/or cryoprecipitate may be required to replace clotting factors and maintain coagulability.
Establish a history of bleeding, including information on location of bleeding, estimated duration, amount of total blood lost, and occult bleeding sites.	

NURSING DIAGNOSIS: IMPAIRED GAS EXCHANGE

Related To decreased oxygen-carrying capacity

Defining Characteristics
Hypoxia (PaO_2 < 60 torr; SaO_2 < 90%)
Hypercapnia ($PaCO_2$ > 45 torr)
Inability to remove secretions
Confusion, somnolence, restlessness, irritability
Cyanosis

Patient Outcomes
Gas exhange between alveoli and lung and vascular system will be adequate as evidenced by:
- PaO_2 > 80 torr or return to baseline
- SaO_2 > 90%
- $PaCO_2$ 35–45 torr
- absence of cyanosis
- absence of restlessness, confusion, irritability, and dizziness
- airways clear of mucous

Nursing Interventions	Rationales
Assess respiratory system: respiratory rate, depth, and use of accessory muscles; symptoms of dyspnea, fatigue, drowsiness, headache, and apathy; sudden change or absence of breath sounds, rales or crackles, rhonchi, wheezing, stridor, and pleural rubs; sudden changes in temperature and vital signs.	Ongoing assessment allows determination of early problems with airway clearance and oxygenation.
Assess for changes in level of consciousness or anxiety.	Decreased level of consciousness or anxiety may indicate oxygen desaturation.
Assess nailbeds.	Nailbed color indicates the adequacy of peripheral perfusion.
Monitor hemoglobin, PaO_2 and SaO_2.	Hemoglobin is the major oxygen-carrying compound. PaO_2 reflects how much oxygen is in the blood. Saturation of hemoglobin is reflected by SaO_2. Oxygen transport is compromised with oxygen saturations of less than 90%.

Nursing Interventions | Rationales

Nursing Interventions	Rationales
Administer oxygen as prescribed and make changes as needed according to blood gas analysis or pulse oximeter changes.	Supplementary oxygen may be necessary for adequate gas exchange.
Determine cardiac output.	Cardiac output is an essential component of oxygen delivery.
Encourage patient to turn, cough, and deep breathe.	Position changes, coughing, and breathing deeply maximize alveolar ventilation.
Tracheal suction as needed.	Endotracheal suctioning removes secretions and debris from the tracheobronchial tree and promotes airway patency, facilitating ventilation.
Limit patient activities. Provide an environment conducive to rest. Provide uninterrupted rest periods.	Activity and inadequate rest may increase oxygen consumption.

NURSING DIAGNOSIS: DECREASED CARDIAC OUTPUT

Related To decreased venous return

Defining Characteristics

Hypotension
CO < 4 L/min
CVP < 2 mmHg
Urine output < 30 ml/hour
Cardiovascular collapse

Dysrhythmias
CI < 2.5 L/min/m^2
PCWP < 8 mmHg

Patient Outcomes

Cardiac output will be maintained/restored, as evidenced by
- blood pressure return to patient baseline
- heart rate 60–100 bpm
- urine output > 30 mL/hr
- CVP 2–10 mmHg; PCWP 8–12 mmHg
- CO 4–8 L/min; CI 2.5–4.0 L/min/m^2
- absence of dysrhythmias
- absence of cardiovascular collapse

Nursing Interventions	Rationales
Assess and document cardiovascular status: heart rate and blood pressure, hemodynamics (CVP, PCWP, CO, CI, MAP), peripheral pulses, cardiac rhythm, and signs of cardiovascular collapse (bradycardia, hypotension, decreased CO/CI, decreased MAP, weak peripheral pulses).	
Administer fluids as prescribed and monitor response.	Hypovolemia can precipitate decreased cardiac output.
Elevate lower extremities 20°–30° from horizontal position.	Elevation of the lower extremities causes increased venous return.
Administer inotropic agents as prescribed and monitor response.	Inotropic agents may be necessary to increase cardiac output via increased contractility.

NURSING DIAGNOSIS: ALTERED TISSUE PERFUSION

Related To decreased circulating blood volume

Defining Characteristics
Confusion or change in level of consciousness
CO < 4 L/min; CI < 2.5 L/min/m^2 SVR > 1200 dyn/s/cm^{-5}
Hypotension   Cool, clammy skin
CVP < 2 mmHg   PCWP < 8 mmHg
Urine output < 30 mL/hr SvO_2 < 70%
Tachycardia   Weak, thready peripheral pulses

Patient Outcomes
Central and peripheral perfusion is stable, as evidenced by
- MAP > 60 mmHg
- CO 4–8 L/min; CI 2.5–4 L/min/m^2
- CVP 2–10 mmHg; PCWP 8–12 mmHg
- SVR 800–1200 dyn/s/cm^5
- SvO_2 > 70 %
- mental status return to baseline
- warm and dry skin
- urine output > 30 mL/hr

Nursing Interventions	Rationales
Monitor heart rate, respiratory rate, and blood pressure.	Blood pressure will remain low until volume is corrected by administration of colloids and/or crystalloids. Heart rate and respiratory rate will be elevated as long as tissue perfusion is inadequate.
Monitor and record CO/CI and SVR.	Low CO/CI may result from hypovolemia. Increased SVR indicates inadequate tissue perfusion.
Monitor CVP, PCWP and SvO_2 if available.	Low CVP and PCWP indicate hypovolemia. A low SvO_2 indicates inadequate tissue perfusion.
Monitor for changes in mental status.	Hypovolemia may produce changes in mental status due to decreased cerebral perfusion.
Monitor urine output every hour.	Decreased urine output is an early sign of decreased perfusion to the kidneys.
Monitor peripheral circulation. Inspect skin, noting color and temperature. Check quality of peripheral pulses and capillary refill time (CRT).	Cool, clammy, pale skin, weak peripheral pulses, or increased CRT indicate decreased circulating volume and decreased peripheral perfusion.
Provide preventive skin care: 1. Change patient's position regularly. 2. Keep skin clean and dry. 3. Inspect skin for erythema/blanching with each position change. 4. Gently massage vulnerable areas with each position change. 5. Utilize specialized mattress or beds in patients on bedrest and/or with decreased spontaneous movement. 6. Provide range-of-motion exercises and consult with physical therapy.	Decreased tissue perfusion puts the patient at risk for skin breakdown. Frequency of nursing interventions should be increased if any reddened areas do not resolve within 1 hr.

DISCHARGE PLANNING/CONTINUITY OF CARE

- Assess need for/type of long-term care and follow-up.
- If the discharge destination is home, assess existing supports and the need for assistance.
- Determine coping deficits/support needs and institute assistance measures.
- Determine knowledge deficits/teaching needs and document and institute a teaching plan.
- Refer patient to social services as appropriate.
- Communicate coping deficits/support needs and knowledge. deficits/teaching needs to unit accepting patient on transfer.

REFERENCES

Duchick, R., Martin, P., & Friedman, L. J. (1991). Management of bleeding ulcers. *Medical Clinics of North America, 75*(4), 946–965.

Fried, S. J., Satiani, B., & Zeeb, B. P. (1986). Normothermic rapid volume replacement for hypovolemic shock. *Journal Trauma, 26,* 183.

Hoyt, K. S. (1988). Massive transfusion therapy. *Emergency Nursing Reports, 3*(9), 1–8.

Moore, E. E., Mattox, K. L., & Feliciano, D. V. (1991). *Trauma* (2nd ed.) Norwalk, CT: Appleton.

Rabinovici, R., Gross, D., & Krausz, M. M. (1989). Infusion of small volume of 7.5 percent sodium chloride in 6 percent dextran 70 for the treatment of uncontrolled hemorrhagic shock. *Surgical Gynecology and Obstetrics, 169,* 137.

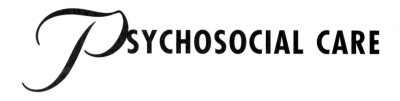

PSYCHOSOCIAL CARE

Critical illness and the critical care environment create multiple unique stresses on the patient not only physically but also psychologically. The patient's psychological response will depend on the level of stress/threat, the patient's coping mechanisms and support systems, previous experiences with hospitalization/critical care units, age and physical condition. Although the tendency and possible priority in this highly technical environment may be to focus on the patient's physical condition, ignoring psychological concerns and needs can have a significant impact on the patient's physical recovery.

ETIOLOGIES

- Threat of death
- Sensory overload
- Sensory deprivation
- Sleep deprivation
- "Foreign" environment
- Medications
- Previous hospital experiences/losses
- Threat of permanent disability/change in life style
- Change in patient/significant other roles
- Lack of knowledge about illness/condition
- Physical condition

CLINICAL MANIFESTATIONS

- Psychological signs
  - irritability
  - depression
  - hallucinations
  - restlessness
  - confusion
  - withdrawal
  - delusions
  - crying

- uncooperative
- combative
- expressions of anger
- expressions of anxiety
- expressions of hopelessness
- expressions of powerlessness
- expressions of increased psychological/physical pain
- expressions of spiritual distress
- Physical signs
  - tachycardia
  - dilated pupils
  - hyperventilation
  - diaphoresis
  - elevated systolic blood pressure

CLINICAL/DIAGNOSTIC SIGNS

There are no definitive tests for psychological disturbances. However, physical derangements that might contribute to and/or aggravate psychological disturbances (e.g., hypoxia, electrolyte disturbances) should be ruled out.

NURSING DIAGNOSIS: ANXIETY

Related To
- Admission/transfer from critical care area
- Lack of knowledge about condition/prognosis
- Loss of control
- Disruption of normal roles and activity
- Threat of death or permanent life style changes

Defining Characteristics

Apprehension
Shakiness
Irritability
Insomnia
Voice quivering
Increased systolic blood pressure
Diaphoresis
Nausea/vomiting

Fearfulness
Restlessness
Withdrawal
Facial tension
Tremors
Tachycardia
Hyperventilation
Palpitations

Patient Outcomes
The patient will express a decrease in anxiety.

Nursing Interventions	Rationales
Assess for physical and/or behavioral signs of anxiety on an ongoing basis.	Anxiety is a common reaction to any stressful situation with reactions ranging from mild to severe. Interventions will be most effective if anxiety is diagnosed early.
Assess for cause of anxiety.	Without determining the specific source of the anxiety it is difficult to institute interventions that will effectively alleviate it.
Assess coping mechanisms used successfully in the past and encourage patient to use them.	Patients come with an array of established coping mechanisms but due to anxiety may not be able to apply them to the current situation without assistance.
Provide information regarding diagnosis, treatments, and procedures in amount and terms patient can understand. Repeat explanations as needed and obtain feedback to corroborate patient's understanding.	Anxiety is frequently due to lack of knowledge regarding the diagnosis and its implications. Anxiety can also interfere with learning so information must be repeated and feedback obtained.
Develop supportive/empathetic relationship with patient by encouraging patient to ask questions; allowing patient to express fears, concerns, and anger; clarifying misconceptions; and staying with the patient while anxiety is present.	Verbalization acts as a form of release of anxiety. The nurse's presence, empathetic attitude, and active listening will help develop a supportive relationship between the nurse and the patient.
Orient patient to critical care routines and environment.	The equipment, strange noises, loss of control, and fear of the unknown may be sources of anxiety.
Encourage significant others to visit.	The use of normal support systems can provide comfort and reduce fear.
Teach the patient relaxation techniques.	Relaxation has been shown to have a positive effect on stress levels and anxiety.

Nursing Interventions	Rationales
Administer sedation/antianxiety medications as prescribed and monitor/record response.	Short-term use of medication may be necessary to reduce severe anxiety so the patient can utilize coping skills more effectively.
Allow patient as much control over immediate environment and cares as possible.	Anxiety may be due to feelings of powerlessness and loss of control.
Provide consistent caregivers as much as possible.	Consistent caregivers allow the patient and nurse to establish a rapport and develop a supportive relationship.
Avoid blanket reassurances, such as "You're doing just fine." Provide specific indicators of current condition and progress.	Blanket reassurances may cause feelings of isolation or lack of understanding. Honest discussion of the patient's condition and prognosis provides reassurance and enables the patient to be an active participant in decision making.
Assist patient in focusing on the present and establishing short-term goals.	Patients may become discouraged by the long-term picture. Getting the patient to focus on realistic short-term goals helps the patient maintain a realistic perspective.

NURSING DIAGNOSIS: SLEEP PATTERN DISTURBANCE

Related To
- Stress of illness
- Anxiety
- Strange environment
- Frequent interruptions/procedures
- Physical condition: pain, immobility

Defining Characteristics
Complaints of inability to sleep
Complaints of not feeling rested
Changes in behavior: irritability, restlessness, lethargy, combativeness, anxiety
Changes in thought content: delusions, hallucinations, illusions, paranoia, disorientation
Frequent yawning

Sleepiness during the day
Frequent wakenings/interventions

Patient Outcomes
- The patient reports being able to sleep and feeling rested.
- The patient's total sleep time approximates the patient's normal.
- The patient is alert and oriented.

Nursing Interventions	Rationales
Assess patient's normal sleep patterns: hours per night, time of retiring, time of rising, presleep routines, normal position used to fall asleep, and use of sleep medications.	Sleep patterns/habits vary from patient to patient and must be assessed. Incorporation of normal sleep patterns/habits into the patient's care routine will facilitate adequate and restful sleep.
Assess for presence of sleep deprivation (see Defining Characteristics) and try to determine cause.	Due to physical discomfort, the frequency of interventions and procedures, and/or anxiety, the patient may have difficulty getting enough sleep. Normal sleep consists of four to five 90-min sleep cycles per night; less than this over a period of time can produce behavioral and mental status changes as well as interfere with the patient's physiological recovery.
Assess for modifiable factors contributing to inability to sleep: anxiety, pain, noise and lights.	
Allow uninterrupted periods of at least 90 min as much as possible.	The average complete sleep cycle [non-REM (rapid eye movement) and REM sleep] requires at least 90 min.
Administer sleep medications as appropriate and monitor response.	Sleep medications affect patients differently and may actually contribute to sleep deprivation by depriving patients of REM sleep.

Nursing Interventions	Rationales
Create an environment that is conducive to sleep: 1. Accommodate patient's normal sleep patterns/sleep rituals as much as possible. 2. Eliminate extraneous noise as much as possible. 3. Darken room at night if possible. 4. Group interruptions and/or treatments. 5. Assist patient to a comfortable position.	
Encourage increased activity during day hours.	
Administer pain medication as appropriate and monitor response.	

NURSING DIAGNOSIS: INEFFECTIVE INDIVIDUAL COPING

Related To
- Critical illness
- Ineffective support system
- Inadequate psychological resources

Defining Characteristics
Verbalization of inability to cope
Inability to meet basic needs
Inappropriate use of defense mechanisms
Verbal manipulation
Inability to make decisions or participate in decision making

Patient Outcomes
- The patient exhibits effective coping mechanisms.
- The patient verbalizes feelings indicating ability to cope with illness.
- The patient shows an interest in the environment or illness.

Nursing Interventions	Rationales
Identify coping mechanisms patient has used successfully in the past.	Past coping mechanisms may be transferable to the current situation.

Nursing Interventions	Rationales
Assess current coping mechanisms being utilized.	This enables the nurse to identify adaptive/maladaptive patient responses.
Assist patient in identifying strengths and positives in current situation.	This shows respect for the patient and provides the patient with a sense of control and hope.
Provide explanations in terms patient can understand.	
Reinforce use of distractions, that is, TV, radio, and hobbies.	
Provide encouragement to patient regarding progress.	
Set realistic short-term goals with patient.	This provides the patient with a greater sense of control over the current situation and helps the patient focus energy in a realistic direction.

NURSING DIAGNOSIS: HOPELESSNESS

Related To
- Severity of illness/poor prognosis
- Prolonged hospital stay
- Prolonged dependence on equipment for life support
- Significant changes in life style/established roles

Defining Characteristics
Decreased verbalization Decreased affect
Lack of involvement in care Decreased appetite

Patient Outcomes
- The patient will express feelings of optimism about the present and future.
- The patient will become involved in self-care activities.

Nursing Interventions	Rationales
Determine situations from which patient derives hope.	The nurse may be able to apply this information to the current situation.

Nursing Interventions	Rationales
Determine what it is about the current situation that creates feelings of hopelessness.	
Determine patient's strengths and emphasize these.	This focuses on the positive rather than the negative, giving the patient indications of hope.
Provide patient with information regarding physical condition and progress.	This enables the patient to take a part in decision making and provides realistic information on which to base hope for the future.
Listen to patient's concerns and fears.	This supports the patient's feelings of self-worth.
Encourage patient to participate in care as he or she is able.	This provides the patient with the sense that he or she can have an influence on the outcome of the illness.
Clarify and modify the patient's perceptions of reality. Correct misinformation.	Hopelessness may be based on misperceptions of the patient's condition and/or prognosis.
Assist patient in developing realistic short-term goals.	Focusing on short-term goals provides the patient with more immediate signs of progress and thus reasons for hope.
Provide consistent caregivers as much as possible.	
Encourage significant others to visit as much as possible.	

NURSING DIAGNOSIS: POWERLESSNESS

Related To
- Loss of control
- Lack of knowledge
- Lack of motivation
- Physical condition

Defining Characteristics
Verbal expression of having no control over situation or outcome
Apathy, fatigue, withdrawal

Depression over physical deterioration
Nonparticipation in care or decisions about care

Patient Outcomes

- The patient will participate in decision making regarding care and treatment.
- The patient will verbalize feeling increased control over the situation.

Nursing Interventions	Rationales
Assess situation that generates feelings of powerlessness	
Provide patient with feedback regarding physical progress	Feedback on progress provides the patient with hope and with encouragement to participate in care and treatment.
Provide information regarding diagnosis and treatment as patient is able.	This shows respect for the patient and allows the patient to participate in decision making with adequate information.
Allow patient control over environment as he or she is able: placement of personal belongings, time of bath, and time to get out of bed.	This will reduce anxiety and support feelings of control over the patient's physical well-being.
Encourage patient to ask questions and participate in decision making regarding care.	This shows respect for the patient and supports the patient's control.
Work with patient to establish realistic goals.	This helps the patient focus on elements of care within the patient's control. Setting unrealistic goals will reinforce the patient's feelings of powerlessness.
Listen to patient's concerns, fears, and anxieties.	
Provide consistent staffing as much as possible.	

NURSING DIAGNOSIS: ALTERED SENSORY PERCEPTION
Related To sensory overload

Defining Characteristics
Hallucinations/delusions
Confusion
Restlessness
Mood alterations
Disorientation
Agitation
Anger
Sleep disturbance

Patient Outcomes
The patient will demonstrate decreased signs of sensory overload, as evidenced by absence of defining characteristics.

Nursing Interventions	Rationales
Assess for factors contributing to sensory overload.	In order to minimize sensory overload, the nurse must identify modifiable factors that may cause it, such as unneeded lights, loud conversation, or inadequate pain control.
Assess for behaviors indicating sensory overload.	
Provide information regarding cares, procedures, and treatments.	This lessens anxiety and attaches meaning to activities.
Orient to equipment/tubes and explain purpose. Place supportive devices out of patient's line of sight when possible, that is, ventilator, monitor, and IV pumps.	Most supportive devices have little meaning for the patient, contributing to sensory overload and adding a source for anxiety.
Provide meaningful stimuli: clocks and calendars.	This helps maintain the patient's orientation.
Minimize excess stimuli as possible, that is, lights and loud talking.	
Determine patient's interpretation of incoming stimuli and clarify misperceptions. Orient as needed.	Misinterpretation of stimuli can create anxiety and fear.

Nursing Interventions	Rationales
Provide for uninterrupted sleep as much as possible.	Sleep deprivation can contribute to disorientation and make the patient more vulnerable to sensory overload.
Promote movement as much as possible, that is, change in position, out of bed, and isometric exercises.	This keeps the patient in touch with normal sensations and the patient's own body.
Control pain/discomfort with medications/relaxation measures and monitor response.	This will minimize pain/discomfort as a source of sensory overload.
Encourage appropriate visiting by significant others.	Significant others can help maintain the patient's reality orientation.
Consider the use of head phones with the patient's favorite music.	This can help mask the unfamiliar noises of the critical care environment.
Provide continuity of care as much as possible.	

NURSING DIAGNOSIS: ALTERED SENSORY PERCEPTION

Related To sensory deprivation

Defining Characteristics
Confusion
Restlessness
Anxiousness
Hallucinations/delusions
Agitation
Anger

Patient Outcomes
The patient will demonstrate decreased symptoms of sensory deprivation, as evidenced by absence of defining characteristics.

Nursing Interventions	Rationales
Assess for sources/signs of sensory deprivation.	In order to minimize/prevent sensory deprivation, the nurse must identify modifiable sources.

Nursing Interventions	Rationales
Assess for other causes/contributing factors to confusion, that is, medications, electrolyte imbalance, and hypoxia.	
Provide explanations of all cares and procedures.	This helps the patient find meaning in these experiences.
Explain environment, that is, equipment, machines, and their purpose.	The unfamiliarity of the critical care environment can contribute to sensory deprivation.
Place familiar items of meaning within patient's sight, that is, pictures, cards, letters, clocks, calendars.	This helps maintain orientation.
Provide meaningful stimuli, that is, favorite music, favorite TV shows, and tapes of significant others.	
Encourage significant others to visit.	The patient is deprived of normal contact and interaction with significant others because of hospitalization. Maintaining normal contacts helps minimize this as a source of sensory deprivation.
Encourage patient to participate in decision-making process.	This helps attach meaning to care activities and treatments.

NURSING DIAGNOSIS: ALTERED THOUGHT PROCESSES

Related To acute brain failure/delirium secondary to hypoxia
- Drug withdrawal
- Electrolyte imbalance
- Drug intoxication
- Nutritional imbalance
- Acid-base imbalance
- Endocrine dysfunction
- Sepsis
- Intracranial pathology
- Hepatic encephalopathy
- Cardiac arrest

Defining Characteristics
Clouding of consciousness
Incoherent speech
Inability to maintain attention
Perceptual disturbances (illusions, hallucinations)
Disturbance of sleep-wakefulness cycle
Increased or decreased psychomotor activity
Disorientation and memory impairment

Patient Outcomes
The patient will return to baseline mentation.

Nursing Interventions	Rationales
Determine baseline mental status.	
Monitor current mental status continuously for signs of delirium and notify physician.	
Identify possible contributing/causative factors (see related to statement).	
Avoid confrontations with patient. Maintain simple, clear, calm communications.	Confrontation will not resolve acute brain failure and will only increase anxiety.
Administer sedation as ordered and monitor response.	Research has shown the most effective medications are a combination of haloperidol and lorazepam. Haloperidol is especially useful because of its lack of respiratory depression.
Reorient as necessary. Deal with hallucinations in a matter-of-fact manner, pointing out reality.	Reorientation and reinforcement of reality encourages the patient to focus on what is actually occurring rather than focusing on misperceptions.
Protect patient from injury: siderails up, bed in low position; padded siderails; extremity restraints, posey as needed; and visually monitor patient continuously.	Restraints may be necessary, but try to avoid their use as they tend to make patients with acute brain failure more agitated.
Allow significant others to stay with patient if they have a calming effect. Consider restricting the number of visitors.	Visitors may provide reality orientation but also cause patient fatigue. Fatigue contributes to/worsens brain failure.
Allow adequate sleep periods.	Sleep deprivation can contribute to/worsen brain failure.
Control stimuli that can startle the patient: Keep alarm volumes to a minimum and avoid sudden bright lights or noises.	

NURSING DIAGNOSIS: ALTERED FAMILY PROCESSES
Related To critical illness of family member

Defining Characteristics
Family system is unable to meet physical/emotional needs of members.
Patient expresses concern regarding significant others' response to illness.
Family system does not adapt constructively to the crisis.
Family expresses inadequate understanding/knowledge of patient condition.
The family decision-making process is unhealthy.
The level and direction of energy are inappropriate.

Patient Outcomes
The family will be able to
- verbalize thoughts/feelings to other family members and professional nurse.
- seek appropriate assistance/resources when needed.
- participate in the care of the ill member.
- maintain a system of mutual support within the family.

Nursing Interventions	Rationales
Assess for presence of family dysfunction.	
Assess for causative/contributing factors to family dysfunction.	
Provide family with regular updates regarding patient condition and progress. Evaluate comprehension	Families want to be kept informed and have their questions answered honestly. Misconceptions need to be addressed immediately.
Allow family to express feelings, anxieties, and concerns.	This lets the family know their feelings are valued and respected and helps establish a therapeutic/supportive relationship between the family and nurse. Ventilation of feelings also enables the family to put current events in perspective.

Psychosocial Care

Nursing Interventions	Rationales
Encourage family to participate in patient cares as appropriate.	This enables the family to feel they can make a contribution to the patient's well-being.
Discuss with family ways they can contribute to patient's progress and recovery.	Family members need to feel helpful to the patient to minimize feelings of powerlessness and inadequacy.
Accompany family to bedside on first visit.	This provides emotional support and allows nurse to evaluate family response and provide additional explanations as needed.
Provide consistent caregivers as much as possible.	
Provide flexible visiting hours if possible.	Family members have a need to be with the patient yet may have other obligations that conflict with established visiting hours.
Reassure family members it is alright to leave hospital and they will be contacted immediately with any changes in the patient's condition.	Family members may be torn between staying with the patient and taking care of themselves and/or the family unit. Supporting their decision and assuring them they will be contacted can minimize feelings of guilt and anxiety.
Encourage family members to touch and talk to the patient even if unconscious.	This promotes normal contact between the family and the patient, relieving family anxiety.
Identify/anticipate areas of family concern and provide information.	This shows the family members they are being respected and assures them they will be kept informed.
Refer family to social services or other resources for assistance as needed.	

NURSING DIAGNOSIS: SPIRITUAL

Related To
- Suffering
- Separation from religious/cultural ties
- Challenged belief and value systems

Defining Characteristics
Expression of concern with meaning of life/death and/or belief systems
Anger toward God
Verbalizes spiritual concerns
Verbalizes inner conflict about beliefs
Seeks spiritual assistance
Questions meaning of own existence
Unable to participate in usual religious practices
Alteration in behavior/mood

Patient Outcomes
The patient will express satisfaction with the meaning and purpose of illness/suffering/death.

Nursing Interventions	Rationales
Assess for importance of religious beliefs.	This enables the nurse to determine appropriate interventions.
Assess for interference of hospitalization/illness with religious beliefs/values.	
Assess affect, attitude, verbalization, interpersonal relationships, and environment for signs of spiritual distress.	
Arrange for clergy to visit as appropriate.	The patient may feel most comfortable expressing spiritual concerns to hospital or personal clergy.
Allow patient to express concerns and feelings without judgment.	
Utilize therapeutic touch as appropriate.	Touch can provide emotional comfort and support.

Nursing Interventions	Rationales
Offer to pray/read scripture with patient as appropriate.	The patient may find strength and hope in these activities.
Provide patient with appropriate signs of hope and progress.	
Provide for privacy for reflection or spiritual expression.	

DISCHARGE PLANNING/CONTINUITY OF CARE

- Assess need for/type of long-term care and follow-up.
- If the discharge destination is home, assess existing supports and the need for assistance.
- Determine coping deficits/support needs and institute assistance measures.
- Determine knowledge deficits/teaching needs and document and institute a teaching plan.
- Refer patient to social services or other support systems as appropriate.
- Communicate coping deficits/support needs and knowledge deficits/learning needs to unit accepting patient on transfer.

REFERENCES

AACN. (1990). *AACN Outcome standards for nursing care of the critically ill.* Laguna Niguel, CA: American Association of Critical-Care Nurses.

Compton, P. (1991). Critical illness and intensive care: What it means to the client. *Critical Care Nurse, 11*(1), 50–56.

Hickey, M. (1990). What are the needs of families of critically ill patients? A review of the literature since 1976. *Heart & Lung, 19*(4), 401–415.

Inaba-Roland, K. E. & Maricle, R. A. (1992). Assessing delirium in the acute care setting. *Heart & Lung, 21*(1), 48–55.

Koller, P. A. (1991). Family needs and coping strategies during illness crisis. *AACN Clinical Issues in Critical Care Nursing, 2*(2), 338–345.

Ludwig, L. M. (1989). Acute brain failure in the critically ill patient. *Critical Care Nurse, 9*(10), 62–75.

Meijs, C. A. (1989). Care of the family of the ICU patient. *Critical Care Nurse, 9*(8):42–45.

Morath, J. M. & Lynch M. K. (1989). Intensive care psychosis. In M. S. Sommers, (Ed.), *Difficult Diagnosis in Critical Care Nursing* (pp. 193–211), Rockville, MD: Aspen.

Sampson, T. (1991). The family as a source of support for the critically ill adult. *AACN Clinical Issues in Critical Care Nursing, 2*(2), 229–235.

Shaffer, J. L. (1991). Spiritual distress and critical illness. *Critical Care Nurse, 11*(1), 42–49.

Stanik, J. A. (1990). Caring for the family of the critically ill surgical patient. *Critical Care Nurse, 10*(1), 43–47.

▼

SEPTIC SHOCK

Septic shock results from a systemic response to microorganisms in the blood resulting in vasodilatation with selective vasoconstriction causing maldistribution of blood flow. The principal element responsible for development of septic shock is thought to be endotoxin, which is released from the cell wall of gram-negative bacteria. Endotoxin activates neuroendocrine, complement, kinins, coagulation, and immune system defense mechanisms. Bacterial killing mechanisms such as cytokines, proteases, and toxic oxygen species (free radicals) are released. The most damaging results are myocardial depression, vasodilation, and increased capillary permeability with shunting of fluids into the interstitial space causing distributional hypovolemia and decreased tissue perfusion. The initial presentation is a hyperdynamic state (septic syndrome) that may be reversed with early recognition and aggressive therapy. Progression to a hypodynamic state (septic shock) is much more difficult to reverse and can lead to multiorgan system failure and death.

ETIOLOGIES

- Microorganisms associated with sepsis (asterisk indicates the most common ones)

    Gram-negative bacteria
    - *Escherichia coli**
    - *Klebsiella enterobacter**
    - *Pseudomonas aeruginosa**
    - *Proteus mirabilis*
    - *Serratia marcescens*
    - *Neisseria meningitidis*

    Gram-positive bacteria
    - *Staphylococcus*
    - *Streptococcus*
    - *Clostridium*
    - *Pneumococcus*
    - viruses
    - fungi

- Common access sites for microorganisms
    - urinary tract: Foley catheters, suprapubic catheters, cystoscopic exam
    - respiratory tract: suctioning, aspiration, endotracheal tubes, tracheostomy tubes, respiratory therapy

- gastrointestinal tract: peritonitis, cirrhosis, abdominal abscess, ascites
- skin: surgical wounds, burns, intravenous/invasive monitoring catheters, trauma
- Risk factors
  - extremes of age
  - malnutrition
  - prolonged hospitalization
  - chronic illness
  - pregnancy
  - traumatic/thermal injuries
  - surgical procedures
  - alcohol/IV drug abuse
  - invasive procedures
  - drugs: antibiotics, steroids, antineoplastics

CLINICAL MANIFESTATIONS

- Cardiovascular: Vasodilatation and decreased force of contraction produce the following:

  Septic Syndrome
  - hypotension
  - tachycardia
  - SVR < 800 dyn/s/cm^{-5}
  - CVP < 2 mmHg
  - PCWP < 8 mmHg
  - CO > 8 L/min
  - CI > 4 L/min/m^2
  - widened pulse pressure
  - warm flushed skin

  Septic Shock
  - hypotension
  - tachycardia
  - SVR > 1200 dyn/s/cm^{-5}
  - CVP < 2 mmHg
  - PCWP < 8 mmHg
  - CO < 4 L/min
  - CI < 2.5 L/min/m^2
  - decreased pulse pressure
  - cool pale skin

- Renal: Vasodilatation and decreased renal perfusion produce a urine output below 30 mL/hr.
- Pulmonary: Interstitial edema, atelectasis, and decreased tissue oxygenation produce
  - tachypnea
  - rales
  - PVR > 250 dyn/s/cm^{-5}
  - decreased breath sounds
  - SvO_2 < 70%
- Neurological: Decreased cerebral perfusion produces
  - confusion
  - obtundation
  - agitation
  - lethargy
  - restlessness
- Gastrointestinal: Decreased perfusion and bowel motility produce
  - nausea
  - diarrhea
  - abdominal distention
  - vomiting
  - decreased bowel sounds

CLINICAL/DIAGNOSTIC FINDINGS

- Positive cultures: blood, urine, sputum
- Arterial hypoxemia (PaO_2 < 80 torr)
- Plasma lactate > 2.2 mEq/L

- Respiratory alkalosis ($PaCO_2$ < 35 torr, pH > 7.45)
- Neutrophilic leukocytosis with a left shift and eosinopenia
- Thombocytopenia
- Serum iron < 42 mg/dL
- Metabolic acidosis (HCO_3 < 22 mEq/L; pH < 7.35)
- BUN > 18 mg/dL
- Creatinine > 1.2 mg/dL
- Hypoglycemia (< 70 mg/dL)
- Hypertriglyceridemia (> 150 mg/dlL)

NURSING DIAGNOSIS: ALTERED TISSUE PERFUSION

Related To vasodilation and redistribution of blood flow

Defining Characteristics
Hypotension
SvO_2 < 60%
Warm/pink skin or cool/pale skin
SVR < 800 $dyn/s/cm^{-5}$
Urine output < 30 mL/hr

Patient Outcomes
Tissue perfusion will be maintained/restored, as evidenced by
- blood pressure within 10 mmHg of patient baseline
- SvO_2 60–80%
- SVR 800–1200 $dyn/s/cm^{-5}$
- urine output > 30 mL/hr
- normal skin temperature and color

Nursing Interventions	Rationales
Assess neurological status: level of consciousness and dizziness.	Changes in neurological status may indicate decreased cerebral perfusion.
Assess skin color, temperature, and character.	In the early phase of septic shock skin may be pink, warm, and dry due to vasodilation. Cool, pale, diaphoretic skin is indicative of a later, vasoconstrictive phase of septic shock.
Assess for site of infection: obtain urine, sputum, blood, and wound cultures.	This will help determine the source of infection and infectious agent.

Nursing Interventions	Rationales
Assess/monitor renal function: urine output, urine specific gravity, and serum BUN and creatinine.	A decrease in urine output and increased specific gravity may indicate decreased renal perfusion. If not corrected, this can lead to ATN.
Administer fluids as prescribed and monitor response.	Vasodilatation and redistribution of fluids into the interstitial space produce a distributional hypovolemia requiring fluid resuscitation.
Institute measures to control temperature.	An increased temperature will produce more vasodilation and increase the metabolic rate and demand and possibly worsen tissue perfusion and ischemia.
Maintain adequate oxygenation.	Decreased pulmonary perfusion can produce a ventilation/perfusion mismatch producing hypoxemia. Decreased tissue perfusion can produce inadequate delivery of oxygen to tissues.
Maintain adequate cardiac output. Administer fluid as prescribed and monitor response.	Cardiac output determines tissue perfusion and oxygenation and must be maintained to prevent progression of shock and complications of shock. During septic syndrome, when vasodilation occurs, large volumes of fluids may be required to compensate for vascular pooling. As septic shock progresses, excess fluid may precipitate cardiac and ventilatory failure.
Administer antibiotics as ordered and monitor response.	
Minimize sites for infection: 1. Remove foley catheter if possible. 2. Change intravenous sites regularly and culture catheter tips. 3. Utilize sterile technique when changing dressings. 4. Provide regular catheter care.	

Nursing Interventions	Rationales
Monitor laboratory studies for indications of inadequate tissue perfusion: increased BUN, increased creatinine, increased serum amylase, and decreased platelet count.	

NURSING DIAGNOSIS: IMPAIRED GAS EXCHANGE

Related To
- Altered alveolar-capillary membrane permeability
- Ventilation/perfusion mismatch
- Alveolar edema

Defining Characteristics
Hypoxia ($PaO_2 < 60$ torr; $SaO_2 < 90\%$)
Pulse oximetry $< 90\%$
Rales
$PaCO_2 > 45$ torr
Tachypnea
Confusion, restlessness, somnolence, irritability
$PVR > 250$ dyn/s/cm^{-5}

Patient Outcomes
Gas exchange will be maintained/restored, as evidenced by
- $PaO_2 > 80$ torr or return to baseline
- pulse oximetry/$SaO_2 > 90\%$
- absence of adventitious lung sounds
- absence of restlessness, confusion, irritability
- PVR 100–250 dyn/s/cm^{-5}

Nursing Interventions	Rationales
Assess/record respiratory status: rate, depth, and rhythm of respirations; use of accessory muscles; breath sounds; symptoms of dyspnea, fatigue, drowsiness, headache, and apathy; ability to handle secretions; and color of nail beds/mucous membranes	Interstitial edema, atelectasis, and decreased tissue oxygenation can produce changes in respiratory status.

Nursing Interventions	Rationales
Administer oxygen and make changes as needed according to blood gas analysis or oximeter changes.	This will ensure the provision of adequate oxygen for gas exchange.
Maintain/protect airway. Assess need for intubation and have equipment and ventilator on standby. Suction as needed.	Septic shock can produce ARDS, requiring intubation and mechanical ventilation to ensure adequate oxygenation.
Monitor determinants of oxygen delivery: CO/CI, PaO_2, SaO_2, hemoglobin, and pulse oximetry.	Cardiac output, hemoglobin, and oxygen saturation are the major determinants of tissue oxygen delivery.
Monitor SvO_2 continuously.	The SvO_2 directly reflects oxygen delivery and usage at the tissue level. During the hyperdynamic phase of septic shock SvO_2 is usually increased, reflecting increased oxygen delivery due to increased cardiac output and decreased SVR. During the hypodynamic phase of septic shock SvO_2 will decrease, reflecting inadequate oxygen delivery.
Turn and reposition patient every 2 hr.	Position changes reduce pooling of secretions in dependent areas of the lung.
Encourage patient to cough and deep breath.	
Monitor PVR and pulmonary compliance (if mechanically ventilated).	Decreased compliance may indicate impending/worsening ARDS.
Monitor fluid balance closely.	Patients in septic shock generally receive large amounts of fluid which could aggravate leakage of fluid into the alveoli.
Position patient for ease of respiratory effort, that is, HOB elevated. Assess effect of positioning on pulse oximetry and SvO_2.	

NURSING DIAGNOSIS: ALTERED CARDIAC OUTPUT

Related To
- Myocardial depression
- Fluid redistribution
- Decreased afterload

Defining Characteristics
Increased/decreased CO/CI
Increased/decreased CVP/PCWP
SVR < 800 dyn/s/cm^{-5}

Patient Outcomes
Cardiac output will be maintained/restored, as evidenced by
- CO 4–8 L/min; CI 2.5–4 L/min/m^2
- CVP 2–10 mmHg; PCWP 8–12 mmHg
- SVR 800–1200 dyn/s/cm^{-5}
- blood pressure within 10 mmHg of baseline

Nursing Interventions	Rationales
Assess/monitor cardiovascular status: blood pressure, heart rate, respirations, temperature, hemodynamics (CVP/PCWP, CO/CI, SVR), peripheral pulses, and skin color/temperature.	Hemodynamic measurements will assist in the diagnosis and staging of septic shock.
Monitor for cardiac dysrhythmias and treat according to protocols.	Dysrhythmias can indicate myocardial ischemia and decrease cardiac output.
Administer volume and/or pressors as ordered and monitor response.	Volume is used to correct the distributional hypovolemia and pressors such as epinephrine may be used to increase SVR to normal range.

DISCHARGE PLANNING/CONTINUITY OF CARE

- Assess need for/type of long-term care and follow-up.
- If the discharge destination is home, assess existing supports and the need for assistance.

- Determine coping deficits/support needs and institute assistance measures.
- Determine knowledge deficits/teaching needs and document and institute a teaching plan.
- Refer patient to social services as appropriate.
- Communicate coping deficits/support needs and knowledge deficits/learning needs to unit accepting patient on transfer.

REFERENCES

Bone, R. C. (1991). Gram-negative sepsis: Background, clinical features and intervention. *Chest, 100*(3), 802–808.

Hoyt, N. J. (1990). Preventing septic shock: Infection control in the intensive care unit. *Critical Care Nursing Clinics of North America, 2*(2), 287–298.

Klein, D. M. & Witek-Janusek, L. (1992). Advances in immunotherapy of sepsis. *Dimensions of Critical Care Nursing, 11*(2), 75–89.

Littleton, M. T. (1988). Pathophysiology and assessment of sepsis and septic shock. *Critical Care Nursing Quarterly, 11*(1), 30–47.

Norwood, S., Ruby, A., Civetta, J., & Cortes, V. (1991). Catheter-related infections and associated septicemia. *Chest, 99*(4), 968–975.

Roach, A. C. (1990). Antibiotic therapy in septic shock. *Critical Care Nursing Clinics of North America, 2*(2), 179–186.

Schumann, L. L. (1990). The use of maloxone in treating endotoxic shock. *Critical Care Nurse, 10*(2), 63–71.

Sommers, M. S. & Russell, A. C. (1989). Septic shock. In M. S. Sommers, (Ed.), *Difficult diagnoses in critical care nursing* (pp. 48–74), Rockville, MD: Aspen.

Stroud, M., Swindell, B., & Bernard, G. R. (1990). Cellular and humoral mediators of sepsis syndrome. *Critical Care Clinics of North America, 2*(2), 151–160.

▼

Appendices

▼

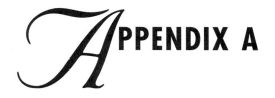
APPENDIX A

NURSING DIAGNOSIS: ALTERED NUTRITION—LESS THAN BODY REQUIREMENTS

Related To
- Metabolic disturbances
- Dysfunction of GI system
- Protracted nutrient loss
- Drugs with antinutrient or catabolic properties
- Prolonged hypocaloric IV solutions
- Increased metabolic need
- Neurological dysfunction
- Surgery

Defining Characteristics

Weight loss
Decreased appetite
Muscle weakness
Tachycardia
Diarrhea
Edema
Muscle wasting
Loss of hair
Anorexia
Activity intolerance
Abdominal pain
Nausea and vomiting
Decreased bowel sounds
Delayed healing
Brittle nails
Alopecia
Thrombocytopenia (platelets < 150,000/mm^3)
Serum albumin < 3.5 g/dL
Transferrin < 200 mg/dL
Lymphocyte count < 1000/mm^3
Negative nitrogen balance

Patient Outcomes

The patient's nutritional intake meets metabolic requirements as evidenced by
- absence of physical signs of inadequate nutrition
- albumin 3.5–5 g/dL

- transferrin 200–360 mg/dL
- lymphocytes 1000–4000/mm^3
- platelet count 150,000–400,000/mm^3

Nursing Interventions	Rationales
Assess/document patient dietary history, including dietary intake and special diet, appetite, GI disturbances, difficulty chewing or swallowing, food allergies/intolerance, medications that interfere with nutrient uptake or cause GI problems, and food likes/dislikes.	A dietary history provides information related to the patient's nutritional state on admission, dietary habits, and knowledge about diet. This provides vital data needed to plan current needs and future dietary teaching.
Assess for risk factors for nutritional deficit and document: 1. inability/unwillingness to eat 2. increased metabolic need (surgery, fever, trauma, infection, extensive burns) 3. grossly underweight (below 80% standard) 4. recent weight loss (10% or more of usual) 5. chronic debilitation (alcoholism, chronic illness, cancer) 6. chronic disease (diabetes mellitus, obesity, endocrine imbalance) 7. NPO 8. protracted nutrient loss (malabsorption; short gut syndromes/fistulas, draining abscesses, wounds; renal dialysis) 9. IV support with dextrose or saline alone for more than 5 days.	
Determine admission serum albumin, serum transferrin, and lymphocyte count.	A serum albumin below 3.5 g/dL, serum transferrin less than 200 mg/dL, and/or total lymphocyte count below 1,000/mm^3 indicate chronic undernutrition and increase the need for early replenishment in critical illness. Sudden critical illness can decrease albumin another 1–1.5 g/dL in 3–7 days.

Nursing Interventions	Rationales
Note admission height/weight and daily weight.	Calculating appropriate weight for patient height assists in evaluating caloric needs and establishing weight goals. Daily weights assist in evaluation of adequate nutrition by tracking weight gain or loss.
Assess for clinical manifestations of malnutrition (see Defining Characteristics).	
Assess GI system and document: bowel sounds; abdominal distention, firmness, and tenderness; ability to swallow; gag and cough reflexes; and diarrhea, vomiting, or GI bleeding.	Gastrointestinal function will determine the patient's ability to ingest adequate oral intake, tolerate enteral feedings, and/or need for TPN. The enteral route is preferred because it is less expensive, is more physiological, and has fewer complications than TPN.
In patients able to eat, monitor oral intake and calorie counts.	Monitoring current oral intake and calorie counts assists in evaluating the need for supplementary intravenous or enteral nutrition.
During the first few days of feeding, monitor for signs of refeeding syndrome, in particular hypophosphatemia and hypomagnesemia.	When chronically malnourished patients receive carbohydrate or protein anabolic enzymes and pathways are activated and may deplete electrolytes, particularly phosphate and magnesium.
Monitor laboratory studies. Twice a week: CBC, platelet count, magnesium, calcium, electrolytes, phosphate, glucose, BUN, creatinine, total protein, and albumin. Once a week: SGOT, SGPT, total bilirubin, PT, alkaline phosphatase, iron, and uric acid.	These laboratory studies reflect electrolyte balance, adequacy of nutrition, nitrogen balance, and the body's response. Adjustments in oral intake and/or enteral or parenteral solutions can be made based on these results.
Monitor for occult signs of GI bleeding: hematest stools and NG drainage or emesis; monitor Hgb and Hct.	Enteral feeding may actually prevent GI bleeding in critically ill patients. However, critically ill patients receiving TPN may be susceptible to stress ulcers.

Nursing Interventions	Rationales
Encourage institution of nutrition as soon as feasible after admission.	Critical illness creates a state of hypermetabolism, increased protein breakdown, and a tendency for lipid oxidation and insulin resistance. Unless adequate calories and protein are provided, muscle catabolism and weight loss will result, especially in patients already malnourished. In addition, in NPO patients, decreased gut stimulation can result in atrophy of intestinal mucosa within 3 days.
Initiate referral to a nutritional team/registered dietitian to determine needed calories, protein, and fat intake.	
For patients able to eat normally, provide optimal environment during attempts at oral intake, assistance with eating as necessary, and small frequent meals.	Meal presentation and amounts can affect appetite, especially if the patient has anorexia.
Assure parenteral nutrition solutions are delivered as prescribed and monitor for response and complications.	
Monitor glucose meter every 4–6 hr.	High concentrations of dextrose can cause excessive stress on pancreatic insulin production and high blood sugars requiring supplementary insulin.
If administration must be interrupted, hang 10% dextrose in water in the interim.	Interruption of high concentration glucose solutions can produce hypoglycemia due to high production of insulin by the pancreas.
Institute measures to prevent sepsis. Administer via dedicated IV line. Utilize strict aseptic technique when changing tubings or dressing. Allow only pharmacist to mix or add to solution. Assess the catheter insertion site for signs of inflammation or phlebitis.	High concentration glucose solutions are excellent mediums for bacterial growth and interruption of the line increases the risk for sepsis.

Nursing Interventions	Rationales
Administer parenteral nutrition via central line or peripherally utilizing a fine-bore (23-gauge) 15-cm silicone catheter.	Central lines eliminate the risk of thrombophlebitis from the hyperosmolar solution. Recent research shows that thrombophlebitis, a frequent complication of peripheral administration, is minimized by using longer fine-bore silicone catheters.
Monitor for complications of central line insertion: pneumothorax, hemothorax, hydrothorax, chylothorax, and air embolism.	
Increase infusion rate gradually.	This allows time for the pancreas to adjust insulin release based on the new high glucose load.
Administer lipid solutions as prescribed and monitor for response and complications.	
During lipid administration assess for alopecia, thrombocytopenia, poor wound healing, increased capillary fragility, brittle nails, and increased susceptibility to infection.	These signs and symptoms may indicate a fatty acid deficiency.
During lipid administration, monitor for chills, fever, dizziness, headache, allergic reactions, back pain, nausea and vomiting, chest pain, sleepiness, abdominal pain, and irritability.	These signs and symptoms may indicate fat overload.
During lipid administration, monitor serum triglycerides and liver function tests.	These indicate the ability of the liver to metabolize and clear lipids from the blood.
Administer enteral nutrition solutions and monitor for complications.	
During enteral nutrition administration, assess bowel sounds. Monitor for nausea, vomiting, abdominal distension, abdominal cramping, inadequate gastric emptying, and malabsorption.	These are the most frequent complications of enteral therapy.

Nursing Interventions	Rationales
During enteral nutrition administration, monitor for diarrhea, assess for cause, and institute corrective measures.	Diarrhea can result from the high osmolality or bacterial contamination of the tube feeding, lactose intolerance, low serum albumin and/or transferrin levels, and concurrent use of antibiotics. Consider the use of premixed sterile bags of tube feeding and bulk-forming cathartics to control diarrhea.
During enteral nutrition administration, check tube feeding placement and residuals every 4 hr or before each feeding. If residuals exceed 100–150 mL, hold tube feeding and check residual again in 2 hr before reinstituting feeding.	This prevents aspiration due to movement of the tube or vomiting.
Obtain chest x-ray to verify feeding tube placement after insertion.	It may not be easy to assess the position of a feeding tube, especially if it has a small bore. A chest x-ray is essential to confirm positioning prior to starting feedings.
Add food color to enteral tube feeding.	This enables early detection of silent aspiration.
Keep HOB elevated at least 20° during feedings and for 1 hr after. Turn off feeding if lying patient flat.	This can prevent vomiting and aspiration.
Maintain enteral tube patency. Flush tube with 30–50 mL of water every 4 hr for continuous feeding. Avoid giving medications via a tube, but when necessary, use liquid form or finely crushed tablet, flushing tube before and after. Attempt to unclog tube using water or soda. Utilize continuous feeding pump when possible.	

Nursing Interventions	Rationales
Initiate and increase administration gradually, starting with a dilute solution at a slow rate.	This allows the GI system to adjust to the hyperosmolar solution and enables early detection of intolerance.
Ensure adequate free water administration during enteral tube feedings.	High protein content and electrolyte concentrations can cause a high renal solute load resulting in dehydration in patients receiving inadequate free water.
Monitor serum glucose at least every 6 hr when initiating enteral feedings.	The high glucose content of enteral feedings may stress the pancreas beyond its ability to produce insulin, causing hyperglycemia and requiring the use of supplementary insulin.
Monitor for metabolic complications of enteral feeding: fluid overload, dehydration, and electrolyte abnormalities.	
Provide antacids/histamine antagonists as ordered and assess response.	The stress of illness and/or drugs such as corticosteroids can increase production of acids in the stomach, leading to stress ulcers, and prevent utilization of the GI tract for feeding.

REFERENCES

Buckner, M. M. (1990). Perioperative nutrition problems: Nursing management. *Critical Care Nursing Clinics of North America*, 2(4), 559–566.

Champagne, M. T. & Ashley, M. L. (1989). Nutritional support in the critically ill elderly patient. *Critical Care Nursing Quarterly*, 12(1), 15–25.

Edes, T. E. (1991). Nutrition support of the critically ill patient: Guidelines for optimal management. *Postgraduate Medicine*, 89(5), 193–200.

Farley, J. M. (1991). Nutritional support of the critically ill patient. In J. T. Dolan (Ed.), *Critical care nursing: Clinical management through the nursing process* (pp. 1125–1150). Philadelphia, PA: Davis.

Heather, D. J., Howell, L., Montana, M., Howell, M., & Hill, R. (1991). Effect of bulk-forming cathartic on diarrhea in tube-fed patients. *Heart & Lung*, 20(4), 409–413.

Madan, M., Alexander, D., & McMahon, M. (1992). Influence of catheter type on occurrence of thrombophlebitis during peripheral intravenous nutrition. *Lancet, 339*(8785), 101–103.

Miskschi, D. B., Davidson, L. J., Flournoy, D. J., & Parker, D. E. (1990). Contamination of enteral feedings and diarrhea in patients in intensive care units. *Heart & Lung, 19*(4), 362–370.

Stotts, N. A. & Washington, D. F. (1990). Nutrition: A critical component of wound healing. *AACN Clinical Issues in Critical Care Nursing, 1*(3), 85–592.

▼

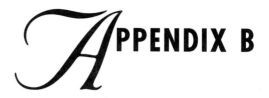

NURSING DIAGNOSIS: KNOWLEDGE DEFICIT

Related To
- New diagnosis
- Prevention of complications
- Therapeutic regimen
- Disease process

Defining Characteristics
Patient expresses a lack of understanding regarding diagnosis, therapeutic regimen, and/or long term therapy.
Patient is unable to verbalize understanding of diagnosis, therapy, and follow-up.

Patient Outcomes
The patient will be able to verbalize an understanding of the illness, prescribed treatment, and prevention of complications.

Nursing Interventions	Rationales
Assess patient readiness to learn. Avoid extensive teaching when patient is still critically ill.	Information provided before a patient indicates he or she is ready is not absorbed. During critical illness, the patient's attention will be directed primarily toward physiological needs.
Assess patient knowledge base of disease process, medications, and complications.	This provides baseline data for the development of an individualized teaching plan. The patient may become bored/disinterested if information is repeated.

Nursing Interventions	Rationales
Assess patient psychomotor and interpretive skills if needed, that is, for use of glucose meter or self-administration of injections.	The patient must have the physical ability to perform psychomotor skills and the ability to understand the skill being taught.
Design a teaching program which includes information on 1. pathophysiology and causes of disease 2. signs and symptoms of disease, including rationale for interventions 3. signs and symptoms associated with crisis states 4. situations that require physician notification 5. medications: name, action, dose, schedule, administration, importance of adherence, potential side effects	
Provide written materials/audiovisual materials to supplement/reinforce teaching.	Most learners absorb information better visually rather than just auditory.
Demonstrate any psychomotor skills required and provide time for return demonstration.	
Create environment conducive to learning: 1. Provide ample time to answer questions. 2. Encourage participation of significant other. 3. Break up instruction into small parts. 4. Provide praise and build success. 5. Use a variety of teaching strategies. 6. Provide opportunity to apply new knowledge and practice skills while still in hospital. 7. Use frequent repetition. 8. Do not force teaching on patient. If he or she is not receptive, find out why.	

Nursing Interventions	Rationales
If patient is cognitively impaired, limit teaching to significant other or to what patient wants/needs to know.	
Consult/coordinate teaching with ancillary personnel, that is, dietitian and physical therapist.	This will ensure consistency of the information being provided.
Instruct patient to inform all health care providers of disorders/carry ID card/wear ID bracelet.	
Provide means for patients to get questions answered after discharge.	This reassures patients that if unanticipated situations/needs/questions come up after discharge, someone will be available to assist them.
Schedule follow-up teaching session after discharge.	The stress of hospitalization may have an effect on retention of information. Once in their normal environment/normal routine, patients may need reinforcement/reconfirmation of learned information.
Provide referral to agencies/support groups that can reinforce/support learning after discharge.	There frequently are support/educational groups in the community for patients to utilize.

REFERENCES

Armstrong, M. L. (1989). Orchestrating the process of patient education: Methods and approaches. *Nursing Clinics of North America*, 24(3), 597–604.

Gessner, B. A. (1989). Adult education: The cornerstone of patient teaching. *Nursing Clinics of North America*, 24(3), 589–596.

Hussey, L. C. & Gilliland, K. (1989). Compliance, low literacy and locus of control. *Nursing Clinics of North America*, 24(3), 605–612.

Rakel, B. A. (1992). Interventions related to patient teaching. *Nursing Clinics of North America*, 27(2), 397–424

Ruzicki, D. A. (1989). Realistically meeting the educational needs of hospitalized acute and short-stay patients. *Nursing Clinics of North America*, 24(3), 629–638.

Smith, C. E. (1989). Overview of patient education: Opportunities and challenges for the twenty-first century. *Nursing Clinics of North America*, 24(3), 583–588.

▼

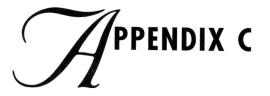

APPENDIX C

NURSING DIAGNOSIS: HIGH RISK FOR INJURY

Risk Factors
- Paralysis
- Elderly
- Bed/chair bound
- Incontinence
- Poor skin turgor
- Muscle weakness
- Fractures
- Critical illness
- Immobility
- Poor nutrition
- Edema
- Hematological alterations
- Altered level of consciousness/mental status

Patient Outcomes
- The patient will remain free of injury.
- The patient will remain free from skin breakdown.

Nursing Interventions	Rationales
Monitor level of consciousness, orientation, and spontaneous movement with every vital sign check.	If the patient's level of consciousness and ability to move is diminished, this demands more active intervention by the nurse to prevent injury or skin breakdown.

Nursing Interventions	Rationales
Institute protective measures to prevent falls: 1. bed in lowest position 2. call light within reach 3. padded siderails, siderails up 4. water, kleenex, urinal, and so on, placed within easy reach 5. assessment of need for support with activity and assist or standby assist provided as needed 6. utilization of bed check, posey restraint, and/or soft restraints as necessary 7. sedated as necessary and response monitored	Multiple factors such as altered mental status or orientation, an unfamiliar environment, equipment, muscle weakness, and age can contribute to or cause injury and falls in critically ill patients. Sedation may be necessary but in turn cause increased confusion and risk for falls.
Turn and reposition every 2 hr. Assess pressure points for redness, blanching, or breakdown with each position change.	Decreased tissue perfusion, bedrest, and decreased spontaneous movement put the patient at risk for skin breakdown. The frequency of position changes and skin inspection should be increased if any reddened areas do not resolve within 1 hr.
Cleanse skin regularly. Avoid hot water. Use mild cleansing agent. Avoid dry skin. Minimize force and friction applied to skin.	During cleansing, some of the skin's natural barrier is removed and the skin becomes drier and more susceptible to irritants.
Minimize skin contact with moisture from incontinence, perspiration, or wound drainage by using pads that absorb moisture and topical barrier agents.	
Provide frequent mouth care.	
Provide pressure relief measures: eggcrate or air mattress, heel protectors, and specialized beds.	
Use lifting devices to move patients who are unable to assist with movement.	Friction from dragging patients can decrease the amount of external pressure required to produce pressure ulcers.

Nursing Interventions	Rationales
Avoid positioning directly on trochanter when side lying.	Higher interface pressures and lower transcutaneous oxygen tension occurs when directly lying on trochanter.
Maintain head of bed (HOB) at lowest degree consistent with medical condition and/or limit amount of time with HOB elevated.	The HOB elevation increases shear forces and causes blood vessels in the sacral area to be twisted and distorted, increasing the likelihood for tissue ischemia and necrosis.
Assess extent of edema and document.	Edema makes the skin more friable and prone to pressure ulcers.
Avoid massage of bony prominences.	Massage of bony prominences may lead to deep-tissue trauma.
Ensure active or passive range-of-motion exercises and encourage early mobility.	Range-of-motion exercise and early mobility can prevent muscle weakness and/or complications of immobilization such as thromboemboli.
Apply elastic hose and/or intermittent pneumatic compression devices to lower extremities.	Elastic hose and pneumatic compression devices help prevent formation of thromboemboli.
Elevate HOB 30°–45° if patient condition permits.	The patient with altered level of consciousness is at risk for vomiting and aspiration. Elevating the head of the bed will minimize this risk.
Obtain order for nasogastric tube in patients with altered level of consciousness.	The patient with altered level of consciousness is at risk for vomiting and aspiration. Inserting a nasogastric tube and keeping the stomach empty will minimize this risk.

Nursing Interventions	Rationales
Assess for signs of bleeding and institute preventive measures; monitor/minimize puncture sites for signs of bleeding; assess stools, gastric secretions, pulmonary secretions, and urine for blood; assess for easy bruising and protect patient; and administer antacids and/or histamine antagonists as prescribed and monitor effect.	Disorders that affect hematological factors such as platelets put the patient at risk for bleeding, especially in the subcutaneous tissues or on mucosal surfaces such as the gastric and pulmonary tracts.

REFERENCES

Agency for Health Care Policy and Research. (1992). How to predict and prevent pressure ulcers. *American Journal of Nursing, 92*(7), 52–60.

Cullen, L. (1992). Interventions related to circulatory care. *Nursing Clinics of North America, 27*(2), 445–476.

Glavis, C. & Barbour, S. (1990). Pressure ulcer prevention in critical care: State of the art. *AACN Clinical Issues in Critical Care Nursing, 1*(3), 602–613.

Kanak, M. F. (1992). Interventions related to patient safety. *Nursing Clinics of North America, 27*(2), 371–396.

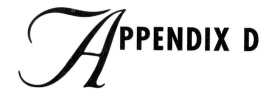

APPENDIX D

Normal Laboratory Values

Activated clotting time (ACT)	70–120 s
Adrenocorticotropic hormone (ACTH)	a.m. 15–100 pg/mL p.m. <50 pg/mL
Albumin	3.5–5 g/dL
Alkaline phosphate	35–100 IU/L
Ammonia	15–45 µg/dL
Amylase	25–85 IU/L
Anion gap	6–16 mEq/L
Antidiuretic hormone (ADH)	1–5 pg/mL
Antithrombin III	80–120% of normal activity
Bilirubin: Total	0.3–1.0 mg/dL
Direct	0.1–0.4 mg/dL
Indirect	0.2–0.8 mg/dL
Bleeding time	3–10 min
Blood urea nitrogen (BUN)	5–20 mg/dL
Calcium	8.5–10.5 mg/dL
Chloride	95–105 mEq/L
Cholesterol	100–210 mg/dL
Cortisol	a.m. 6–28 µg/dL; p.m. 2–12 µg/dL
Creatinine phosphokinase (CPK)	50–180 IU/L
Creatinine	0.6–1.2 mg/dL
D-dimer	<0.5 mg/L
Eosinophils	50–350/mm^3
Erythrocyte sedimentation rate (ESR)	0–15 mm/hr men; 0–25 mm/hr women
Fibrinogen	200–400 mg/dL
Fibrin split products	negative
Folic acid	5.9–21 µg/mL
Glucose	60–115 mg/dL
Hemoglobin (Hgb)	13–18 g/dL
Hematocrit (Hct)	35–47% women; 42–52% men
Iron	42–135 µg/dL
Isoamylase	S (salivary) 50%; P (pancreatic) 50%
Lactic acid	0.5–2.2 mEq/L (venous)

Lactic dehydrogenase (LDH)	62–155 U/L
Lipase	4–24 IU/dL
Lymphocytes	1000–4000/mm^3
Magnesium	1.5–2.5 mg/dL
Osmolality	275–295 mOsm/kg
Phosphate	2.5–4.5 mg/dL
Platelets	150,000–400,000/mm^3
Potassium	3.5–5.0 mEq/L
Prolactin	0–23 ng/dL women; 0–20 ng/dL men
Prothombin time (PT)	10–13 s
Partial thromboplastin time (PTT)	30–45 s
Red blood cells (RBCs)	4.4–5.9 10 million/mm^3
Resin T_3 uptake	25–35% uptake
SGOT/AST	0–36 IU/L
SGPT/ALT	4–24 IU/L
Sodium	135–145 mEq/L
Thrombin time	15 s or control ±5 s
Thyroid stimulating hormone	1.9–5.4 μ-IU/mL
Thyroxine (T_4)	5–12.5 μg/dL
Total protein	6–8 g/dL
Transferrin	200–360 mg/dL
Triglycerides	40–150 mg/dL
Triiodothyromine (T_3)	110–230 ng/100 mL
Uric acid	2.4–6 mg/dL women; 3.4–7 mg/dL men
Urine amylase	2–15 IU/hr
Urine bilirubin	negative or 0.02 mg/dL
Urobilinogen	0.1–1 Ehlich unit/dL
Vitamin B_{12}	100–250 pg/mL
White blood cells (WBCs)	5000–10,000/mm^3

NOTE: Normals may vary somewhat depending on the facility and techniques used.

REFERENCES

Fischbach, F. (1988). *A manual of laboratory diagnostic tests.* (3rd ed.). Philadelphia, PA: Lippincott.

Jacobs, D. S., Kasten, B. L., Demott, W. R., & Wolfson, W. L. (1990). *Laboratory test handbook* (2nd ed.). Baltimore, MD: Williams & Wilkins.

▼

Normal Hemodynamic Values

Central venous pressure (CVP)	2–10 mmHg
Pulmonary artery pressure (PAP)	25–30/8–12 mmHg
Pulmonary capillary wedge pressure (PCWP)	8–12 mmHg
Cardiac output (CO)	4–8 L/min
Cardiac index (CI)	2.5–4 L/min/m^2
Systemic vascular resistance (SVR)	800–1200 dyns/s/cm^{-5}
Pulmonary vascular resistance (PVR)	100–250 dyns/s/cm^{-5}
Mean arterial pressure (MAP)	70–90 mmHg
Left ventricular stroke work index (LVSWI)	35–85 g/mL
Right ventricular stroke work index (RVSWI)	8.5–12 g/mL
Saturation of venous oxygen (SvO$_2$)	70–90%

From "Data acquisition from the cardiovascular system" by J. Vitello-Cicciu and J. S. Eagan, in *AACN's Clinical Reference for Critical Care Nursing* (2nd ed., p. 559) by M. R. Kinney, D. R. Packa, and S. B. Dunbar (Eds.), 1988, New York, NY: McGraw-Hill.

Normal Arterial Blood Gas (ABG) Values

pH	7.35–7.45
PaCO$_2$	35–45 torr
PaO$_2$	80–100 torr
HCO$_3$	21–28 mEq/L
SaO$_2$	95–100%
Base excess	±3 mEq/L
A-a DO2	5–20 mmHg

INDEX

Note: Page numbers followed by t indicate tables

A

Abdominal aortic aneurysm, 63–68
 acute pain and, 67
 altered tissue perfusion and, 64–65
 aneurysmal rupture and, 65–66
 clinical findings, 64
 clinical manifestations, 63–64
 continuity of care, 68
 diagnostic findings, 64
 discharge planning, 68
 emboli and, 66–67
 etiologies, 63
 knowledge deficit and, 67–68
Abdominal surgery, 70–77
 acute pain and, 72–73
 altered nutrition and, 77
 clinical findings, 71–72
 clinical manifestations, 71
 continuity of care, 77
 diagnostic findings, 71–72
 discharge planning, 77
 etiologies, 70–71
 fluid volume deficit and, 73–74
 impaired gas exchange and, 74–76
 infection risk and, 76
Ace inhibitors, in abdominal aortic aneurysm, 66
Acetaminophen, in thyroid storm, 56
Acetazolamide
 in hyperphosphatemia, 376
 in metabolic alkalosis, 420
Acid-base balance, and acute respiratory failure, 251
Acid-base imbalance
 and metabolic alkalosis, 419–421
 and respiratory alkalosis, 304–305
 and status asthmaticus, 314
Acquired immunodeficiency syndrome (AIDS). See Human immunodeficiency virus

Activated charcoal, in drug overdose, 430
Activity intolerance
 and acute adrenal crisis, 10–11
 and acute renal failure, 346–347
 and human immunodeficiency virus, 144–145
 and hyperkalemia, 389–390
 and hyperphosphatemia, 377
 and hypokalemia, 394–395
 and hypophosphatemia, 383–383
 and myxedema coma, 49
 and thyroid storm, 57–58
Acute adrenal crisis, 3–11
 activity intolerance and, 10–11
 altered thought processes and, 9–10
 altered tissue perfusion and, 7–9
 clinical findings, 4–5
 clinical manifestations, 4
 continuity of care, 11
 diagnostic findings, 4–5
 discharge planning, 11
 etiologies, 3–4
 fluid volume deficit and, 5–7
Acute gastrointestinal bleed, 86–95
 altered tissue perfusion and, 92–93
 clinical findings, 88
 clinical manifestations, 87
 continuity of care, 95
 diagnostic findings, 88
 discharge planning, 95
 etiologies, 86–87
 fluid volume deficit and, 88–91
 impaired gas exchange and, 91–92
 knowledge deficit and, 94
Acute pain
 and abdominal aortic aneurysm, 67
 and abdominal surgery, 72–73
 and acute pancreatitis, 99–100
 and chest trauma, 264–265

495

496 Index

and peritonitis, 80–81
and pulmonary embolism, 293–294
and thoracic surgery, 322–323
Acute pancreatitis, 96–103
   acute pain and, 99–100
   altered nutrition and, 100–101
   clinical findings, 97
   clinical manifestations, 97
   continuity of care, 103
   diagnostic findings, 97
   discharge planning, 103
   electrolyte imbalance and, 101–102
   etiologies, 96–97
   fluid volume deficit and, 97–99
   impaired gas exchange and, 102–103
Acute renal dialysis, 329–336
   continuous renal replacement therapy injury and, 334–336
   contraindications, 330–331
   fluid volume deficit and, 331–332
   hemodialysis injury and, 334–336
   indications, 330
   peritoneal dialysis injury and, 332–334
Acute renal failure, 338–348
   activity intolerance and, 346–347
   altered urinary elimination and, 341–343
   clinical findings, 341
   clinical manifestations, 340–341
   continuity of care, 348
   diagnostic findings, 341
   discharge planning, 348
   etiologies, 339–340
   fluid volume deficit and, 344–345
   fluid volume excess and, 343–344
   impaired skin integrity and, 347–348
   infection risk and, 345–346
Acute respiratory distress syndrome, 237–244
   clinical findings, 238
   clinical manifestations, 237–238
   continuity of care, 244
   decreased cardiac output and, 243–244
   diagnostic findings, 238
   discharge planning, 244
   etiologies, 237
   impaired airway clearance and, 242–243
   impaired gas exchange and, 238–240
   ineffective breathing pattern and, 240–241
Acute respiratory failure, 246–256
   acid-base balance and, 251
   altered nutrition and, 255–256
   anxiety and, 254–255
   clinical findings, 247
   clinical manifestations, 247
   continuity of care, 256
   diagnostic findings, 247
   discharge planning, 256
   etiologies, 246–247
   impaired gas exchange and, 250–251
   ineffective airway clearance and, 252–254
   ineffective breathing pattern and, 247–249
   nutrition and, 256
Acute spinal cord injury, 151–163
   altered tactile perception and, 158–159
   bowel incontinence and, 160–161
   clinical findings, 153
   clinical manifestations, 152, 153
   continuity of care, 163
   decreased cardiac output and, 153–155
   diagnostic findings, 153
   discharge planning, 163
   etiologies, 151
   impaired physical mobility and, 156–158
   ineffective breathing pattern and, 155–156
   ineffective individual coping and, 162–163
   ineffective thermoregulation and, 159–160
   levels of, 152t
   types of, 152t
   urinary retention and, 161
Acute tubular necrosis, 338. See also Acute renal failure
Acyclovir, in human immunodeficiency virus, 143
Adrenal crisis. See Acute adrenal crisis
Adrenal gland, diseases of. See Acute adrenal crisis
AIDS. See Human immunodeficiency virus

Airway clearance
  impaired, and acute respiratory
    distress syndrome, 242–243
  ineffective
    and acute respiratory failure,
      252–254
    and chest trauma, 262–264
    and increased intracranial
      pressure, 204–205
    and mechanical ventilation, 275–
      277
    and myasthenia crisis, 221–222
    and thoracic surgery, 321–322
Alkali, oral
  in acute renal failure, 343
  in metabolic acidosis, 416
Aluminum hydroxide, in
  hyperphosphatemia, 376
Amicar. See Aminocaproic acid
Amiloride, in hypomagnesemia, 371
Aminocaproic acid (Amicar)
  in cerebral aneurysm, 168
  in disseminated intravascular
    coagulation, 130
Aminophylline
  in anaphylaxis, 121
  in mechanical ventilation, 277
  in status asthmaticus, 310
  in thoracic surgery, 319
Amitriptyline, in human
  immunodeficiency virus, 141
Amphetamines, overdose of, 425, 426.
  See also Drug intoxication
Amphotericin, in human
  immunodeficiency virus, 143
Analgesics
  in cerebral aneurysm, 168
  in chest trauma, 264
  in peritonitis, 80
Anaphylaxis, 119–123
  clinical findings, 120
  clinical manifestations, 120
  continuity of care, 123
  decreased cardiac output and, 122–
    123
  diagnostic findings, 120
  discharge planning, 123
  etiologies, 119
  ineffective breathing pattern and,
    120–121
Anesthetics, in status asthmaticus,
  311

Aneurysm
  abdominal aortic. See Abdominal
    aortic aneurysm
  cerebral. See Cerebral aneurysm
Aneurysmal rupture, and abdominal
  aortic aneurysm, 65–66
Antacids
  in acute gastrointestinal bleed, 90
  in acute spinal cord injury, 161
  in altered nutrition, 481
  in hypercalcemia, 355
  in hypocalcemia, 359
Anterior cord syndrome, 152t. See also
  Acute spinal cord injury
Antianxiety drugs, in psychosocial
  care, 450
Antibiotics
  in acute respiratory distress
    syndrome, 242
  in acute respiratory failure, 253
  in chest trauma, 263
  in head trauma, 188
  in human immunodeficiency virus,
    140
  in increased intracranial infections,
    213
  in mechanical ventilation, 276,
    283
  in peritonitis, 83
  in septic shock, 468
  in status asthmaticus, 311
  in thoracic surgery, 322
  in thyroid storm, 56
Anticholinergics
  in acute respiratory distress
    syndrome, 242
  in acute respiratory failure, 253
  in chest trauma, 263
  in mechanical ventilation, 276
  overdose of, 425, 426. See also
    Drug intoxication
Anticholinesterase drugs, in myasthenia
  crisis, 220, 221, 222
Anticoagulant therapy, in pulmonary
  embolism, 292
Anticonvulsants, in drug intoxication,
  432
Antidiuretic hormone disturbances,
  22–29
  continuity of care, 29
  diabetes insipidus, 22–25
  discharge planning, 29

syndrome of inappropriate antidiuretic hormone, 25–29
Antifibrinolytics, in cerebral aneurysm, 168
Antihypertensives
　in abdominal aortic aneurysm, 66
　in acute renal dialysis, 336
　in acute spinal cord injury, 155
Anti-inflammatory agents, in acute respiratory distress syndrome, 240
Antimicrobial therapy, in acute renal failure, 346
Antiplatelet substances, in pulmonary embolism, 293
Antipsychotics, overdose of, 425, 426–427. See also Drug intoxication
Antithrombin concentrate, in disseminated intravascular coagulation, 129
Anxiety
　and acute respiratory failure, 254–255
　and mechanical ventilation, 283–284
　and psychosocial care, 448–450
　and status asthmaticus, 313–314
Aortic aneurysm, abdominal. See Abdominal aortic aneurysm
Arborvirus, 209. See also Intracranial infections
Aspirin
　in pulmonary embolism, 293
　in thyroid storm, 56
Ativan. See Lorazepam
Atropine
　in acute spinal cord injury, 155
　in anaphylaxis, 121
　in myasthenia crisis, 221
　in status asthmaticus, 310
Autonomic dysreflexia, 151. See also Acute spinal cord injury

B

Bactrim, in human immunodeficiency virus, 138
Barbiturates
　in increased intracranial pressure, 199
　overdose of, 426, 427. See also Drug intoxication

Benzodiazepines
　in human immunodeficiency virus, 140
　overdose of, 427. See also Drug intoxication
　in status epilepticus, 230
Beta-adrenergics
　in acute respiratory distress syndrome, 242
　in acute respiratory failure, 253
　in chest trauma, 263
　in mechanical ventilation, 276
Beta blockers
　in abdominal aortic aneurysm, 66
　in drug intoxication, 433
Bleeding. See also Acute gastrointestinal bleed; Hemorrhage
　risk of, 490
Bowel elimination, altered, and Guillain-Barré syndrome, 183–184
Bowel incontinence, and acute spinal cord injury, 160–161
Brain abscesses, 209–210. See also Intracranial infections
Breathing pattern, ineffective
　and acute respiratory distress syndrome, 240–241
　and acute respiratory failure, 247–249
　and acute spinal cord injury, 155–156
　and anaphylaxis, 120–121
　and chest trauma, 261–262
　and diabetic ketoacidosis, 18–19
　and drug intoxication, 428–429
　and fulminant hepatic failure, 112–113
　and Guillain-Barré syndrome, 176–177
　and hypokalemia, 395–396
　and hypophosphatemia, 381–382
　and mechanical ventilation, 270–273
　and metabolic alkalosis, 421–422
　and myasthenia crisis, 219–221
　and myxedema coma, 47–48
　and peritonitis, 83–84
　and respiratory acidosis, 298–300
　and respiratory alkalosis, 305–306
　and status asthmaticus, 309–311
　and thoracic surgery, 317–319
　and thyroid storm, 56–57

Bronchodilators
 in acute respiratory failure, 252
 in anaphylaxis, 121
 in chest trauma, 263
 in mechanical ventilation, 277, 279
 in respiratory acidosis, 300
 in status asthmaticus, 310
 in thoracic surgery, 319
Brown-Séquard syndrome, 152t. See also Acute spinal cord injury

C

Calcitonin, in hypercalcemia, 354
Calcium
 in hypermagnesemia, 365
 in hyperphosphatemia, 376
 in hypocalcemia, 359
Calcium blockers. See Calcium channel blockers
Calcium channel blockers
 in abdominal aortic aneurysm, 66
 in cerebral aneurysm, 169
 in hypercalcemia, 353
 in thyroid storm, 55
Calcium chelators, in hypercalcemia, 353
Calcium disturbances. See Hypercalcemia; Hypocalcemia
Calcium gluconate
 in hyperphosphatemia, 388
 in hypocalcemia, 358
Carbamazepine, in diabetes insipidus, 25
Cardiac output
 altered, and septic shock, 471
 decreased
  and acute respiratory distress syndrome, 243–244
  and acute spinal cord injury, 153–155
  and anaphylaxis, 122–123
  and chest trauma, 266–267
  and disseminated intravascular coagulation, 131
  and drug intoxication, 432–433
  and Guillain-Barré syndrome, 179–180
  and human immunodeficiency virus, 138–139
  and hyperkalemia, 386–389
  and hyperphosphatemia, 375–376
  and hypocalcemia, 359–360
  and hypokalemia, 392–393
  and hypophosphatemia, 379–381
  and hypovolemic shock, 443–444
  and mechanical ventilation, 280–281, 281–282
  and metabolic acidosis, 414–416
  and myasthenia crisis, 224
  and myxedema coma, 44–45
  and pulmonary embolism, 294–295
  and respiratory acidosis, 300–301
  and thyroid storm, 53–55
Cardiopulmonary tissue perfusion, altered, and status epilepticus, 228–230
Cardiovascular tissue perfusion, altered, and acute adrenal crisis, 7–9
Cation exchange resins, in hyperphosphatemia, 388
Central cord syndrome, 152t. See also Acute spinal cord injury
Cerebral aneurysm, 165–172
 altered cerebral tissue perfusion and, 166–170
 clinical findings, 166
 clinical manifestations, 165–166
 continuity of care, 172
 diagnostic findings, 166
 discharge planning, 172
 etiologies, 165
 fluid volume excess and, 170–171
 impaired physical mobility and, 171–172
Cerebral angioplasty, in cerebral aneurysm, 169
Cerebral tissue perfusion, altered
 and cerebral aneurysm, 166–170
 and head trauma, 187–189
 and increased intracranial pressure, 193–200, 200t–202t
 and intracranial infections, 213–214
 and status epilepticus, 228–230
Chest physiotherapy
 in chest trauma, 263
 in mechanical ventilation, 276, 279
 in thoracic surgery, 321
Chest trauma, 258–268
 acute pain and, 264–265

clinical findings, 259
clinical manifestations, 258–259
continuity of care, 267–268
decreased cardiac output and, 266–267
diagnostic findings, 259
discharge planning, 267–268
etiologies, 258
fluid volume deficit and, 265–266
impaired gas exchange and, 259–261
ineffective airway clearance and, 262–264
ineffective breathing pattern and, 261–262
Chlorpromazine, in human immunodeficiency virus, 140
Chlorpropamide (Diabinese), in diabetes insipidus, 25
Clindamycin, in human immunodeficiency virus, 138
Clotrimazole, in human immunodeficiency virus, 143
Cocaine, overdose of, 426. See also Drug intoxication
Coma. See Hyperglycemic hyperosmotic nonketotic coma; Myxedema coma
Continuous arteriovenous hemodialysis, 330. See also Acute renal dialysis
Continuous arteriovenous hemofiltration, 330. See also Acute renal dialysis
Continuous renal replacement therapy, 329–330. See also Acute renal dialysis
    contraindications, 331
    indications, 330
    injury risk and, 334–336
Convulsive status epilepticus, 226. See also Status epilepticus
Coping, ineffective individual. See Individual coping, ineffective
Corticosteroids
    in anaphylaxis, 121
    in increased intracranial pressure, 205
Cryoanalgesia, in thoracic surgery, 323

D

Dapsone (diaminodiphenylsulfone), in human immunodeficiency virus, 138

Decadron. See Dexamethasone
Demeclocycline, in diabetes insipidus, 29
Depressant drugs, overdose of, 426. See also Drug intoxication
Dexamethasone (Decadron)
    in acute adrenal crisis, 5
    in increased intracranial pressure, 199
Dextran
    in cerebral aneurysm, 168
    in pulmonary embolism, 293
Dextrose
    in acute adrenal crisis, 7
    in altered nutrition, 478
    in drug overdose, 430
    in hypoglycemic crisis, 38
    in status epilepticus, 229
Diabetes insipidus, 22–25
    clinical findings, 23
    clinical manifestations, 23
    diagnostic findings, 23
    etiologies, 22–23
    fluid volume deficit and, 24–25
Diabetes mellitus. See Diabetic ketoacidosis
Diabetic ketoacidosis, 13–21
    altered thought processes and, 19–20
    clinical findings, 14
    clinical manifestations, 14
    continuity of care, 21
    diagnostic findings, 14
    discharge planning, 21
    electrolyte imbalance and, 16–18
    etiologies, 13
    fluid volume deficit and, 15–16
    ineffective breathing pattern and, 18–19
Diabinese (chlorpropamide), in diabetes insipidus, 25
Diaminodiphenylsulfone (Dapsone), in human immunodeficiency virus, 138
Diarrhea, and human immunodeficiency virus, 143–144
Diazepam (Valium), in status epilepticus, 230
Digoxin
    effects, and hypophosphatemia, 393
    in hypophosphatemia, 393
    in thyroid storm, 55
    toxicity

and hyperphosphatemia, 388
and hypocalcemia, 360
and hypomagnesemia, 370
Dilantin (phenytoin), in status epilepticus, 230
Discharge planning
  and abdominal aortic aneurysm, 68
  and abdominal surgery, 77
  and acute adrenal crisis, 11
  and acute gastrointestinal bleed, 95
  and acute pancreatitis, 103
  and acute renal failure, 348
  and acute respiratory distress syndrome, 244
  and acute respiratory failure, 256
  and acute spinal cord injury, 163
  and anaphylaxis, 123
  and antidiuretic hormone disturbances, 29
  and cerebral aneurysm, 172
  and chest trauma, 267–268
  and diabetic ketoacidosis, 21
  and disseminated intravascular coagulation, 133
  and drug intoxication, 436
  and fulminant hepatic failure, 114–115
  and Guillain-Barré syndrome, 184–185
  and head trauma, 190
  and human immunodeficiency virus, 146
  and hypercalcemia, 361
  and hyperglycemic hyperosmotic nonketotic coma, 34
  and hyperkalemia, 396
  and hypermagnesemia, 372–373
  and hypernatremia, 404
  and hyperphosphatemia, 383
  and hypocalcemia, 361
  and hypoglycemic crisis, 40
  and hypokalemia, 396
  and hypomagnesemia, 372–373
  and hyponatremia, 404
  and hypophosphatemia, 383
  and hypovolemic shock, 446
  and intracranial infections, 216
  and intracranial pressure, increased, 208
  and mechanical ventilation, 285
  and metabolic acidosis, 417
  and metabolic alkalosis, 422
  and myasthenia crisis, 224–225
  and peritonitis, 84–85
  and primary water deficit, 412
  and primary water excess, 412
  and psychosocial care, 463
  and pulmonary embolism, 295–296
  and respiratory acidosis, 301–302
  and septic shock, 471–472
  and status asthmaticus, 314–315
  and status epilepticus, 233
  and thoracic surgery, 325
  and thyroid storm, 60
Disseminated intravascular coagulation, 125–133
  altered tissue perfusion and, 126–128
  clinical findings, 126
  clinical manifestations, 126
  continuity of care, 133
  decreased cardiac output and, 131
  diagnostic findings, 126
  discharge planning, 133
  etiologies, 125–126
  impaired gas exchange and, 132–133
  impaired tissue integrity and, 130
  injury risk and, 128–130
Diuretics
  in acute renal failure, 344
  in acute spinal cord injury, 155
  in chest trauma, 261
  in diabetes insipidus, 28
  in drug overdose, 431
  in fulminant hepatic failure, 113
  in hypernatremia, 400
  in hyperphosphatemia, 376, 389
  in hypocalcemia, 353
  in hypomagnesemia, 371
  in increased intracranial pressure, 198, 204
  in primary water excess, 408
Dobutamine, in chest trauma, 267
Dopamine
  in chest trauma, 267
  in drug intoxication, 431
Drug intoxication, 425–436
  altered thought processes and, 429–432
  clinical findings, 427–428
  clinical manifestations, 426–427
  continuity of care, 436
  decreased cardiac output and, 432–433

diagnostic findings, 427–428
discharge planning, 436
etiologies, 425–426
ineffective breathing pattern and, 428–429
ineffective individual coping and, 433–434
injury risk and, 434
violence risk and, 435–436

E

Electrolyte imbalance
  and acute pancreatitis, 101–102
  and diabetic ketoacidosis, 16–18
  and hypercalcemia, 352–355
  and hyperglycemic hyperosmotic nonketotic coma, 33
  and hypocalcemia, 357–359
Electrolytes. *See also specific types*
  in abdominal surgery, 74
  in acute gastrointestinal bleed, 90
  in diabetic ketoacidosis, 16–18
Emboli, and abdominal aortic aneurysm, 66–67
Embolism, pulmonary. *See* Pulmonary embolism
Encephalitis, 209. *See also* Intracranial infections
Endotracheal suctioning
  in acute respiratory distress syndrome, 240
  in acute respiratory failure, 249, 251
  in chest trauma, 261
  in disseminated intravascular coagulation, 132
  in hypovolemic shock, 443
  in mechanical ventilation, 272, 275
Enteral nutrition therapy, 479–481
Epinephrine
  in anaphylaxis, 121, 123
  in septic shock, 471
  in status asthmaticus, 310
Ethylenediaminetetraacetic acid (EDTA), in hypercalcemia, 353
Exogenous surfactant, in acute respiratory distress syndrome, 240
Expectorants
  in acute respiratory distress syndrome, 242
  in acute respiratory failure, 253
  in mechanical ventilation, 276

F

Family processes, altered, and psychosocial care, 460–462
Fasting hypoglycemia, 35–36. *See also* Hypoglycemic crisis
Fibrinolytics, in pulmonary embolism, 292
Fluconazole, in human immunodeficiency virus, 143
Fludrocortisone
  in cerebral aneurysm, 169
  in human immunodeficiency virus, 139
Fluid volume
  deficit
    and abdominal surgery, 73–74
    and acute adrenal crisis, 5–7
    and acute gastrointestinal bleed, 88–91
    and acute renal failure, 344–345
    and chest trauma, 265–266
    and diabetes insipidus, 24–25
    and diabetic ketoacidosis, 15–16
    and fulminant hepatic failure, 106–108
    and hyperglycemic hyperosmotic nonketotic coma, 32–33
    and hypernatremia, 398–400
    and hypovolemic shock, 440–441
    and peritonitis, 81–82
    and primary water deficit, 410–411
  excess
    and acute renal failure, 343–344
    and cerebral aneurysm, 170–171
    and hyponatremia, 402–403
    and mechanical ventilation, 280–281
    and myxedema coma, 43–44
    and primary water excess, 407–408
    and syndrome of inappropriate antidiuretic hormone, 27–29
Foscarnet, in human immunodeficiency virus, 143
Fulminant hepatic failure, 104–115
  altered nutrition and, 109–110
  altered thought processes and, 110–112
  clinical findings, 105–106
  clinical manifestations, 105
  continuity of care, 114–115

diagnostic findings, 105–106
discharge planning, 114–115
etiologies, 104
fluid volume deficit and, 106–108
impaired skin integrity and, 114
ineffective breathing pattern and, 112–113
Furosemide, in acute spinal cord injury, 155

G

Ganciclovir, in human immunodeficiency virus, 143
Gas exchange, impaired
and abdominal surgery, 74–76
and acute gastrointestinal bleed, 91–92
and acute pancreatitis, 102–103
and acute respiratory distress syndrome, 238–240
and acute respiratory failure, 250–251
and chest trauma, 259–261
and disseminated intravascular coagulation, 132–133
and human immunodeficiency virus, 136–138
and hypocalcemia, 360–361
and hypovolemic shock, 442–443
and increased intracranial pressure, 203–304
and mechanical ventilation, 273–275
and peritonitis, 83–84
and primary water excess, 408–409
and pulmonary embolism, 289–291
and septic shock, 469–470
and status asthmaticus, 312–313
and status epilepticus, 230–231
and thoracic surgery, 319–320
Gastrointestinal bleeding. *See* Acute gastrointestinal bleed
Gastrointestinal surgery. *See* Abdominal surgery
Glasgow Coma Scale, 201t
Glucagon, in anaphylaxis, 123
Glucocorticoids
in acute adrenal crisis, 9
in hypercalcemia, 354

in increased intracranial pressure, 199
in status asthmaticus, 311
Glucose
in diabetic ketoacidosis, 18
in hyperphosphatemia, 388
in hypoglycemic crisis, 38
Guillain-Barré syndrome, 174–185
altered bowel elimination and, 183–184
altered sensory perception and, 181–182
altered urinary elimination and, 183–184
clinical findings, 175
clinical manifestations, 175
continuity of care, 184–185
decreased cardiac output and, 179–180
diagnostic findings, 175
discharge planning, 184–185
etiologies, 174
impaired physical mobility and, 178–179
impaired skin integrity and, 184
ineffective breathing pattern and, 176–177

H

Hallucinogens, overdose of, 425, 427. *See also* Drug intoxication
Haloperidol
in human immunodeficiency virus, 140
in psychosocial care, 459
H_1 antihistamines, in anaphylaxis, 121
Head trauma, 186–190
altered cerebral tissue perfusion and, 187–189
clinical findings, 187
clinical manifestations, 186–187
continuity of care, 190
diagnostic findings, 187
discharge planning, 190
etiologies, 186
impaired physical mobility, 189
injury risk and, 189–190
Hemodialysis, 329. *See also* Acute renal dialysis
contraindications, 330–331
in drug intoxication, 432
indications, 330

injury risk and, 334–336
Hemofiltration
    in drug intoxication, 432
    in hyponatremia, 403
Hemoperfusion, in drug intoxication, 432
Hemorrhage, and thoracic surgery, 323–324
Heparin
    in acute spinal cord injury, 158
    in disseminated intravascular coagulation, 130
    in pulmonary embolism, 292
Hepatic failure. See Fulminant hepatic failure
Herpes simplex infections, 209. See also Intracranial infections
Histamine antagonists
    in acute gastrointestinal bleed, 90
    in acute spinal cord injury, 161
    in altered nutrition, 481
    in hypercalcemia, 355
HIV. See Human immunodeficiency virus
Hopelessness, and psychosocial care, 453–454
Human immunodeficiency virus, 134–146
    activity intolerance and, 144–145
    altered nutrition and, 142–143
    altered sensory perception and, 140–141
    clinical findings, 136
    clinical manifestations, 135–136
    continuity of care, 146
    decreased cardiac output and, 138–139
    diagnostic findings, 136
    diarrhea and, 143–144
    discharge planning, 146
    etiologies, 134–135
    impaired gas exchange and, 136–138
    impaired skin integrity and, 141–142
    ineffective individual coping and, 145–146
    infection risk and, 139–140
Hydrochloric acid, in metabolic acidosis, 420
Hydrocortisone, in acute adrenal crisis, 9
Hypercalcemia, 350–356
    altered urinary elimination and, 355–356
    clinical findings, 351–352
    clinical manifestations, 351
    continuity of care, 361
    diagnostic findings, 351–352
    discharge planning, 361
    electrolyte imbalance and, 352–355
    etiologies, 350–351
Hyperglycemic hyperosmotic nonketotic coma, 30–34
    altered thought processes and, 33–34
    clinical findings, 31
    clinical manifestations, 31
    continuity of care, 34
    diagnostic findings, 31
    discharge planning, 34
    electrolyte imbalance and, 33
    etiologies, 30–31
    fluid volume deficit and, 32–33
Hyperkalemia, 385–390
    activity intolerance and, 389–390
    clinical findings, 386
    clinical manifestations, 386
    continuity of care, 396
    decreased cardiac output and, 386–389
    diagnostic findings, 386
    discharge planning, 396
    etiologies, 385–386
Hypermagnesemia, 363–368
    activity intolerance and, 367–368
    clinical findings, 364
    clinical manifestations, 363–364
    continuity of care, 372–373
    decreased cardiac output and, 364–365
    diagnostic findings, 364
    discharge planning, 372–373
    etiologies, 363
    ineffective breathing pattern and, 366–367
Hypernatremia, 397–401
    altered thought processes and, 400–401
    clinical findings, 398
    clinical manifestations, 398
    continuity of care, 404
    diagnostic findings, 398
    discharge planning, 404
    etiologies, 397–398
    fluid volume deficit and, 398–400

Hyperosmolar agents, in increased intracranial pressure, 198
Hyperphosphatemia, 374–377
    activity intolerance and, 377
    clinical findings, 375
    clinical manifestations, 374–375
    continuity of care, 383
    decreased cardiac output and, 375–376
    diagnostic findings, 375
    discharge planning, 383
    etiologies, 374
Hyperthermia, in thyroid storm, 55–56
Hyperthyroidism. See Thyroid storm
Hypocalcemia, 356–361
    clinical findings, 357
    clinical manifestations, 356–357
    continuity of care, 361
    decreased cardiac output and, 359–360
    diagnostic findings, 357
    discharge planning, 361
    electrolyte imbalance and, 357–359
    etiologies, 356
    impaired gas exchange and, 360–361
Hypoglycemic crisis, 35–40
    altered nutrition and, 37–38
    altered thought processes and, 39–40
    clinical findings, 36
    clinical manifestations, 36
    continuity of care, 40
    diagnostic findings, 36
    discharge planning, 40
    etiologies, 35–36
Hypokalemia, 390–396
    activity intolerance and, 394–395
    clinical findings, 391
    clinical manifestations, 391
    continuity of care, 396
    decreased cardiac output and, 392–393
    diagnostic findings, 391
    discharge planning, 396
    etiologies, 390–391
    ineffective breathing pattern and, 395–396
Hypomagnesemia, 368–373
    activity intolerance, 371–372
    clinical findings, 369
    clinical manifestations, 369
    continuity of care, 372–373
    decreased cardiac output and, 369–371
    diagnostic findings, 369
    discharge planning, 372–373
    etiologies, 368
Hyponatremia, 401–404
    altered thought processes and, 403–404
    clinical findings, 402
    clinical manifestations, 401–402
    continuity of care, 404
    diagnostic findings, 402
    discharge planning, 404
    etiologies, 401
    fluid volume excess and, 402–403
Hypophosphatemia, 378–383
    activity intolerance and, 382–383
    clinical findings, 379
    clinical manifestations, 378–379
    continuity of care, 383
    decreased cardiac output and, 379–381
    diagnostic findings, 379
    discharge planning, 383
    etiologies, 378
    ineffective breathing pattern and, 381–382
Hypothermia, and myxedema coma, 45
Hypothyroidism. See also Myxedema coma
Hypotonic solutions, in abdominal surgery, 74
Hypovolemic shock, 438–446
    altered tissue perfusion and, 444–446
    clinical findings, 439–440
    clinical manifestations, 439
    continuity of care, 446
    decreased cardiac output and, 443–444
    diagnostic findings, 439–440
    discharge planning, 446
    etiologies, 438–439
    fluid volume deficit and, 440–441
    impaired gas exchange and, 442–443

I

Individual coping, ineffective
    and acute spinal cord injury, 162–163
    and drug intoxication, 433–434

and human immunodeficiency
    virus, 145–146
and psychosocial care, 452–453
Indomethacin, in hypercalcemia, 354
Infection risk
    and abdominal surgery, 76
    and acute renal failure, 345–346
    and human immunodeficiency
        virus, 139–140
    and mechanical ventilation, 282–283
    and peritonitis, 82–83
Injury risk, 487–490
    and acute renal dialysis, 332–336
    and disseminated intravascular
        coagulation, 128–130
    and drug intoxication, 434
    and head trauma, 189–190
    and increased intracranial pressure,
        207–208
    and intracranial infections, 215–216
    and status epilepticus, 232–233
    and thoracic surgery, 323–324
Inocur, in chest trauma, 267
Inotropic agents
    in abdominal aortic aneurysm, 65
    in acute respiratory distress
        syndrome, 243
    in anaphylaxis, 123
    in cerebral aneurysm, 168
    in chest trauma, 267
    in disseminated intravascular
        coagulation, 131
    in hypovolemic shock, 444
    in mechanical ventilation, 282
Insulin
    in diabetic ketoacidosis, 18
    in hyperphosphatemia, 388
Insulin-dependent diabetes mellitus. *See*
    Diabetic ketoacidosis
Intracranial infections, 209–216
    altered cerebral tissue perfusion
        and, 213–214
    altered thought processes and,
        212–213
    clinical findings, 211
    clinical manifestations, 210–211
    continuity of care, 216
    diagnostic findings, 211
    discharge planning, 216
    etiologies, 210

impaired physical mobility and,
    214–215
injury risk and, 215–216
Intracranial pressure
    increased, 191–208
        altered cerebral tissue perfusion
            and, 193–200, 200t–202t
        altered sensory perception and,
            206–207
        clinical findings, 192–193
        clinical manifestations, 192
        continuity of care, 208
        diagnostic findings, 192–193
        discharge planning, 208
        etiologies, 191–192
        Glasgow Coma Scale and, 201t
        impaired gas exchange and, 203–204
        impaired physical mobility and,
            205–206
        ineffective airway clearance and,
            204–205
        injury risk and, 207–208
        monitoring devices and, 202t
        pathologic reflexes and, 200t
        pressure waveforms and, 202t
        respiratory patterns related to
            brain pathology and, 201t
    monitoring devices, 202t
    waveforms, 202t
Iodide agents, in thyroid storm, 55
Isotonic solutions, in abdominal
    surgery, 74

K

Kayexalate, in hyperphosphatemia,
    388
Ketoacidosis, diabetic. *See* Diabetic
    ketoacidosis
Ketoconazole, in human
    immunodeficiency virus, 143
Knowledge deficit, 483–485
    and abdominal aortic aneurysm,
        67–68
    and acute gastrointestinal bleed, 94

L

Lactulose, in fulminant hepatic failure,
    112
Laxatives
    in cerebral aneurysm, 167

in Guillain-Barré syndrome, 183
Levothyroxine sodium, in myxedema coma, 44
Lithium, in diabetes insipidus, 29
Liver failure. *See* Fulminant hepatic failure
Lorazepam (Ativan)
  in psychosocial care, 459
  in status epilepticus, 230
Lugol's solution, in thyroid storm, 55

M

Magnesium
  in hypomagnesemia, 370, 371
  in status asthmaticus, 311
Magnesium disturbances. *See* Hypermagnesemia; Hypomagnesemia
Mannitol
  in acute spinal cord injury, 155
  in increased intracranial pressure, 198
Mechanical ventilation, 269–285
  in acute respiratory failure, 249
  altered nutrition and, 284–285
  anxiety and, 283–284
  in chest trauma, 262
  clinical findings, 270
  clinical manifestations, 270
  continuity of care, 285
  decreased cardiac output and, 281–282
  diagnostic findings, 270
  discharge planning, 285
  in disseminated intravascular coagulation, 132
  dysfunctional ventilatory weaning response and, 277–280
  etiologies, 269–270
  fluid volume excess and, 280–281
  impaired gas exchange and, 273–275
  ineffective airway clearance and, 275–277
  ineffective breathing pattern and, 270–273
  infection risk and, 282–283
  in pulmonary embolism, 290
  in respiratory alkalosis, 306
  in status asthmaticus, 310
  in thoracic surgery, 318
Meningitis, 219. *See also* Intracranial infections

Metabolic acidosis, 413–417
  altered thought processes and, 416–417
  clinical findings, 414
  clinical manifestations, 414
  continuity of care, 417
  decreased cardiac output and, 414–416
  diagnostic findings, 414
  discharge planning, 417
  etiologies, 413
Metabolic alkalosis, 418–422
  acid-base imbalance and, 419–421
  clinical findings, 419
  clinical manifestations, 419
  continuity of care, 422
  diagnostic findings, 419
  discharge planning, 422
  etiologies, 418
  ineffective breathing pattern and, 421–422
Methylprednisolone, in status asthmaticus, 311
Methylxanthines
  in acute respiratory distress syndrome, 242
  in acute respiratory failure, 253
  in chest trauma, 263
  in mechanical ventilation, 276
Miconazole, in human immunodeficiency virus, 143
Mithramycin, in hypercalcemia, 354
Monamine oxidase inhibitors, overdose of, 425, 426. *See also* Drug intoxication
Morphine, in acute pancreatitis, 99
Mucolytics
  in acute respiratory distress syndrome, 242
  in acute respiratory failure, 253
  in chest trauma, 263
  in mechanical ventilation, 276
  in status asthmaticus, 311
Muscle relaxants, in status asthmaticus, 311
Myasthenia crisis, 218–225
  clinical findings, 219
  clinical manifestations, 218–219
  continuity of care, 224–225
  decreased cardiac output and, 224
  diagnostic findings, 219
  discharge planning, 224–225

etiologies, 218
impaired physical mobility and, 222–223
ineffective airway clearance and, 221–222
ineffective breathing pattern and, 219–221
Myoclonic status epilepticus, 226. *See also* Status epilepticus
Myxedema coma, 41–50
    activity intolerance and, 49
    altered thought processes and, 46–47
    clinical findings, 42–43
    clinical manifestations, 41–42
    decreased cardiac output and, 44–45
    diagnostic findings, 42–43
    etiologies, 41
    fluid volume excess and, 43–44
    hypothermia and, 45
    ineffective breathing pattern and, 47–48

N

Naloxone, in drug overdose, 430
Narcotics, in acute renal dialysis, 336
Nasogastric lavage, in acute gastrointestinal bleed, 90
Nembutal. *See* Pentobarbital
Neomycin sulfate, in fulminant hepatic failure, 111
Neuromuscular blocking agents
    in chest trauma, 262
    in respiratory alkalosis, 306
Nifedipine, in hypercalcemia, 353
Nitrates, long-acting, in acute renal dialysis, 336
Nitroprusside
    in abdominal aortic aneurysm, 66
    in acute respiratory distress syndrome, 243
Nonconvulsive status epilepticus, 226. *See also* Status epilepticus
Nonsteroidal anti-inflammatory drugs, in pulmonary embolism, 294
Nutrition
    and acute respiratory failure, 256
    altered, 475–481
        and abdominal surgery, 77
        and acute pancreatitis, 100–101
        and acute respiratory failure, 255–256
        and enteral nutrition solutions, 479–481
        and fulminant hepatic failure, 109–110
        and human immunodeficiency virus, 142–143
        and hypoglycemic crisis, 37–38
        and mechanical ventilation, 284–285
        and thoracic surgery, 324
Nystatin, in human immunodeficiency virus, 143

P

Pain, acute. *See* Acute pain
Pain medication. *See also specific types*
    in acute pancreatitis, 99
    in chest trauma, 264
    in peritonitis, 84
    in thoracic surgery, 323
Pancreatitis. *See* Acute Pancreatitis
Paracentesis, in fulminant hepatic failure, 113
Paralytic agents, in acute respiratory distress syndrome, 240
Paraplegia. *See* Acute spinal cord injury
Parasympathetic blockers, in status asthmaticus, 310
Partial status epilepticus, 226. *See also* Status epilepticus
Pathologic reflexes, and increased intracranial pressure, 200t
Pentamidine, in human immunodeficiency virus, 138
Pentobarbital (Nembutal)
    in increased intracranial pressure, 199
    in status epilepticus, 230
Peritoneal dialysis, 329. *See also* Acute renal dialysis
    contraindications, 331
    indications, 330
    injury risk and, 332–334
Peritoneal lavage, in acute pancreatitis, 103
Peritonitis, 78–85
    acute pain and, 80–81
    clinical findings, 79–80

clinical manifestations, 79
continuity of care, 84–85
diagnostic findings, 79–80
discharge planning, 84–85
etiologies, 79
fluid volume deficit and, 81–82
impaired gas exchange and, 83–84
ineffective breathing pattern and, 83–84
infection risk and, 82–83
Persantine, in pulmonary embolism, 293
Phenobarbital, in status epilepticus, 230
Phenytoin (Dilantin), in status epilepticus, 230
Phosphate, in hypophosphatemia, 380
Phosphate-binding drugs
in hyperphosphatemia, 376
in hypocalcemia, 359
Phosphate disturbances. See Hyperphosphatemia; Hypophosphatemia
Physical mobility, impaired
and acute spinal cord injury, 156–158
and cerebral aneurysm, 171–172
and Guillain-Barré syndrome, 178–179
and head trauma, 189
and increased intracranial pressure, 205–206
and intracranial infections, 214–215
and myasthenia crisis, 222–223
Pitressin, in acute gastrointestinal bleed, 90
Plasmapheresis
in drug intoxication, 432
in Guillain-Barré syndrome, 179
in myasthenia crisis, 221
Plicamycin, in hypercalcemia, 354
Postprandial hypoglycemia, 36. See also Hypoglycemic crisis
Potassium
in acute pancreatitis, 102
in acute renal dialysis, 334
in hyperphosphatemia, 388
in hypophosphatemia, 393
in metabolic alkalosis, 420
Potassium disturbances. See Hyperkalemia; Hypokalemia

Powerlessness, and psychosocial care, 454–455
Primaquine, in human immunodeficiency virus, 138
Primary water deficit, 409–412
clinical findings, 410
clinical manifestations, 410
continuity of care, 412
diagnostic findings, 410
discharge planning, 412
etiologies, 409–410
fluid volume deficit and, 410–411
Primary water excess, 406–409
clinical findings, 407
clinical manifestations, 406–407
continuity of care, 412
diagnostic findings, 407
discharge planning, 412
etiologies, 406
fluid volume excess and, 407–408
impaired gas exchange and, 408–409
Propranolol, in thyroid storm, 54, 55
Propylthiouracil, in thyroid storm, 55
Prostaglandin E_1, in acute respiratory distress syndrome, 243
Psychosocial care, 447–463
altered family processes and, 460–462
altered sensory perception and, 456–458
altered thought processes and, 458–460
anxiety and, 448–450
clinical manifestations, 447–448
clinical signs, 448
continuity of care, 463
diagnostic signs, 448
discharge planning, 463
etiologies, 447
hopelessness and, 453–454
ineffective individual coping and, 452–453
powerlessness and, 454–455
sleep pattern disturbance and, 450–452
spiritual concerns and, 462–463
Pulmonary embolism, 287–296
acute pain and, 293–294
altered pulmonary tissue perfusion and, 291–293

clinical findings, 288–289
clinical manifestations, 288
continuity of care, 295–296
decreased cardiac output and, 294–295
diagnostic findings, 288–289
discharge planning, 295–296
etiologies, 287–288
impaired gas exchange and, 289–291
Pulmonary tissue perfusion, altered, and pulmonary embolism, 291–293
Pyridostigmine, in myasthenia crisis, 220

Q

Quadriplegia. See Acute spinal cord injury

R

Recombinant t-PA, in pulmonary embolism, 292
Renal dialysis. See Acute renal dialysis
Renal failure, acute. See Acute renal failure
Renal tissue perfusion, altered, and status epilepticus, 231–232
Respiratory acidosis, 297–302
  clinical findings, 298
  clinical manifestations, 298
  continuity of care, 301–302
  decreased cardiac output and, 300–301
  diagnostic findings, 298
  discharge planning, 301–302
  etiologies, 297
  ineffective breathing pattern and, 298–300
Respiratory alkalosis, 303–307
  acid-base imbalance and, 304–305
  clinical findings, 304
  clinical manifestations, 303–304
  diagnostic findings, 304
  etiologies, 303
  ineffective breathing pattern and, 305–306
Respiratory distress syndrome. See Acute respiratory distress syndrome
Respiratory failure. See Acute respiratory failure
Respiratory patterns, related to brain pathology, 201t

S

Saline
  in abdominal surgery, 74
  in cerebral aneurysm, 169
  in diabetes insipidus, 28
  in diabetic ketoacidosis, 16
  in drug overdose, 431
  in hyperphosphatemia, 376
  in hypocalcemia, 353
  in hyponatremia, 403
  in metabolic alkalosis, 421
Sclerotherapy, in fulminant hepatic failure, 108
Sedatives
  in acute respiratory distress syndrome, 240, 249
  in cerebral aneurysm, 167
  in chest trauma, 264
  in disseminated intravascular coagulation, 131
  in drug intoxication, 432
  in mechanical ventilation, 273, 277, 282, 284
  in peritonitis, 80
  in psychosocial care, 450, 459
  in pulmonary embolism, 293
  in respiratory acidosis, 300
  in respiratory alkalosis, 306
  in status asthmaticus, 311
  in thyroid storm, 58
Sensory perception, altered
  and acute spinal cord injury, 158–159
  and Guillain-Barré syndrome, 181–182
  and human immunodeficiency virus, 140–141
  and increased intracranial pressure, 206–207
  and psychosocial care, 456–458
Septic shock, 465–472
  altered cardiac output and, 471
  altered tissue perfusion and, 467–469
  clinical findings, 466–467
  clinical manifestations, 466
  continuity of care, 471–472
  diagnostic findings, 466–467
  discharge planning, 471–472
  etiologies, 465–466
  impaired gas exchange and, 469–470

Septra, in human immunodeficiency virus, 138
Shock
  hypovolemic. *See* Hypovolemic shock
  septic. *See* Septic shock
  spinal. *See* Acute spinal cord injury
Skin integrity, impaired
  and acute renal failure, 347–348
  and fulminant hepatic failure, 114
  and Guillain-Barré syndrome, 184
  and human immunodeficiency virus, 141–142
Sleep medications, in psychosocial care, 451
Sleep pattern disturbance, and psychosocial care, 450–452
Slow continuous ultrafiltration, 329–330. *See also* Acute renal dialysis
Sodium bicarbonate
  in diabetic ketoacidosis, 18
  in drug overdose, 431
  in hypercalcemia, 354
  in hyperphosphatemia, 389
  in metabolic acidosis, 415
Sodium disturbances. *See* Hypernatremia; Hyponatremia
Sodium morrhuate, in fulminant hepatic failure, 108
Sodium tetradeclysulfate, in fulminant hepatic failure, 108
Spinal cord injury. *See* Acute spinal cord injury
Spinal shock, 151. *See also* Acute spinal cord injury
Spiritual concerns, and psychosocial care, 462–463
Spironolactone, in hypomagnesemia, 371
Status asthmaticus, 308–315
  acid-base imbalance and, 314
  anxiety and, 313–314
  clinical findings, 309
  clinical manifestations, 308–309
  continuity of care, 314–315
  diagnostic findings, 309
  discharge planning, 314–315
  etiologies, 308
  impaired gas exchange and, 312–313
  ineffective breathing pattern and, 309–311

Status epilepticus, 226–233
  altered cardiopulmonary tissue perfusion in, 228–230
  altered cerebral tissue perfusion and, 228–230
  altered renal tissue perfusion and, 231–232
  clinical findings, 228
  clinical manifestations, 227–228
  continuity of care, 233
  diagnostic findings, 228
  discharge planning, 233
  etiologies, 227
  impaired gas exchange and, 230–231
  injury risk and, 232–233
Steroids
  in acute spinal cord injury, 155
  in myasthenia crisis, 220, 222
  in thoracic surgery, 322
Stool softeners
  in acute spinal cord injury, 161
  in cerebral aneurysm, 167
  in Guillain-Barré syndrome, 183
  in pulmonary embolism, 293
Streptokinase, in pulmonary embolism, 292
Sucralfate
  in acute spinal cord injury, 161
  in hypercalcemia, 355
Sympathomimetics
  overdose of, 425. *See also* Drug intoxication
  in status asthmaticus, 310
Syndrome of inappropriate antidiuretic hormone, 25–29
  clinical findings, 26
  clinical manifestations, 26
  diagnostic findings, 26
  etiologies, 25–26
  fluid volume excess and, 27–29
Syrup of ipecac, in drug overdose, 431

T

Tactile perception, altered, and acute spinal cord injury, 158–159
Theophylline
  in acute respiratory distress syndrome, 241
  in acute respiratory failure, 249
Thermoregulation, ineffective, and acute spinal cord injury, 159–160

Thiamine, in status epilepticus, 229
Thiazide
   in diabetes insipidus, 25
   in hypomagnesemia, 371
Thoracic surgery, 316–325
   acute pain and, 322–323
   altered nutrition and, 324
   clinical findings, 317
   clinical manifestations, 317
   continuity of care, 325
   diagnostic findings, 317
   discharge planning, 325
   etiologies, 316
   hemorrhage and, 323–324
   impaired gas exchange and, 319–320
   ineffective airway clearance and, 321–322
   ineffective breathing pattern and, 317–319
Thought processes, altered
   and acute adrenal crisis, 9–10
   and diabetic ketoacidosis, 19–20
   and drug intoxication, 429–432
   and fulminant hepatic failure, 110–112
   and hyperglycemic hyperosmotic nonketotic coma, 33–34
   and hypernatremia, 400–401
   and hypoglycemic crisis, 39–40
   and hyponatremia, 403–404
   and intracranial infections, 212–213
   and metabolic acidosis, 416–417
   and myxedema coma, 46–47
   and psychosocial care, 458–460
   and thyroid storm, 59–60
Thrombolytics, in pulmonary embolism, 292
Thyroid drugs, in myxedema coma, 44
Thyroid hormone, in myxedema coma, 45
Thyroid storm, 51–60
   activity intolerance and, 57–58
   altered thought processes and, 59–60
   clinical findings, 52–53
   clinical manifestations, 51–52
   continuity of care, 60
   decreased cardiac output and, 53–55
   diagnostic findings, 52–53
   discharge planning, 60
   etiologies, 51
   hyperthermia and, 55–56
   ineffective breathing pattern and, 56–57
Tissue integrity, impaired, and disseminated intravascular coagulation, 130
Tissue perfusion, altered
   and abdominal aortic aneurysm, 64–65
   and acute adrenal crisis, 7–9
   and acute gastrointestinal bleed, 92–93
   and cerebral aneurysm, 166–170
   and disseminated intravascular coagulation, 126–128
   and head trauma, 187–189
   and hypovolemic shock, 444–446
   and increased intracranial pressure, 193–200, 200t–202t
   and intracranial infections, 213–214
   and pulmonary embolism, 291–293
   and septic shock, 467–469
   and status epilepticus, 228–230, 231–232
Total parenteral nutrition, in acute pancreatitis, 101
Tranquilizers, in respiratory acidosis, 300
Triamterene, in hypomagnesemia, 371
Tricyclic antidepressants, overdose of, 425, 427. *See also* Drug intoxication
Trimethoprim-sulfamethoxazole, in human immunodeficiency virus, 138
Trimetrexate, in human immunodeficiency virus, 138

U

Urinary elimination, altered
   and acute renal failure, 341–343
   and Guillain-Barré syndrome, 183–184
   and hypercalcemia, 355–356
Urinary retention, and acute spinal cord injury, 161
Urokinase, in pulmonary embolism, 292

V

Valium (Diazepam), in status
  epilepticus, 230
Vasoactive drugs
  in acute respiratory distress
    syndrome, 243
  in disseminated intravascular
    coagulation, 131
Vasoconstrictors, in cerebral aneurysm,
  168
Vasodilators
  in acute respiratory distress
    syndrome, 244
  in drug intoxication, 433
Vasopressin
  in acute gastrointestinal bleed, 90
  in diabetes insipidus, 25
  in fulminant hepatic failure, 108
Vasopressors
  in drug intoxication, 433
  in myxedema coma, 45
Ventilatory weaning response,
  dysfunctional, and mechanical
  ventilation, 277–280

Verapamil, in hypercalcemia, 353
Violence risk, and drug intoxication,
  435–436
Vitamin D
  in hyperphosphatemia, 376
  in hypocalcemia, 359
Vitamin supplements, in fulminant
  hepatic failure, 110

W

Warfarin, in pulmonary embolism, 292
Water balance disturbances. *See*
  Primary water deficit;
  Primary water excess
Water deficit, primary. *See* Primary
  water deficit
Water excess, primary. *See* Primary
  water excess

X

Xylocaine, in hypophosphatemia, 393

Z

Zidovudine, in human
  immunodeficiency virus, 141